Pharmaceutical Care
in Digital Revolution

Pharmaceutical Care in Digital Revolution
Insights Towards Circular Innovation

Edited by

Claudia Rijcken

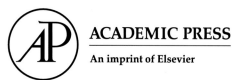

Academic Press is an imprint of Elsevier
125 London Wall, London EC2Y 5AS, United Kingdom
525 B Street, Suite 1650, San Diego, CA 92101, United States
50 Hampshire Street, 5th Floor, Cambridge, MA 02139, United States
The Boulevard, Langford Lane, Kidlington, Oxford OX5 1GB, United Kingdom

Notices
Knowledge and best practice in this field are constantly changing. As new research and
experience broaden our understanding, changes in research methods, professional practices, or
medical treatment may become necessary.

Practitioners and researchers must always rely on their own experience and knowledge in
evaluating and using any information, methods, compounds, or experiments described herein.
In using such information or methods they should be mindful of their own safety and the safety
of others, including parties for whom they have a professional responsibility.

To the fullest extent of the law, neither the Publisher nor the authors, contributors, or editors,
assume any liability for any injury and/or damage to persons or property as a matter of products
liability, negligence or otherwise, or from any use or operation of any methods, products,
instructions, or ideas contained in the material herein.

Library of Congress Cataloging-in-Publication Data
A catalog record for this book is available from the Library of Congress

British Library Cataloguing-in-Publication Data
A catalogue record for this book is available from the British Library

ISBN: 978-0-12-817638-2

For information on all Academic Press publications
visit our website at https://www.elsevier.com/books-and-journals

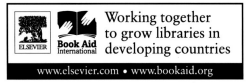

Publisher: Andre Gerhard Wolff
Acquisition Editor: Erin Hill-Parks
Editorial Project Manager: Sandra Harron
Production Project Manager: Punithavathy Govindaradjane
Cover Designer: Victoria Pearson

Typeset by SPi Global, India

Contents

PART 1 WHY: GLOBAL HEALTHCARE SYSTEMS UNDER PRESSURE

PART 2 WHAT: DIGITAL ADVANCES TO INNOVATE PHARMACEUTICAL CARE JOURNEYS

PART 4 HOW: WHAT TO DO TOMORROW AS A PHARMACEUTICAL CARE LEADER

About the editor and
disclosure of conflicts of
interest

Claudia Rijcken

Claudia has an educational background as a pharmacist and obtained a PhD in Pharmacoepidemiology and a Master of Health Administration (eMBA).

After managing community pharmacy roles for 7 years, she moved into clinical drug development and served for 7 years in roles of increasing global responsibility at Organon and Novartis.

In the next 5 years, she acted within Novartis internationally in leadership roles in patient access, key account management, and public affairs. She developed a growing ambition to build more synergy between value-driven pharmaceutical

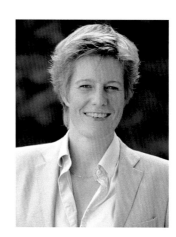

care and the use of digital health technology and invested in learning about business development and health technology at Erasmus University Rotterdam and MIT Sloan and moved into a European digital innovation role within Novartis.

Currently, Claudia is the founder of the company pharmacare.ai BV (digital pharmaceutical care education and strategy) and the startup Pharmi BV (developing digital pharmaceutical care solutions). Both companies are located at the Philips High Tech Campus in Eindhoven, the Netherlands. Claudia has been a mentor and strategic advisor for various digital health startups at the Brightlands Innovation Factory, acts as a volunteer for different health charity organizations, and is a member of the World Healthcare Forum Advisory Board.

Claudia is affiliated to the University of Utrecht, Netherlands to co-develop digital pharmaceutical care education.

Because the author was partially an employee at Novartis during the time of writing of this book, this is to confirm that this book is published under personal title, and the views and opinions expressed in this book are those of the author and do not represent any official policy or position of Novartis and its affiliated companies.

About the authors and disclosure of conflicts of interest

Paul Iske

Paul Iske is professor at the School of Business and Economics, University Maastricht, the Netherlands, focusing on open innovation and business ventures.

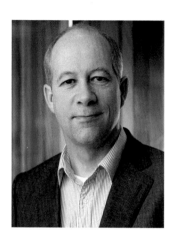

He is a member of the Service Science Factory Advisory Board (www.servicesciencefactory.nl) and is on the boards of the Maastricht Centre for Entrepreneurship (www.mc4e.nl) and the Network of Social Innovation.

As of September 2015, Paul is Chief Dialogues Officer at PNA Group (www.pna-group.com).

From 1997 to 2015 Paul had various functions at ABN AMRO Bank. His last position was Chief Dialogues Officer and Director of the Dialogues Incubator at ABN AMRO Bank. In these roles he was responsible for open, radical, social, and sustainable innovation.

Paul acts as an independent consultant on knowledge-conscious management and supports organizations in the development and implementation of programs focusing on leveraging knowledge as a strategic production factor. He teaches on topics related to new business developments at universities in various countries, including the Netherlands (Rotterdam), South Africa (Stellenbosch), South Korea (Seoul), Norway (Bergen), and Oman.

Since 2014 Paul has been a member of the Scientific Advisory Board of the Dutch Heart Foundation (www.hartstichting.nl) and a member of the Industrial Advisory Board of the Delta Institute for Theoretical Physics (http://www.d-itp.nl/).

Paul was chairman of the Dutch Norwegian Business Network (www.dnbn.nl) from 2012 to 2017.

In 2014 Paul cofounded the International Institute for Serious Optimism (www.iiso.eu), and since 2017 he has also been a member of the international team of the Stanford Peace Innovation Lab (https://peaceinnovation.stanford.edu).

Paul is as well extra-ordinary Professor Knowledge Management at the Stellenbosch University in South Africa.

Rob Peters

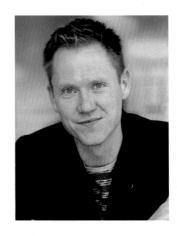

Rob graduated in 2012 as a certified public accountant (CPA) at Nyenrode Business University. After working for 7 years as an accountant, in 2014 Rob began setting up a new business line, Assuring Medical Apps, at Deloitte Innovation. This business line is focused on security and privacy topics in mobile and web healthcare applications. He started this business line due to the exponential growth of technology in healthcare and the growing demand for trust in this technology. Rob is fascinated by exponential technologies in healthcare and wants to collaborate on the shift from healthcare to the prevention of illnesses. In this work Rob has gained significant experience in the field of compliance, privacy, and information security in the healthcare sector. As of June 2017 Rob is cofounder and part of the Digital Health Compliance team at Deloitte Legal. The team's work goes beyond ensuring the compliance of medical applications to focusing on the reliable handling of patient data in the digitization of healthcare. Rob is responsible for setting up new, innovative, compliance-related digital services in the healthcare sector.

Rob is a mentor for various accelerator programs that help startups with early-stage compliance. He is also involved in various innovation juries and committees within the healthcare sector and has been a partner in the annual Dutch Health Hackathon for several years. Rob also writes articles for care-related platforms and professional journals. He speaks on compliance in healthcare at renowned international conferences and regularly gives guest lectures on information security.

As the author is at the time of this writing an employee of Deloitte, this is to confirm that this book is published under personal title, and the views and opinions expressed in this book are those of the author and do not represent any official policy or position of Deloitte and its affiliated companies.

Barry Meesters

Since graduating in business administration at the Erasmus University Rotterdam, Barry has specialized in IT management, IT auditing, and cybersecurity. Since 1997 Barry has worked for various consultancy firms focused on advising and training in IT management and IT system implementation. In 2004 Barry joined Deloitte and also began his postgraduate education in electronic data processing (EDP) auditing at Erasmus University Rotterdam, and was registered as an EDP auditor in 2006. At Deloitte Barry developed an extensive practice in the Southern Netherlands in IT auditing, IT assurance, and cybersecurity.

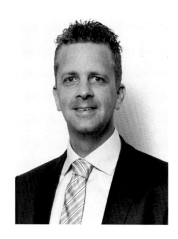

Barry has also been responsible for the development of various innovative assurance services, such as assuring the quality and security of cloud services and medical applications. Digitization in healthcare is his passion; therefore Barry has focused on this area for the last years. Barry is cofounder of the Digital Health Compliance service, in which he helps healthcare and technological organizations deal with security, privacy, and compliance challenges and successfully implement digitization. He also searches for innovative solutions to simplify processes and reduce compliance costs. Barry is at the time of this writing director of Digital Health Compliance with Deloitte Legal B.V.

As the author is at the time of this writing an employee of Deloitte, this is to confirm that this book is published under personal title, and the views and opinions expressed in this book are those of the author and do not represent any official policy or position of Deloitte and its affiliated companies.

Wilma Göttgens

Wilma is a pharmacist and has practiced as a community pharmacist since 1983. She enjoys working directly with patients, doctors, and other professionals in a pharmacy setting.

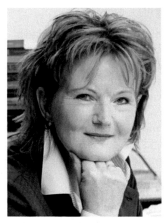

Wilma believes that for long time her profession has been in transition and is adjusting its scope of practice to address societal needs and expectations. Pursuing her passion for philosophy, Wilma received a Master of Philosophy at Radboud University Nijmegen in 2005, while continuing her work as a community pharmacist.

By studying philosophy she became more aware of the uniqueness of the pharmacy practice and the role of the pharmacist from a scientific point of view. The aspects involved in providing pharmaceutical services in increasingly complex situations with increasing time constraints are the primary focus of pharmaceutical specializations, ranging from master degree students to community and hospital pharmacists. Grounded in the philosophy of pharmacy as a value-based practice, her work today is dedicated to further developing the profession of pharmacy and nourishing the professional identity (the heart and soul), skills, and attitudes of pharmacists.

At Radboud University Medical Center Nijmegen, Wilma is PhD researcher on the philosophy and ethics of clinical guidelines. She also teaches ethics and professionalism at the KNMP Advanced Community Pharmacist Education Program. She was founder and chair and is still a member of the Special Interest Group on Ethics and Philosophy of Pharmacy. Wilma is also a member of the Narrative Healthcare Network Advisory Board, which was established in 2017.

Paul Rulkens

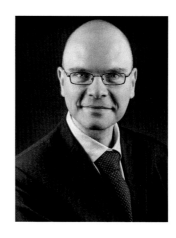

How do the best get better? Companies like McKinsey, KPMG, and ExxonMobil work with Paul Rulkens to raise the bar and quickly bring results to the next level.

Paul knows that doing more is no longer the default answer to too much to do. He is an expert in strategic high performance: the art and science of accelerating bold executive outcomes with the least amount of effort. He is an award-winning professional speaker, international author, and a trusted boardroom advisor who has helped thousands of business executives, managers, and professionals get everything they can out of everything they have. His ideas to improve results and accelerate careers are often described as thought-provoking and counterintuitive, yet highly effective.

You do not have to be sick in order to get better. As an international keynote speaker, Paul annually addresses dozens of successful international audiences about essential mindsets and proven strategies to reap exponential business improvements. His most popular topics cover the secrets of consistent execution, easy innovation, powerful leadership, business growth, career acceleration, and seamless teamwork.

Originally trained as a chemical engineer, Paul's work is based on deep knowledge and extensive experience in the practical business applications of behavioral psychology, neuroscience, and, especially, common sense. His popular TED talks are used frequently in professional training sessions all over the world.

More information about Paul and his work can be found on www.paulrulkens.com.

Foreword

How will humanity prevail in this coming era of exponential disruption in the medical and pharmaceutical sectors? How far would *you* augment yourself with technology in order to "transcend your human limitations"? How will we remain human once technology goes "inside of us," changing our very biology and our consciousness? Once the pharma industry converges with the technology industry, will it be "mission control for humanity"?

While I see much of these coming changes largely as opportunities, we are heading towards many complex and increasingly disturbing ethical dilemmas as technology is becoming almost infinitely capable (and humans may thus become "superhuman," which some fellow futurists seem to see as a worthy goal). During the next 20 years we will witness the advent of global hyper-connectivity and the Internet of Things, the achievement of at least some kind of narrow artificial intelligence, the realization of super/quantum computing, major leaps in material sciences and nano-technology, the rise of 3D printing, and rapid advances in human genome manipulation.

The issue of what I like to call "Digital Ethics" will of course loom large in all industries, worldwide, but will be particularly challenging in the rapidly converging segments of biology and technology. Very soon the question will no longer be IF technology can do something, but WHY it should or WHO will be in charge. It is thus important that we look at all the topics presented in this book in the light of exponential and combinatorial change, as linear thinking will be detrimental!

On the one hand, these waves of digital innovation have had and will have a quite positive impact on our lives. Many of the technologies mentioned in the second part of this book promise vast improvements in how patients receive care, how citizens will experience healthcare, and how equal access to healthcare on a global scale could be achieved. Medical care could be provided fast, cheaply, and timely to every patient, completely customized and contextual, and for a fraction of the cost (an abundance that would be similar to media content where this has already been realized).

On the other hand, these digital transformations boggle the mind as science fiction is increasingly become science fact, and as many tried-and-true societal, cultural, and economic paradigms are being questioned.

Do drug logistics need to be separated from healthcare? Is the future really about blended (human and technology) care, or could some patients be satisfied with only their intelligent digital assistants? Can we rely on deep learning algorithms to determine whether a specific drug dosage is actually correct, even if it contradicts decades of human experience? Will we eventually require that all patients must share (some of) their data to the health cloud so that the combined intelligence—the global brain, so to speak—can save millions of lives?

We will very likely live longer than ever before (70 is already the new 50!), but whether we also will experience our newly won years as satisfying and enriching remains to be seen.

The truly awesome, as well as the sometimes also awful, impact of digitization, automation, virtualization, and cognification is becoming clearer every day, which is why in my book *Technology vs. Humanity* (www.techvshuman.com) I repeatedly pose these questions: Because we can, does it mean we should? Is it a good idea to "transcend human limitations" and increasingly become one with technology? My belief is that we must embrace technology, but not become it, because technology has no ethics, but societies are doomed without it (QR Code 1).

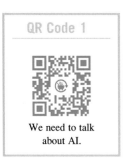

In this book you will find a wealth of ideas on better care opportunities, and may discover some risks as well—it will be all about keeping the balance! In order to master this balance, we must consider the bigger picture of our current healthcare systems that are under significant pressure, as well as the need for what in this book is called "circular pharmaceutical care."

Everything that can be digitized or automated will most probably be treated so, but everything that cannot (human-only skills) will become even more precious. The power of the human "H2H" communication in a situation where a patient needs care will certainly remain of vital importance.

Thus most likely the concept of "digital if possible and human where needed" will offer the optimal approach, where diversity both in the labor force and in patients will provide a panacea for a healthy pharmaceutical future (QR Code 2).

Contemplate the amazing potential you will find in this book, but come back to earth to fuel the pharmaceutical care ecology with the oxygen it needs: that is, enlightened pharmaceutical care stakeholders, who provide a hybrid model of biotic human strengths and abiotic digital innovation in order to create a sustainable symbiosis between digital and human future pharmaceutical care.

Gerd Leonhard

Acknowledgments

To my parents. Because they have always fueled curiosity.

Sometimes one starts an adventure with a Big Hairy Audacious Goal in mind, but without a clear view on where the pathway will lead. This book's adventure started after a reflective sabbatical in 2017, when I had the honor to travel with my husband and dad to a number of inspirational places around the world. Immersed in global cultural experiences and an awakening retreat, I came to realize that with the anticipated, dazzling speed of digital health innovations, society needs true digital innovation frontrunners, including in pharmaceutical care.

These experiences triggered the decision to begin this manuscript. I talked with many peers, but it was my conversations with this book's coauthors in particular that led to our joint goal to merge information on digital health solutions with the daily practice of pharmaceutical care professionals.

Some may consider it as obsolete to write a book about digital innovations, as over time the information will become outdated. However, we believe this book informs interested pharmaceutical care providers about the current state of the digital healthcare industry and why and how it will change over time. We also believe this book can kick-start a serious dialogue on what digitalization means in daily pharmaceutical practices.

However, an initiative is only as good as its first follower. This book would never have been brought to fruition without the coauthors' support, knowledge, and belief in its premise and purposes. Paul Iske, our inspiring conversations about combinatoric innovation, next-generation pharmaceuticals, and brilliant failures really augmented the scope of this book. Wilma, I greatly appreciate our discussions on what is considered good pharmaceutical care, and thank you for alerting me on how to preserve balance, when I was (again and again) distracted by the guilty pleasure of digital gadgets. Rob and Barry, you really made legal and regulatory frameworks an interesting, almost inspiring reason for creating innovation. Keep that enthusiasm for drawing best-ever blueprints! Paul Rulkens, thanks so much for your guidance on how to move smoothly from a corporate to a private entrepreneurial paradigm and how to translate that knowledge into digital perspectives for this book. Gerd Leonhard, your explanation in your book on the required balance between technology and humanity was one of the first times I realized the essential value of understanding and setting the boundaries between digital and human care. All your different perspectives made this book more than complete and made it a synergistic work of art. Thanks so much! Let's continue to collaborate until blended pharmaceutical care pathways truly become a reality.

A special thanks also to the book's many reviewers and contributors. Every insight, every comment, every piece of advice made the book's concepts richer and helped to produce a more mature, collectively intellectual document. Sometimes the comments were tough and made us realize how we could only touch the surface of many topics. As much as we sometimes might have liked to do otherwise, we listened and stayed committed to create an overall, broad perspective. This would not have been possible without the fine input of Lucien Engelen, Han de Gier, Cees Smit, Michelle Putzeist, Raween Kalicharan, Maryse Spapens, Michel van Agthoven, Norbert Schmidt, Samuel Allemann, Bernard Vrijens, Jacob Boersma, Aukje Mantel-Teeuwisse, Nanneke Hendricks, Martina Teichert, Daan Crommelin, Jos Lüers, Berend de Roos, Anna Laven, Sini Eskola, Joris Arts, Maurice Nijssen, Jos van Engelshoven, Esther Abels, Roel Fijn, Patricia van Dijck, Christian Vader, Wouter Kroese, Bert Leufkens, Roman Malina, Ruud van Coolen Brakel, Leon Klinkers, Frank Harmsen, Patrick van der Meer, Bertil van Beusekom, Jos van Oers, Andre Dekker, Stefaan Vancayzeele and many others. I extend profound thanks to each of you.

The discussion about the visuals and aesthetics of this book and its connected animations began more than a year ago. Cathleen, Chris, and Marc, as TIEPES your creativity and ability to transform complex abstract and futuristic matters into accessible, attractive visuals was great to experience. As it was one of your first pharmaceutical projects, I would say you've got talent; you've truly visualized the digital pharmaceutical care movement! Much appreciation and many thanks. We will continue to picture our ambitions.

Animation sponsors, without you the visualization of the concepts in this book would not have been possible. The contributions of Deloitte Digital, Albert Schweitzer Hospital, Service Apotheken, Dutch Innovative Medicine Association, EFPIA, Pharmabrain, and additional partners are reflected in the animations on www.pharmacare.ai. Thank you so much for your support.

Ambassador board of pharmacare.ai, many thanks to you as well. We will continue to collaborate and drive the movement to build circular solutions based on the concepts described in this book.

Novartis and all my former colleagues, thanks for 11 years of global collaboration to reimagine medicine. Being allowed to contribute to so many life-changing innovations with so many brilliant thought leaders was a huge learning experience that is highly lauded throughout this book. Let us keep in touch and walk the innovation pathway together.

On the shoulders of giants. This book would not have become reality if not for the opportunity to learn so much from key opinion leaders, visionaries, futurists, forward thinkers, backward philosophers, and so on. Although this is not an all-inclusive list, here are a number of people and institutions who really influenced the editors' perspectives: Bert Leufkens (for being an epidemiological, regulatory science, and art lighthouse for 25 years), Lucien Engelen (for his verbal inspiration and his interesting written posts), Vas Narasimhan (for blowing the necessary fresh oxygen through pharma), Bertalan Mesko (for his inspirational updates as the medical futurist), Max Tegmark (for his immersive Life 3.0 vision), Gerd Leonhard (for his balanced approach on tech versus humanity), the Singularity University and Exponential Medicine teams (for its, sometimes terrifying, visions of our collective future).

A sincere thanks as well to all dear friends and beloved family for being patient with me and the coauthors all those long days (sometimes holidays) we wrote the manuscript. Thanks for debating, for challenging, for awakening, and for entertaining. This process has once again proven that a social environment is crucial for maintaining well-being (and that wasn't even measured by a wearable).

A last, thank you from the editor to those closest.

Dad, your technical competencies and entrepreneurial spirit drive me through life. It is intensely sad that Mum, whom we already miss for so many years, could not enjoy the journey with us, but I am convinced she would have been so proud of us. I love you. Cristianne, our endeavors as being pharmacists at slightly different ends of the spectrum of the pharmaceutical chain have not prevented us from building synergy. We enjoy life as the Rijcken Pharma sisters, and I hope there will be much more combinatoric innovation in our pipeline. I love you, too. Erik, what an extremely interesting rollercoaster we've ridden in our 25 years together. Thanks from the bottom of my heart for being patient with me. You are honestly my synergistic other half, and I am more than grateful we complement each other in such a heartwarming way. I love you most.

Executive summary

The pharmaceutical ecosystem has always been driven by technology. The discovery, development, manufacturing, and distribution of drugs and other pharmaceutical care services all utilize sophisticated hardware and software applications that facilitate the innovation, accessibility, and usability of drugs.

Medicines themselves have always relied on technology. Although in a less visible and invasive way than surgical interventions can, medications can alter the body significantly, for example, by adjusting neurotransmitter systems or augmenting immune responses. As shown throughout this book, digital health tools can also enhance healthcare; however, before implementing them, both providers and patients need to better understand why and how these tools are used, and they may need to alter their perspectives on use of such tools.

At the same time, due to changing worldviews, demographic profiles, and customers' expectations, the objective of many stakeholders in healthcare systems is to harvest innovative digital technology in order to optimize patient services, to improve management pathways, and to warrant sustainability.

The primary purposes of this book are to create general awareness about impending digital health opportunities, to inspire pharmaceutical care stakeholders to envision the potential future of their profession, and to help frontrunners in the pharmaceutical landscape take an informed, balanced, patient-centric, and structured approach to circular pharmaceutical care.

For these reasons, as well as the space allowed, rather than offering readers a comprehensive scientific reference, the authors' offer an inspirational, thought-provoking book that supports:

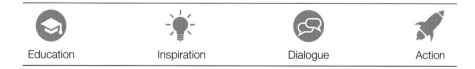

Education   Inspiration   Dialogue   Action

As a forest is a regenerative, symbiotic community of flora and fauna, the authors used a forest analogy throughout the book and compared it metaphorically to the regenerative, symbiotic nature of circular pharmaceutical care systems. Upon finishing this book, we trust readers will have a broad understanding of and will feel engaged with the digital health revolution. Furthermore, readers will be able to move beyond that understanding to taking concrete steps towards implementing circular pharmaceutical care and, more importantly, will feel optimally prepared for the day after tomorrow.

The Foreword

It is expected that over the next 20 years we will witness the advent of global hyper-connectivity and the Internet of Things, the achievement of at least some kind of narrow artificial intelligence, the realization of super/quantum computing, major leaps in material sciences and nano-technology, the rise of 3D printing, and rapid advances in human genome manipulation.

Gerd Leonhard commences the book by writing, "Very soon the question will no longer be IF technology can do something, but WHY it should or WHO will be in charge." He also writes that it will be about keeping a balance between technology and humanity. He also puts forth several questions:

How will humanity prevail in the coming era of exponential disruption in the medical and pharmaceutical sectors? How far would *you* augment yourself with technology in order to "transcend your human limitations"? How will we remain human once technology goes "inside of us," changing our very biology and our consciousness? Once the pharma industry converges with the technology industry, who will be "mission control for humanity"?

You will find a number of answers to these questions in the book. These questions and their answers are intended as stimulants to continuous learning, to adopting strong ethical practices, and to assuring quality and compliance.

Part 1

In Part 1 of the book we focus on the current challenges that healthcare systems are facing. Over the past 200 years, progress in healthcare has significantly increased life expectancy worldwide. As a result, in many countries healthcare expenditures have grown faster than the GDP, mainly due to growing and aging populations, longer survival times of people who are ill, and costlier interventions. Therefore many healthcare systems are under pressure. Within healthcare systems medicines and vaccines are some of the most powerful tools in helping people to live longer and have healthier, more productive lives. The quantity of very promising new medicines is expected to increase exponentially in the coming years. Therefore, ongoing systematic innovation is required to keep healthcare systems affordable, accessible, and secure.

Successful innovation involves creating value and using knowledge and resources in a new way. Because our hyperconnected world is dynamic and complex, we must create environments in which a joint innovation process, one that links different fields of expertise, can flourish. Professor Paul Iske calls this combinatoric innovation in Chapter 2. New skillsets are required to deal with the cultural, strategic, and operational challenges to make this promising form of innovation happen. Crucial skills are an open mindset, trusting and being trusted, and accepting uncertainty. A particular aspect is accepting and learning from brilliant failures. Combinatoric innovation is by definition not an efficient process, in the sense that many of the meetings set up won't produce immediate results. Thus to motivate employees to explore the unknown and initiate disruptive ideas, a failure-and-risk-accepting attitude towards innovation is essential. Additionally, systematic learning from failures is essential to be stimulated.

Looking at innovation in current healthcare systems, we see that many global systems focus on optimizing value-based healthcare, with the goal of generating increased patient value in a cost-effective way. To show ameliorated value, relevant patient outcomes must be proven, and different systems to measure those outcomes are explained in Chapter 3. A trusted, low-threshold relationship between professionals and patients combined with professional expertise and values make pharmaceutical care providers and physicians ideal partners in the delivery of drugs and in a way that achieves the best patient outcomes per money spent.

Also, the upsurge of recent reforms in the payment of medications indicates a shift from activity-based to outcome-based models. Value-based payments in healthcare and in reimbursement of drugs are increasingly facilitated and supported by extensive and interconnected real-world data. Also, broader societal benefits of medicines deserve to be taken into account, such as improved work productivity and reduced time for sick leave. Some of these new models are discussed in Chapter 4, for example, how health impact bonds incentivize stakeholders to merge their strategies on currently siloed healthcare, economic and social budgets, and which opportunities are available to jointly optimize the health of populations. Pharmaceutical care providers are considered essential contributors in outcome-based agreements, as they can optimize patient outcomes by combining (digital) analytic insights with low-threshold, trusted care relationships with patients.

Increasingly engaged and empowered patients want to assume a responsible role in their own healthcare, which is imperative for sustaining future healthcare. Today early patient engagement is driven by consumerism, value-based care, patients' need for adequate information, and regulatory interests, among other factors. Chapter 5 discusses why patient involvement is so imperative in digital pharmaceutical care development and what patients consider to be "good care."

Pharmaceutical care is a philosophy of practice in which the patient is the primary beneficiary of the pharmaceutical professional's actions. Pharmaceutical care providers are value-driven healthcare team members, and by managing the delivery of medications, they are the gatekeepers to facilitating adequate drug use and limiting unintentional harm due to medication, as explained in Chapter 6. In blended care models (digital if possible, human where needed), Digital Pharmaceutical Care can be defined as the digital facilitation of the responsible provision of pharmaceutical care for the purpose of achieving outcomes that improve a patient's quality of life. Blended care models are ideally supported by an integrated personal health record—that is, a digital application that connects all health-related data in one dossier—that is owned and managed by the patient or a patient's representative. Such an integrated system helps to build a circular pharmaceutical care model in which a patient is motivated to adhere to taking medications as prescribed and where waste and avoidable harm are reduced as much as possible.

Part 2

In Part 2 we describe the ecosystem of digital health innovations and its relevance to pharmaceutical care, and we also highlight a number of technologies in more detail. In Chapter 7 we discuss the wealth of upcoming digital health solutions, the various classification systems, and how categories of digital health tools can offer promise in different stages of patient treatment pathways. Mobile applications like smartphones are expected to play an increasing role, and principles of persuasive technology and serious gaming may stimulate adoption and retention of digital health applications. We note that adoption of these tools faces a significant number of hurdles that must be overcome to prove the full potential and economic benefits of digital health and to convince providers, governments, and payers to invest in further development and integration.

Fundamental to the future's data-driven healthcare environment is data tracking in the Internet of Things, the fast-growing internet of health, and the opportunities these data can bring, for example, pharmacy and health records, digital biomarkers, and other digital determinants of health. Because at least 25000 peta (10^{15}) bytes of health data are predicted to be available in 2020, we explain the dimensions of these big data sets (Volume, Veracity, Velocity, Variety, and Value) in Chapter 8. We also talk about why data need to be FAIR and how interconnected health data sets can turn data into value. Integrated Personal Health Applications (PHA) offer huge potential for future pharmaceutical care as they can give a holistic insight into the effects of or tolerance for drugs. A crucial condition for effective PHAs will be to facilitate interoperability of healthcare applications, for example, by adoption of HL7-FHIR standards.

This is particularly relevant for the more than 300,000 health-related apps now available. In Chapter 9 the different objectives, scopes, and functionalities of health apps relevant to the pharmaceutical care ecosystem are explained, including apps that have a specific focus, such as logistic, administrative, reference, and optimized use of drugs. In this fertile jungle of health applications, it is easy to get lost; therefore we offer thoughts on how a pharmaceutical care provider can link the right app with the right patient, how to find your way through app review platforms, how to stay cognizant of certification requirements, and how to determine the efficacy of future health apps.

Apps are crucial for digesting the data that wearables and insideables (the next phase after external wearables) track. We discuss the "quantified self" and how the concept becomes reality through a holistic set of digital biomarker data that are analyzed in applications that convert data into actionable health management advice. Chapter 10 delves into why a Bring Your Own Health Device strategy may increase continued use of wearables, as well as thorough device certification and ethical considerations when wearables are used. Given the exponential growth of the wearable market, we suggest that there is an urgent need for a structured comparison platform for wearables and insideables and their respective features. Such a platform would enable care providers and patients to be well informed about how to select the most appropriate device to augment clinical and pharmaceutical care plans.

We discuss how artificial intelligence (AI) technologies can offer pharmaceutical care providers smart support systems, given that they have access to complete, adequate, and holistic health data sets. AI, as shown in Chapter 11, can support trend analysis and decision making that augment pharmaceutical care expertise. This is what we call *apothecary intelligence*. We provide inspirational examples of how big platforms and AI are now augmenting healthcare providers, both of which are promising as long as they offer transparency in how algorithms are developed, in how they detect data bias, in their literacy and competency building, and in their ethical considerations. With AI-driven pharmacy-as-a-service platforms, augmented pharmaceutical care providers can spend more time doing on what they do best: using human judgment, empathy, and consideration to provide good patient care.

Chatbots are one example of technology built on AI, and they are fast becoming virtual personal assistants in today's healthcare systems, providing clinical triage, diagnosis, and information about healthcare interventions. When a chatbot is implemented in an internal pharmacy environment, it can, for example, reduce administrative burdens and support efficiency. Pharmaceutical bots that act as virtual personal assistants in patient care can be called pharmbots. They can answer pharmaceutical questions or provide treatment advice 24/7 at the convenience of patients. Thus they may enable faster signaling of health issues, nonadherence, and adverse events. Chapter 12 also explains a critical component for the success of pharmbot, that is, a Single Point of Truth (SPOT) platform for medication information, which should be the basis for all digital derivatives, such as electronic patient leaflets and pharmbot-specific algorithms.

In Chapter 13 we explain and provide examples of virtual, augmented, and mixed reality (VR-AR-MR) applications used in medical and pharmaceutical care, which can reduce the need for medication or remove the fear for medical interventions. Visualization, sometimes augmented with aspects of serious gaming in which there is a blend of real and virtual content, can enhance pharmaceutical care in an attractive and interactive way and improve understanding and literacy among medication users. These technologies can be used to support not only efficient pharmaceutical care services but also to augment pharmacy educational programs. The challenges to adopting these technologies are largely related to their feasibility, affordability, and accessibility.

Transfer of data from these applications into electronic pharmacy records must always be done with the greatest level of safety and security. The blockchain environment, an immutable, decentralized, and transparent record of all transactions throughout a peer network, can enable trusted and secure transactions within healthcare systems, facilitating up-to-date and transparent data flows. Chapter 14 depicts how reliable cradle-to-grave healthcare data set solutions can be developed, allowing patients to lead in facilitating a more efficient, secure, and up-to-date information flow among different healthcare providers. Blockchain applications in pharmaceutical care may result in, among other benefits, more secure personal health applications, improved management of health claims, and faster reimbursement of services. However, blockchain technology by itself will not automatically solve all data-related problems that have plagued healthcare information systems for decades. A number of hurdles, described in Chapter 14, have to be overcome before blockchain applications can help pave the way to a more secure and interconnected healthcare system.

Merging the different technologies described in previous chapters can offer opportunities to develop digital therapeutics (DTx), a fast-growing treatment group that most often consists of a behavioral support app, sometimes combined with biomarker assessments, data from wearables, and virtual reality and AI technologies. DTx utilizes health technology to treat a medical or psychological condition by digitally engaging patients and can lead to clinically relevant outcomes. Certified DTx products, as described in Chapter 15, have undergone rigorous clinical testing through randomized clinical trials and real-world pilots to demonstrate their safety and efficacy. Some DTx claim to be able to reduce the need for medication and thus can be considered as a synergistic combinatory package with medication. In digital health management teams, pharmaceutical care professionals can provide knowledge and expertise on which DTx can augment the impact of drugs. Reimbursement structures for DTx are in their early states, and further regulation should ensure that a comparison of health technology with traditional medication is done appropriately and that the value of DTX is quantified.

In Chapter 16, the final chapter in Part 2, we focus on three additional technologies that are currently available and are expected to reach the broader public and change healthcare paradigms in the years to come. The information in this chapter is not meant to be all-inconclusive but as an inspiring view of what lies ahead. Precision medicine, 3D printing of medicines, and the availability of social companion robots in home settings are expected to have a significant impact on how we provide pharmaceutical care.

Precision medicine tailors procedures and therapeutic interventions at an individual patient level. Computational pharmacotherapy connects multiple sources of raw data (e.g., clinical records, labdata, genomic information, microbiome data, and so on) and uses mathematical models to generate diagnostic inferences and predictions. Computational pharmacotherapy will help healthcare providers to drive precision medicine and adapt drugs to the profile of individual patients.

Multiple techniques for 3D printing can tailor drugs in terms of dosage, size, appearance, and delivery system. It can also reduce waste from counterfeit medications and by making dose adjustments more agile.

Social companion robots come in different shapes, that is, monolithic voice-user interfaces, anthropomorphic devices, and humanoids. Social robots may entertain, perform small household tasks, remind people of drug-related activities, and motivate physical action. Robots also help free up healthcare providers' time so that they can focus more on the human touch, an empathic and compassionate touch that cannot be simulated by robots.

To warrant ethical use of social robotic technology in pharmaceutical care, it is recommended that providers understand the way algorithms are programmed, how machine learning mechanisms work, and how the connection is made to what patients consider to be "good care." Both 3D printing and robotics are prone to privacy and security challenges, and the future challenge is to provide safe systems that can be trusted by both providers and patients.

Part 3

In Part 3 the essential conditions for enhancing pharmaceutical care through the use of digital innovation are described. Experts in their field describe the crucial governance and compliance required for digital pharmaceutical care, the ethical considerations necessary when implementing advanced digital tools, and the continuous educational framework required.

In Chapter 17 Rob Peters and Barry Meesters, experts in digital health compliance, discuss the need to take a structured, risk analysis approach and clarify how principles of data privacy, quality compliance, information security, and organizational rules are impacting the compliance-by-design approach. The concept of making a compliance blueprint is explained, which—if integrated into the design of a product—is the cornerstone of releasing a reliable product that both care providers and patients trust. Compliance blueprints are increasingly supported by what is called RegTech: technology that seeks to provide nimble, configurable, easy to integrate, reliable, secure, and cost-effective regulatory solutions. Thus regulatory requirements no longer have to be seen as taking an oppositional stance towards digital pharmaceutical care, but will become true business enablers to establish a circular business model. The connected Appendix provides more detail on legislation that is relevant to bringing a digital innovation to the marketplace.

The digital revolution is now in its fourth stage, and it is gradually changing worldviews and with that ethical perspectives on what is considered a meaningful life. In Chapter 18 pharmacist-philosopher Wilma Göttgens explains the concepts of a virtue-based practice in the pharmaceutical care ecosystem. She explains that the topics of ethical behavior and autonomy are now especially important to the practice of pharmacy, and why in the digital revolution these values are the guiding beacons for pharmaceutical care practitioners to address the uncertainties inherent in fast-paced innovative environments. Also, the need for an awareness of the ethical considerations in the research and use of data is briefly discussed.

B. F. Skinner is credited with saying, "Education is what survives when what has been learned has been forgotten." In Chapter 19 it is noted that the current knowledge and skills of pharmaceutical care professionals need to be aligned with the needs of the future workforce. The study of pharmacy is expected to continue to be a STEM education. However, as a large part of future pharmaceutical care is expected to be driven by humanistic and social expertise, it has been suggested that digital pharma literacy be added as a seventh knowledge domain, in which case it would be more accurate to say that pharmacy is a STEM+ education. The authors note that not every pharmacist needs to be a pharmacy informatics expert but that all pharmacists should have some interest in data science. Based on the digital revolution, new pharmaceutical care roles will develop, and at this point we can only guess what their formal titles will be.

Part 4

In Part 4 we describe inspirational concepts, visions, and thoughts on the development of innovative digital pharmaceutical care pathways in daily practice. We also give advice on creating an organizational culture that can help ensure an effective transition into the digital epoch.

In Chapter 20 we explain the concept of Digital by Design (DbD), a structured framework inspired by the principles of the Quality by Design approach, which is well known in the pharmaceutical industry. DbD's six-step design process (why, who, what, how, do, and sustain) can be used as a guide to effectively analyze digital innovations and apply them in daily pharmaceutical care pathways. The concept is still new and will be further developed in the years to come.

It is rare that organizations achieve the results they want when they attempt to adopt new innovative pathways, as old behaviors are hard to change. In Chapter 21 high performance transformation expert Paul Rulkens suggests six keys for building a high-performance culture within future-oriented organizations and describes how digital pharmaceutical care providers can immediately start role modeling the behaviors needed to do so. The six keys are creating clarity around goals; practical ways to measure progress; a mindset of playing to win; an attitude of falling in love with clients; using the power laws of time, place, and knowledge; and understanding how to let go in order to reach out.

Final Words

This book ends with nine future thoughts that are meant as inspirational triggers towards identifying what is on the pharmaceutical care menu the day after tomorrow. Those future thoughts are:

 1. The transition to a circular pharmaceutical care model is a matter of education, attitude and process change.

 2. Health data are useless unless converted into value-adding knowledge that drives action.

 3. Patient-centric pharmaceutical care is a blend of medication expertise, holistic data analysis, hammock healthcare, and the unique qualities of the human heart.

 4. Combinatoric innovation between pharmaceutical and medical care providers fuels circular pharmaceutical care and innovative blended care models.

 5. Not all pharmaceutical care providers need to be data scientists, but every pharmaceutical care provider needs to have some interest in data science.

 6. Future pharmaceutical care providers are STEM+ professionals, data analytics translators, as well as trusted service providers, who offer digital care if possible and human care where needed.

 7. Digital health compliance blueprints, Digital by Design frameworks, and high-performance cultural transformations are convenient enablers of digital pharmaceutical care.

 8. Core values and virtues of pharmaceutical care practitioners should serve as the beacons through which patients feel comfortable in making well-informed, autonomous medication choices.

 9. Keeping the balance is the crux for achieving circular pharmaceutical care.

Finally, with technology and the balanced conditions described in this book, apothecary intelligence can be augmented such that circular pharmaceutical care is established and so that people taking medicines are able to live better lives.

Contemplate the amazing potential you will find in this book, but then come back to earth and fuel the pharmaceutical care ecology with the oxygen it needs:

blending human and digital pharmaceutical care to establish apothecary intelligence for optimal patient outcomes.

Introduction

It's funny how day by day nothing changes, but when you look back,
everything is different.
C. S. Lewis

Imagine health-tracking wearables measuring every detail of our lives and giving us continuous feedback on how to stay in *optima forma,* algorithms and artificial intelligence techniques persuading us to follow healthier lifestyles and be more thoughtful about medication use, and voice-and-bot technologies residing in our homes, giving us advice we want (and potentially don't want) on all aspects of pharmaceutical care. In this world we no longer need to visit physical pharmacies for care; instead, we have a menu of digital channels to use in our homecare environments.

Welcome to the epoch of health digitization, and a special welcome to the ecosystem of *Pharmaceutical Care in Digital Revolution.*

This book has a significant objective, that is, to elicit thoughts on how to provide circular pharmaceutical care so that our healthcare systems and the medicines we take help us live better and longer lives. Circular pharmaceutical care is defined as a regenerative system in which medications, tools, knowledge, and services are provided in closed loops or cycles, with the goal of continuously optimizing patient outcomes, reducing waste, and avoiding harm due to the use of medications. This approach is in contrast to a linear pharmaceutical care model, which is a "take-make-dispose" concept and is less focused on ongoing integration of innovations based on new insights in healthcare. Circular pharmaceutical care ensures sustainability, supports improved patient experiences, and prepares us for the "day after tomorrow."

The WHY

For the past 20 years I've had the opportunity and honor to gain international experience in epidemiology, community pharmacy, clinical operations, and the commercial and digital pharmaceutical industries. During the inspiring conversations I had with people around the world and the insightful projects and teams I led, I noticed that many of us foresee digitization as a potential means towards optimizing pharmaceutical care pathways. Many of my colleagues share the expectation that digital tools will make the delivery of pharmaceutical care more efficient, and at the same time significantly improve the outcome of patient treatments and the patients' quality of life, while also reducing the monetary cost for such care as well as the harm derived from inappropriate drug use.

Due to challenges inherent in pharmaceutical ecosystems, patient access to innovative drugs is under pressure in many countries. This is a hard fact to accept, and I, along with every pharmaceutical care stakeholder I encountered, believe that steps to address this issue should be a priority. In light of the booming digital revolution, the healthcare professionals I talked with believe that the primary challenge is knowing how to adequately select and use digitization to optimize pharmaceutical care processes and patient outcomes.

Purpose of Book

The pharmaceutical pathway has always been driven by technology. The discovery, development, manufacturing, administration, and service of drugs all rely on sophisticated hardware and software applications that facilitate the innovation, accessibility, and usability of the drugs.

At the time of this writing, the authors are not aware of a manuscript that describes in a holistic, general way both the digital health opportunities that infuse our pharmaceutical care systems and the conditions required to achieve their optimal integration.

This book highlights digital opportunities as they relate to pharmaceutical care with the intention of inspiring the industry's stakeholders to envision the potential and to help frontrunners take an informed, balanced, patient-centric, and structured approach to circular pharmaceutical care.

This book is not intended to be a scientific reference, but as an inspirational, thought-provoking work that supports the facets shown in the following figure.

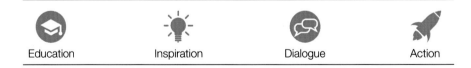

| Education | Inspiration | Dialogue | Action |

Forestry Analogy

This book uses forest metaphors. It is said we are now living in the epoch of the Anthropocene, a term that was widely popularized in 2000 by atmospheric chemist Paul J. Crutzen. The Anthropocene era acknowledges that the strong influence of human behavior on the Earth's atmosphere in recent centuries is so significant as to constitute a new geological epoch. The often irreversible human impact on biodiversity forms one of the primary attributes of the Anthropocene. Humankind has entered into what is sometimes called the Earth's sixth major extinction. It seems to be the first time in the history that humans are deemed to be responsible for this extinctive process.

Unsurprisingly, as in many parts of our flora and fauna, this human footprint has already significantly impregnated our forests. A forest can be characterized as a large area dominated by trees existing within particular relationships that determine the character of the wood. Forest ecosystems contain biotic as well as abiotic elements. The balance between those elements creates the different types of vegetation we see in the world, like rainforests, savannas, sequoia woods, and mangroves.

Human society and forests influence each other in both positive and negative ways. For example, forest ecosystems provide us with oxygen and food. Forests can also positively affect people's health. On the other hand, forests can limit urban expansion and offer a home to dangerous animals.

Humans can foster forests by respecting their ecology and protecting their flora and fauna. Human activities, including harvesting biotic resources, can negatively affect forest ecosystems. This ultimately will harm humans, as environmental disasters and a drop in the level of oxygen produced may occur.

It is this delicate balance that motivates the use of forestial status as a metaphor in this book. Thus digital health opportunities can be seen as a metaphorical forest full of oxygen and resources for the healthcare systems we have built. Mankind definitely needs these resources because, as we explain in this book, our healthcare systems are becoming exhausted under the pressures they face today.

However, without balanced implementation, digitization can result in an abiotic dilemma that will jeopardize the sustainable future of our care systems rather than fuel them.

In other words, this book is about balance: balance between using technology and using human care, balance between digitally augmenting the professional expert and securing the personal touch, and balance between enhancing the impact of drugs based on (digital) data and securing the privacy of patients. We also need the knowledge that will enable us to define the proper balance in future pharmaceutical care, that is, between digital services where possible and human services where needed.

That said, the core values of pharmaceutical care providers are the compass for substantiating the principles of good care. The skills needed to authenticate these values cannot be robotized, and factors that cannot be automated are expected to remain highly valuable.

Scope of Book

As indicated, this book is meant to introduce, educate, inspire, and prepare professionals on the dynamic future in pharmaceutical healthcare services. However, due to the space allowed, we limited the scope of the book as defined in the following sections.

Audience Scope

This book targets professionals who are responsible for providing pharmaceutical care. We frequently write from the stance that the pharmaceutical care provider, which is often a pharmacist, is the central player in this sector. While this may seem logical, and we had to start somewhere, pharmaceutical care is not only provided by pharmacists. Therefore we propose that this book is also relevant for other stakeholders who drive pharmaceutical care, such as physicians, pharmacy chains' employees, payers, regulatory affairs associates, governmental entities, and patients. Additionally, the book may attract those who want to transform pharmaceutical care by successful implementation of smart technology. You don't need to be a digital expert to understand the content of this book. In the domain of pharmaceutical care providers, the core knowledge areas relate to understanding drugs and how they work in the human body and to effectively coaching people on how to use the drugs. Even if you have reservations about the value of such technology and some mistrust about sharing data, this book can still offer you a fundamental, "helicopter" view of the future role technology can play in the industry.

In all cases enabling an informed point of view is what this book is about.

Geographical Scope

In the interest of brevity, this book focuses to a large extent on the pharmaceutical care situation in Western-oriented countries and their healthcare systems.
Some of the earliest digital concepts described in this book may not be integrated in all countries yet and in such countries may represent innovative, cutting-edge healthcare situations. The authors trust that dissemination of these concepts will drive cross-fertilization in different regions, cultures, and systems.

Time Scope

This book primarily focuses on developments over the next five years, in large part because making predictions in the digital sector's fast-paced environment is rather tricky. Because of this speed, at the time of publishing, some of the book's content may already be slightly outdated. In light of this fact, the authors provided links to dynamic QR codes and animations and made every attempt to present a book that will retain its value for readers over time.

Content Scope

The book starts with a broad view on the challenges healthcare systems are facing and how pharmaceutical care will be affected, followed by a more focused discussion on how a number of digital health technologies can be used to address these challenges. The book ends with a description of the conditions and steps needed to initiate circular pharmaceutical care. Thus the book is ideal for innovation-minded generalists who want to understand the bigger picture first and then perhaps study more deeply specific areas relative to the topic.

The authors' hope is that after reading this book pharmaceutical care providers, and related stakeholders, will feel engaged and enabled to move from a having a general understanding of the digital revolution to taking concrete steps to implement digital innovations in daily practice.

This book will never be complete or one hundred percent accurate. First, it is meant as a holistic and inspirational insight into future digital opportunities and only hits the outer circle of knowledge about a number of key technologies.

Second, as addressed before, completeness is a challenge due to the speed of the digital revolution. Thus some concepts may be obsolete in years to come and some examples mentioned in the book may cease to exist. Others may go faster or be completely different than expected, and information in the book may become outdated sooner rather than later.

Third, as this book looks into the future, interpretations of digital opportunities may change due to ongoing insights. What is considered as a promising development in 2019 may be overhauled in 2020. The future will tell.

Readers are cordially invited to send comments, additions, and notation of errors or ideas to the editor so that together we can make the second edition of this book even better.

How This Book is Organized

In Part 1 of this book we zoom in on the current challenges that healthcare systems are facing. Without exception, in both developed and low- and middle-income countries, healthcare costs are rising due to a growing and aging population, the availability of increasingly more expensive technology, higher survival rates in chronic diseases, and inefficient healthcare systems. This part describes how healthcare systems are facing pressure, gives options for structural solutions, explains how the role of patients in those systems is changing, and defines what the global definition and context of pharmaceutical care might be in this respect.

In Part 2 Chapters 7 and 8 describe in general the ecosystem of technological health innovation and its relevance to pharmaceutical care, whereas Chapters 9–16 provide more detail on individual digital solutions and their relationship to supporting efficiency, personalization, and self-management in pharmaceutical care.

Promising digital technologies are described in Chapters 9–16 in a fixed format of four key items:

- Explanation of the individual digital technology
- Impact on the five core responsibilities in pharmaceutical care, as described in Chapter 6
- Implementation in daily practice
- Considerations for use of the technology

In Part 3 of the book essential conditions for enhancing pharmaceutical care by digital innovation are described. Experts in their field have laid out the crucial governance and compliance required for digital pharmaceutical care, the ethical considerations necessary to make when implementing advanced digital tools, and the (continuous) educational framework required.

Finally, in Part 4 practical tips and tricks are provided on implementing technology in daily practice and transforming your way of working into a culture that is ready for the future.

Every chapter of this book ends with a summary of the most important priorities for creating a circular pharmaceutical pathway.

A number of QR codes are included in this book. Simply hover over the code with the QR reader on your smartphone or tablet, and you will be linked to inspiring materials, such as websites and videos, that support the topic you are reading about. If you are reading this book as an e-book, you've got it easy; just click the link and you will be directed to the web page.

To help you visualize some of the challenges you may face in daily practice, this book is connected to 10 inspirational, 1.5- to 2-minute animated videos that explain a number of themes. Just connect via the QR code or click the web link to be directed to the animations' web page: www.pharmacare.ai. Many of the animations have been adopted by supporters of the digital pharmaceutical care movement; you will find more information about these supporters in the book's acknowledgments.

Most important, you don't need to read the book from beginning to the end. You can instead just turn to the subjects you're interested in and read the individual chapters in any order you like.

Assumptions Made

To help ensure that readers derive the full potential of this book, the authors made a few assumptions about a reader:

- You are interested in focusing on how pharmaceutical care providers can use upcoming technology to improve drug use and balance healthcare costs.

- You are aware that digitalization, among other fields, is changing drug development, clinical trial execution, pharmaceutical regulation, and more, although a detailed discussion of these fields is beyond the scope of this book.
- You know the basics on how healthcare systems and pharmaceutical care pathways are organized.
- You have access to and know how to use a computer, tablet, or smartphone with an internet connection.
- You are open to learning about new technologies that go beyond your area of competency and are willing to invest time in identifying its opportunities.

Icons Used in This Interactive Book

 Tip: Marks tips and shortcuts that you can use to integrate digital knowledge and tools in daily practice

 Remember: Marks information that is especially important for pharmaceutical care practice and that bears repeating

 Examples: Includes general trend updates, best practices, company information, digital-pharma collaborations, partnerships, and synergies

 Warning: Signals where things could go wrong. This may be in terms of privacy, regulations, and governmental or other barriers related to going digital

 Ethical Consideration: Gives a recommendation on when to make a balanced decision to protect the well-being of the patient

 QR code: Refers to an illustrated website or video or other online information relevant to the topic of the respective paragraph. To be read with a QR code reader

Beyond the Book

The editor was an employee of Novartis Pharma during some time in which this book was written. Thus the editor wants to confirm that the book is published under a personal title. The views and opinions expressed in this book are those of the editor and do not represent any official policy or position of Novartis and its affiliated companies.

Nine future thoughts for the day after tomorrow

Don't think about why you question, simply don't stop questioning.
Albert Einstein

The following inspirational thoughts can help us understand tomorrow's pharmaceutical care landscape.

Nine future thoughts for every pharmaceutical care provider

 1. The transition to a circular pharmaceutical care model is a matter of education, attitude and process change.

 2. Health data are useless unless converted into value-adding knowledge that drives action.

 3. Patient-centric pharmaceutical care is a blend of medication expertise, holistic data analysis, hammock healthcare, and the unique qualities of the human heart.

 4. Combinatoric innovation between pharmaceutical and medical care providers fuels circular pharmaceutical care and innovative blended care models.

 5. Not all pharmaceutical care providers need to be data scientists, but every pharmaceutical care provider needs to have some interest in data science.

 6. Future pharmaceutical care providers are STEM+ professionals, data analytics translators, as well as trusted service providers, who offer digital care if possible and human care where needed.

 7. Digital health compliance blueprints, Digital by Design frameworks, and high-performance cultural transformations are convenient enablers of digital pharmaceutical care.

 8. Core values and virtues of pharmaceutical care practitioners should serve as the beacons through which patients feel comfortable in making well-informed, autonomous medication choices.

 9. Keeping the balance is the crux for achieving circular pharmaceutical care.

Why: Global healthcare systems under pressure

Oxygen required

Claudia Rijcken

Under pressure everything becomes fluid
Unknown

Our forests are our lifelines. They provide us with resources and produce the oxygen we need to survive. Therefore, although mankind benefits from harvesting wood and needs it as a resource, a balanced approach to the use of our forests is required to ensure that sufficient oxygen remains available.

We might say that humans in healthcare systems are like trees in forests. That is, we need to come up with better options to treat and maintain our bodies, particularly as we age, just as we need to preserve the forests to maintain them for future generations.

In this chapter you will read about the impressive progress in global healthcare systems, the pressure they are experiencing, the value of medicine in these systems, and the global ambition to innovate in order keep sustainable access.

Over the past 200 years, people around the world have achieved impressive progress in terms of their health, which has led to a significant increase in life expectancy. In the United Kingdom life expectancy doubled and is now higher than 80 years of age. In Japan health started to improve later, but the country quickly caught up with the United Kingdom and surpassed it in the late 1960s. In South Korea health started to improve later still, but the country achieved even faster progress than the United Kingdom and Japan. The life expectancy in South Korea now has surpassed that of the United Kingdom (Ourworldindata, 2018). By 2025 it is expected that 1.2 billion of the 8 billion people worldwide will be elderly, which is equivalent to the population of India.

These demographic trends are driven by a stronger focus on hygiene, improved options for the prevention of disease, and higher-quality care. However, these trends also provide a set of challenges for modern healthcare systems, as growing demand for care and changing age ratios have dramatically increased financial expectations, as shown in Figure 1.1. For example, today in the United States treating people with one or more chronic conditions consumes 90 cents of every dollar spent on healthcare (PHMRA, 2018).

Pharmaceutical Care in Digital Revolution. https://doi.org/10.1016/B978-0-12-817638-2.00001-8

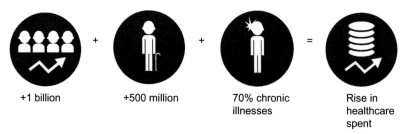

FIGURE 1.1

Pressure on healthcare systems over the next 10 years.

According to OECD (Organisation for Economic Co-operation and Development) data, spending in 2017 on healthcare was about $4000 per person on average (adjusted for purchasing power). The data show that the United States spent almost $10,000 per person on healthcare. Healthcare spending in 2017, according to the OECD, was on average 9% of countries' Gross Domestic Product (GDP), ranging from 4.3% in Turkey to 17.2% in the United States. Hospitals accounted for nearly 40% of healthcare spending (OECD, 2017). In more than 50 countries healthcare expending per capita is still less than $300 (Dieleman et al., 2016).

By 2040 global spending on healthcare is forecasted to grow from $6 trillion to $18 trillion. In the majority of developed countries, healthcare expenses have grown faster than the GDP for decades, mainly due to the previously mentioned increase in population and interventions

Should this trend continue, total health expenditures may more than double as a share of GDP, increasing to an average of about 14% of GDP among the OECD member countries in 2060, resulting in percentages above 20% in high-income countries (QR Code 1.1).

Even in cost-containment scenarios, based on the assumption that policy actions are undertaken to curb pressures on expenditures, the ratio would still increase by more than half and reach 9.5% (OECD, 2013).

This ratio is not considered sustainable by most policymakers, as well as citizens.

QR Code 1.1

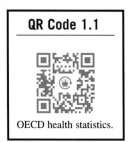

OECD health statistics.

Sustainability Focus

Assuring sustainability is not an easy task: changes to healthcare systems are often considered to be complex in terms of policy and are politically sensitive. Affordable and accessible healthcare systems require a unified approach within developed as well as low and middle-income countries (LMIC), a principle that is broadly debated in our secularized, individualized, and siloed societies.

This situation stresses the need for creative, innovative solutions to attain access to care in optimized future-proof systems. It also emphasizes the push for patients, providers, governments, and payers to share the responsibility for healthcare, as will be explained in more detail in this book.

Given the complexity of healthcare's social and economic impact and the strong links between health, workability, employment, and social care (including people's individual preferences), a broad range of disciplines, sectors, and ministries must work together closely to ensure that policies and practices are consistent, strategically aligned, and focused on future needs of individuals and the population as a whole. Effective cross-sectorial collaboration is required to minimize waste in resources while maximizing outcomes for patients, workforces, and societies.

Patients Are in General Positive, But Expect Better

Although changes in healthcare have long been needed, due to nonradical reforms, siloed budgets, and limited cross-collaborations, the changes have not come either fast or efficiently enough. This state of affairs has created a combination of high costs, unsatisfactory quality, and limited access to healthcare, which has created anxiety and frustration for participants in healthcare systems (Porter, 2006).

However, according to recent OECD data, over 80% of patients report positive experiences in terms of time spent with a doctor, easy-to-understand explanations, and involvement in treatment decisions (OECD, 2017).

Nevertheless, optimization is needed to improve access to care, transparency, speed and to address the issues of payers no longer allowing all innovations to enter the system, doctors unable to select all the therapies they want to use, and pharmacists feeling that drug budgets are being squeezed.

Patients are demanding a better experience, friendlier treatment, and assured outcomes in return for their substantial personal investment, as well as data sharing in healthcare, as is further explained in Chapter 5.

System Change Required to Create Future Oxygen

Given the global ambition to prevent healthcare systems from collapsing under the weight of their own success, that is, the provision of better treatment and extension of longevity, there is a strong need to bring increased healthcare expenditures more in line with the rate of economic growth, or even below that rate.

For years healthcare systems promised transformations, and in many cases they have been successful, for example, by promoting prevention and healthier lifestyles (which are broad determinants of health), reducing waiting times for care, restructuring the delivery of care to make it more efficient, and implementing cost-containment measurements.

 For the first time since 1973, in 2010 health-related spending in Europe declined by 0.6% per capita. A sustainability strategy in many countries has focused on treatment and prevention for the 5% of people with complex medical needs; for example, in the United States this group is responsible for at least 50% of the healthcare costs (Mitchell, 2016).

Healthcare budgets and spending today are to some extent still a mysterious black box, and there is in general a lot of waste. According to the OECD around one-fifth—no one knows the exact figure—of healthcare expenditures are wasted. Some of the waste might be attributed to excessive administration costs or even downright fraud, but a lot of money is also wasted on low-value care, that is, healthcare interventions that don't necessarily result in the best health outcomes for patients (EFPIA, 2018a).

Therefore policymakers increasingly agree that we need to move towards a model where every dollar spent goes towards producing the best outcomes. For many decades systems generally kept the incentive systems for care interventions firmly planted in fee-for-service models, also called activity-based costing. Not until the past decade did charges reach beyond the horizon. The proposed approach is called value-based healthcare, perhaps better stated as value-driven healthcare; the principles are explained in Chapter 3.

The Benefits and Budgets of Drugs in Healthcare Systems

Medicines and vaccines are some of the most powerful tools in helping people to live longer and healthier and have more productive lives. Since the 1980s we have seen death rates from HIV fall by over 80%, since the 1990s death from cancer has fallen by 20%, and recent pharmaceutical innovations mean that 90% of people living with Hepatitis C can be cured through a 12-week course of medicines (EFPIA, 2018b).

Over the past 10 years a significant number of specialty drugs have reached the healthcare market. Moreover, between 2011 and 2015 an impressive number of 226 new biological or chemical entities entered many developed markets (EFPIA, 2016) (QR Code 1.2).

Through 2021 numerous new drugs are expected to reach patients, with 2240 drugs in the late-stage pipeline and an expected 45 new active substances (NASs) forecast to be launched on average per year (in the years prior to 2018, this number was around 25 per year).

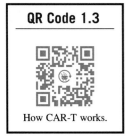

These new drugs will address significant unmet needs in cancer and autoimmune diseases and diseases related to metabolism and the nervous system, among others. In addition to continued research on the mechanisms at work in existing drugs, now drug innovation means, for example, drugs made from living cells, or targeting a specific genetic makeup, or focusing on immunotherapy that harnesses the body's own immune system to fight diseases. Also, using techniques to change genetic materials to treat diseases, such as Chimeric Antigen Receptor T-Cell (CAR-T) therapy (QR Code 1.3) or Clustered Regularly Interspaced Short Palindromic Repeats (CRISPR) to edit genomes, is expected to disruptively change the prognosis for a number of disorders in the coming years.

Value for Medication Money

Ample discussions have been held about the expected increase in drug budgets, as it is now 10%–15% of healthcare costs in most high-income countries.

Most of these drugs have been able to reduce other costs, such as avoiding clinical and surgical interventions, shorter hospital stays, less need for caregivers, or improved working productivity (which are referred to as broader societal benefits, as explained in Chapter 4).

In 2018 global drug budgets were estimated at approximately $1.2 trillion, whereas spending is expected to grow by about 3% and will reach nearly $1.5 trillion by 2021. This figure excludes the significant list-price reductions that are rebated back to payers, governments, and other stakeholders in many countries, which can comprise as much as one-third of a medication's price.

The relative growth of budgets for medicine began slowing in 2016, declining from nearly 9% growth in 2014 and 2015 to an expected 4%–7% CAGR (compound annual growth rate) over the next five years (Aitken, 2016).

The reduction in the growth rate of drug budgets has been achieved by many ways. First, the introduction of generics and biosimilars has led to an 85% switch from branded medicines during the past 10 years, leading to significant price drops, as generics are only a fraction of the cost of branded medicines and biosimilars are also less costly.

Also, companies that develop drugs are modernizing drug discovery and development processes in order to hasten developmental and regulatory approval timelines, which is reflected in the price of drugs. Moreover, new access models driven by value-based healthcare principles (Chapter 3) and innovative payment models based on outcomes (Chapter 4) are co-developed by governments, physicians, patients, and manufacturers to ensure that future healthcare systems pay as much as possible for optimal patient outcomes, rather than purely for product delivery.

However, such approaches won't happen spontaneously. They require a joint effort among all parties involved in the care process. When parties join forces and live up to the principles of value-based healthcare, the value for money spent on medication will increase, as such principles are basically meant to ensure that medication reaches the right patients, at the right time, in the right way.

This foundation will be the new "pharmaceutical forest" that will create clouds of oxygen that will guarantee future sustainable pharmaceutical care.

Principles on how to anchor innovation in existing systems are discussed in Chapter 2.

This means for circular pharmaceutical care:

- Healthcare systems are under serious pressure due to aging populations, longer survival rates from illnesses, and more costly innovative treatment options.
- Ongoing system innovation is required to keep healthcare systems affordable, accessible, and unified.
- Medicines and vaccines are some of the most powerful tools in helping people to live longer, be healthier, and have more productive lives.
- The coming years will introduce a wealth of innovative measures that will make medicines once again the cornerstone for changing the prognosis of many serious conditions.
- Generic introductions and innovative approaches in access models, like value-driven payment models, are concepts that support sustainability of healthcare systems.

An animation on the topic "Changing Healthcare Systems" can be found at www.pharmacare.ai.

QR Code Animation

Changing Healthcare Systems.

Innovation biotopes required

2

Paul Louis Iske

The alchemists in their search for gold discovered many other things of greater value.
Arthur Schopenhauer

Innovation is a much-discussed and written-about subject that always seems to be at the forefront of everyone's minds. This is not surprising: the world is changing rapidly and as addressed in the previous chapter, an innovative biotope is required to create more oxygen in healthcare forests. Some call the current spectrum of forces a "perfect storm," in which technology, economy, and society undergo drastic changes that make new business models possible and necessary.

In this chapter you will read about the principles of innovation and how to effectively implement them, what combinatoric innovation between pharmaceutical and digital technology providers is, and why the concept of brilliant failures is essential to drive digital transformation.

There are many different definitions of innovation in the literature, and based on experiences in many different companies in various industries, the following general description of innovation seems suitable for the purpose of this book:

"Innovation is a process in which ideas and knowledge are applied to achieve new ways of value creation."

Several words in this definition are relevant for this book:

1. **Process:** Innovation is a process in the sense that there is input (ideas, experiences, resources), activities (R&D, technical implementation, product launch, etc.), and output (product, service, new business model, etc.). This process usually consists of identifiable steps.
2. **Innovation:** Innovation always has something to do with "new." This becomes clear when we look at the meaning of the Latin word "innovare," which means "to renew" or "to change." However, innovation is not just something new, but involves a development with a certain value to those involved. This value is not necessarily financial; it can also be

related to happiness, health, convenience, a better society, a cleaner environment, expansion of knowledge, new relationships, and so on.

3. **Use of knowledge and other resources:** Point 1 establishes that innovation is a process in which input is converted to output. The input often consists largely of ideas, information, and insights; these are the constituents of knowledge. But innovation can also be driven by (re-)use of new and/or existing resources, including technology.

Knowledge might be found within an organization, but it might also be (partly) brought in from the outside. It might even come from another industry. No matter which organization one works for, there will always be considerably more knowledge on the outside than on the inside (unless one works for an organization with 7.4 billion colleagues).

From Innovation to Value

Innovation is not just about new products and services. Each new implementation within and around an organization that has value for its stakeholders can be considered an innovation. New revenue models, new partnership models, developments in staff management, (social) innovation, and so on are just as much innovations as innovations resulting from hard-value propositions (products and services). Thus in healthcare new medications (or administration forms) as well as new ways to interact with patients or different working processes in hospitals are considered as innovations, as long as they create additional value.

Technological developments can greatly accelerate the pace of innovation, but more is needed to maximize value creation. In several editions of the Erasmus Innovation Monitor, it was found that technological innovation contributes less than half to the realization of disruptive innovations; the remaining, bigger part is contributed by "social innovation," that is, innovative ways of managing, organizing, working, and collaborating.

In spite of the opportunities for social innovation, organizations frequently invest in technological innovation and subsequently make little to no changes in terms of communication, adapting work processes, or driving cultural transformation in order to work with this new technology (as described in Chapter 21). Sometimes this is even the case when new technologies are introduced to customers.

In these cases the well-known formula $NT + OO = EOO$ applies. It says: New Technology in an Old Organization results in an Expensive Old Organization (Iske, 2016a). It is obvious that this is not the most optimal way for integrating innovative concepts, as one of the big ambitions for our healthcare systems is to make the systems financially sustainable.

In order to determine the essence and value of an innovation, it may be helpful to map the innovation against the value blocks of an organization via the Business Model Canvas (BMC; see Figure 2.1), a framework that captures the essential building blocks of an organization, including health institutes.

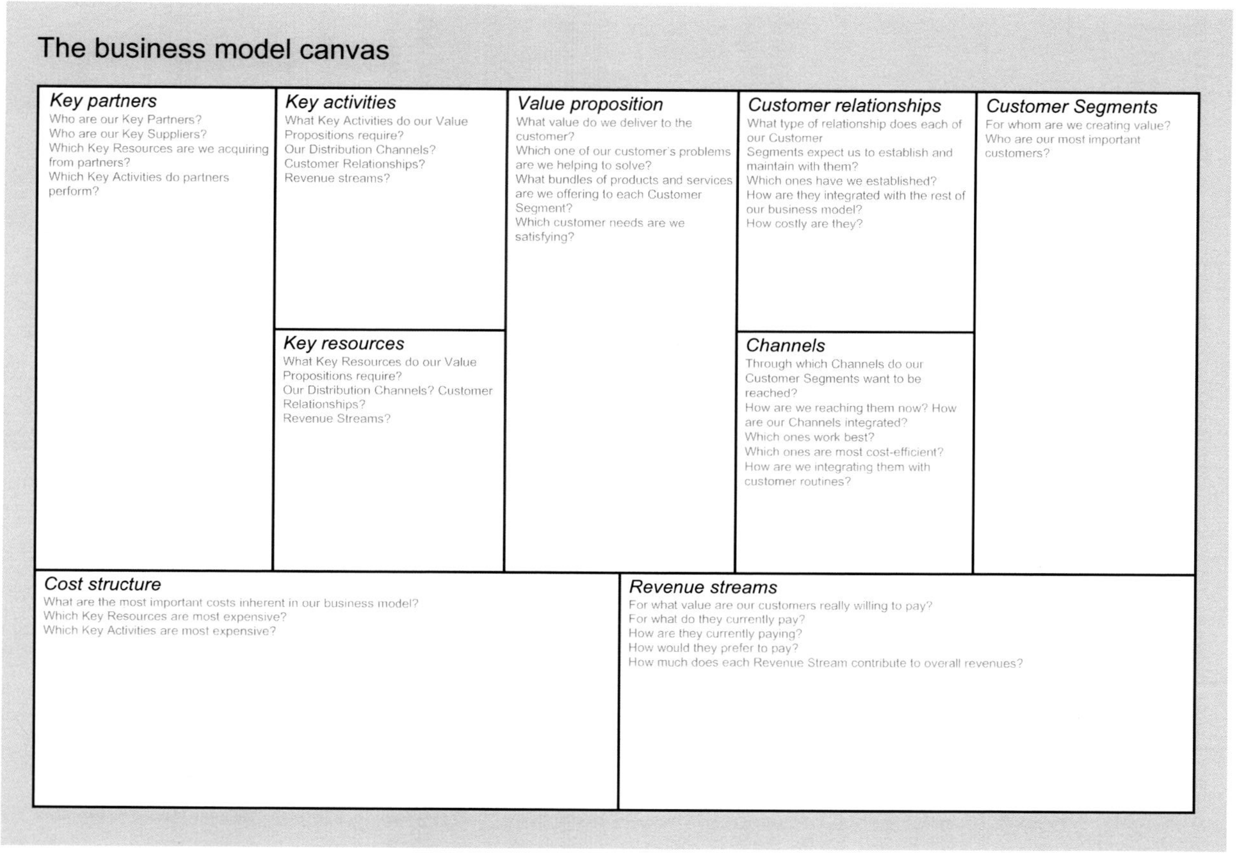

The business model canvas

Key partners

Who are our Key Partners?
Who are our Key Suppliers?
Which Key Resources are we acquiring from partners?
Which Key Activities do partners perform?

Key activities

What Key Activities do our Value Propositions require?
Our Distribution Channels?
Customer Relationships?
Revenue streams?

Key resources

What Key Resources do our Value Propositions require?
Our Distribution Channels? Customer Relationships?
Revenue Streams?

Value proposition

What value do we deliver to the customer?
Which one of our customer's problems are we helping to solve?
What bundles of products and services are we offering to each Customer Segment?
Which customer needs are we satisfying?

Customer relationships

What type of relationship does each of our Customer Segments expect us to establish and maintain with them?
Which ones have we established?
How are they integrated with the rest of our business model?
How costly are they?

Channels

Through which Channels do our Customer Segments want to be reached?
How are we reaching them now? How are our Channels integrated?
Which ones work best?
Which ones are most cost-efficient?
How are we integrating them with customer routines?

Customer Segments

For whom are we creating value?
Who are our most important customers?

Cost structure

What are the most important costs inherent in our business model?
Which Key Resources are most expensive?
Which Key Activities are most expensive?

Revenue streams

For what value are our customers really willing to pay?
For what do they currently pay?
How are they currently paying?
How would they prefer to pay?
How much does each Revenue Stream contribute to overall revenues?

FIGURE 2.1

Business Model Canvas (Osterwalder and Pigneur, 2010).

The Business Model Canvas is a great tool for communicating with and among stakeholders and for addressing the most important aspects of business development. For readers of this book, all building blocks are relevant, especially the ones referring to value proposition, channel, customer relationship, revenue model, and key activities. It goes beyond the scope of this book to explain the different compartments of this grid, as they need to be worked out in more detail; however, for those interested in systematically introducing value-adding innovations, the instructions on how to use this grid (which can be found on the internet or in books about the BMC) may be considered as valuable.

General Principles of Successful Innovation

Successful innovators spot opportunities for industry revolution just a bit faster than the rest of the pack. They apparently seem to visualize how new practices will fundamentally change customer expectations and behaviors or break long-established industry paradigms. Simply put, they challenge the status quo and strive to find ways of doing things better while also having the competency of actually implementing the changes.

An interesting book for those who aim to become top-notch innovators is *The Four Lenses of Innovation* by Rowan Gibson (Gibson, 2015). The book identifies four key business perspectives that enable readers to discover groundbreaking opportunities as the keys to successful innovation.

As a reader, one has probably already started using the first and second lens from the left, shown in Figure 2.2, in order to challenge the current pharmaceutical care dogmas. Picking up this book to understand what's going on is an important step, and after reading it and understanding the trends changing the healthcare landscape, you will be halfway to innovation leadership.

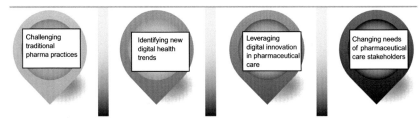

FIGURE 2.2

The four lenses of innovation in pharmaceutical care. Adapted from Gibson (2015).

One of the outcomes of reading this book or individual chapters may be that new ideas will inspire pharmaceutical care providers (PCPs) to build new concepts for reorganizing patient care. This would lead to the blue lens of innovation, meaning getting followers of the new ideas and resources to put new concepts into practice. But first the ideas need to be validated thoroughly to ensure that they truly meet the needs of the targeted audience (red lens) and have the potential to "disruptively" change and direct pharmaceutical care towards improvement and sustainability.

About disruptive innovation

In general, if we look at the current understanding of what real disruptive innovation is, we see that it consists of three basic elements (Christensen, 2009):

1. **Technological enabler:** Typically, this refers to sophisticated technology whose purpose is to simplify; it routinizes the solution to problems that previously required unstructured processes of intuitive experimentation.
2. **Business model innovation:** This model can deliver simplified solutions to customers in ways that make the innovations affordable and easily accessible.
3. **Value network:** This model is most often a commercial infrastructure in which constituent organizations have consistently disruptive, mutually reinforcing socioeconomic models.

Complexity and paradigm shifts are especially, but not exclusively, found in these transformative innovations. Clayton Christensen's *The Innovator's Dilemma* (Christensen, 2016) provides a good description as well as many examples of disruptive innovations with a large impact on established companies and even on entire industries. For decades almost every field has seen disruptive innovations that led to dramatic increases in quality of knowledge, resulting in a high level of expertise and high-quality knowledge centers, networks, and institutions.

Developments in such systems lead to emergent phenomena, that is, disruptive developments that cannot be controlled but instead require "navigation" skills such as agility and learning capacity; the impact of these new skill needs on pharmaceutical care are described in Chapters 19 and 21.

Disruptive changes usually don't come from within an industry, but from the outside. The taxi industry was not disrupted by a taxi company but by the Uber IT platform. AirBnB introduced a new hotel model without owning any hotels. Banks no longer look to each other but to tech companies such as Google, FinTech startups, crowdfunding platforms, and so on. Former IT companies now produce phones. The oil industry is about to share the playing field with sustainable energy sources, and street retailers are competing with internet parties. In short, it turns out that the world is bigger and more complex than just the limited environment in which we've always operated and competed.

Increasingly, we hear the term "kodakized," a verb reflecting the fact that the photo company Kodak did not adjust fast enough to the upcoming digitalization of the photo world and completely lost its market leadership to new entrants in the digital picture arena. Societies' big challenge is determining whether healthcare systems in general and pharmaceutical care processes in particular are deemed to be kodakized under the pressure of sustainability and by new entrants that adjust faster to innovation than the traditional systems can.

The Innovation Funnel

In general, the innovation process consists of several stages (see Figure 2.3): ideation (generation of ideas), concept (developed idea), quick scan (validated concept), business case (substantive reporting, including planning for development and implementation), prototype (development of products and services to the point where those involved have a representative image and are able to give feedback), and last but not least the launch (market introduction).

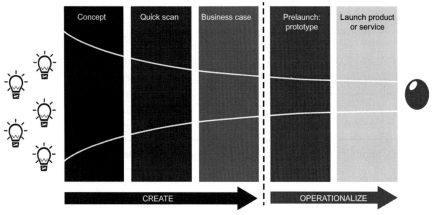

FIGURE 2.3

The funnel approach to the innovation process (Iske, 2016a).

It's becoming increasingly more common to organize processes in an agile (flexible, adaptive) way, allowing for adjustments during and especially in between the stages. This requires a type of decision making that does not determine all goals and milestones in advance, but allows decisions to be made and resources to be allocated based on intermediate results and trial and error.

That said, innovation always starts with a promising idea. How to get to that idea is the question.

Open Innovation

The idea of using knowledge and inspiration from outside an organization is not new. Organizations already know that it is often more effective not to develop all required knowledge themselves, but to search for external parties that already have complementary knowledge or that are more capable of developing it. This is known as "open innovation." This type of innovation is logically positioned on the opposite side of the more traditional "closed innovation" model, which involves parties developing and marketing their own internal ideas and knowledge.

An essential aspect of open innovation is that it requires the ability to use one's own knowledge internally as well find it externally and expand the relevant knowledge elsewhere. For pharmaceutical care this means that PCPs must develop a number of additional skills, including

- the ability to find knowledge outside the organization;
- the ability to assess that knowledge;
- the ability to integrate external knowledge into the existing knowledge;
- the ability to connect to other parties; and
- the ability to determine how the combination can successfully market the results.

An organization must therefore have a minimal knowledge of other parties and be prepared to share its success, in line with the phrase, "A small piece of a large pie is better than a large piece of a small pie." In short, existing knowledge is joined with another ability: interface management (see Figure 2.4).

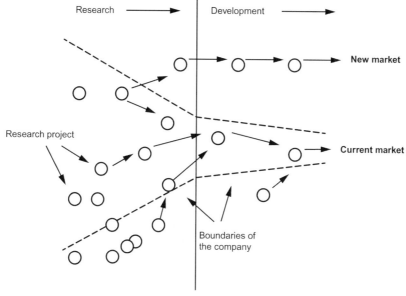

FIGURE 2.4

Open innovation requires looking into other industries (Chesbrough, 2003).

Therefore it is crucial to the success of open innovation that organizations and professionals have the alliance skills (as explained later in this book) needed to bridge the digital and pharmaceutical sectors, but also between the various stakeholders in the healthcare system (professionals, patients, managers, payers, government, industry, science). These skills are crucial to finding a fit between the potential partners in the innovation alliance.

Three areas are essential for establishing a fruitful collaborative climate: a cultural fit, a strategic fit, and an operational fit.

1. **Cultural fit:** It is important to acknowledge and work with the different backgrounds, needs, and viewpoints of stakeholders in an innovation network. If parties cannot agree on the basic, most important paradigms, collaboration and joint innovation may be very problematic.
2. **Strategic fit:** In an alliance the parties work on a joint goal. However, most often they will also have to deal with individual ambitions and targets, and if these do not match well, the alliance will probably suffer, making it difficult to achieve a sustained commitment.
3. **Operational fit:** Even when parties have the ambition and will to cooperate and jointly develop new propositions, practical issues may create challenges. These issues include availability, communication (between people, but possibly also between systems that use different data models), finance, and so on.

Examples of open innovation are everywhere. The business world collaborates with knowledge institutions (e.g., pharmaceutical companies collaborates with academia), larger organizations collaborate with smaller, specialized companies (e.g., pharmaceutical chains collaborate with specialized digital companies), and some companies leverage the knowledge of their suppliers and partners.

The challenge in this open innovation setting is to bring together unfamiliar parties (e.g., the pharmaceutical sector and digital health providers) that are able to create synergy in their business propositions.

Combinatoric Innovation

Combinatoric innovation is a methodological approach to multidisciplinary value creation. It emphasizes diversity and presupposes that it is worthwhile to bring together parties with diverse skills, backgrounds, ideas, customers, and interests in order to let them explore and discover how they can create value together in an innovative way.

Combinatoric innovation is also a creative process that combines trial and error, learning, and renewal. It is by definition nonlinear and to a certain extent unpredictable. It often cannot be captured in quick, short-term outcomes that have a positive influence on profit and loss margins.

Moreover, a combinatoric innovation process can unveil new forms of value creation by combining and applying previously unrelated intellectual capital (Iske, 2016a). This discovery process can result in serendipity, which is the skill to find something important by coincidence. It indeed is a skill to create an environment of trust, understanding, and ambition in which parties together are motivated to find new opportunities for value creation for themselves and for others.

Combinatoric innovation is in large part a social innovation, as it's often about a new way of organizing, collaborating, and innovating.

Creating the Best Environment for Combinatoric Innovation

The dynamics of successfully innovating together can to a certain extent be compared to managing successful alliances.

In addition to cultural, operational, and strategic fits, for an organization to be innovative and thrive, a number of environments are essential:

- Social space
- Process and organization space
- Virtual and digital space
- Physical and real space

In this book we do not delve into the details on optimizing these four environments, but for a more detailed description of their characteristics, refer to the book *Combinatoric Innovation* (Iske, 2016a). The point we want to make is that although we cannot always manage or control the process of (open, combinatoric) innovation, we can manage interventions in the environment that support it.

An interesting healthcare example of combinatoric innovation testing can be found in the United Kingdom's National Health Service (NHS). The NHS's *Five Year Forward View,* published in October 2014, described the NHS's intention to develop a small number of "test bed" sites. These projects will serve as real-world sites for evaluating "combinatorial" innovations that integrate new technologies and other novel approaches that offer the prospect for better care and better patient experiences at the same or lower overall cost. Upon opening QR Code 2.1, you will find an explanation about how innovators can express interest, as well as the process the NHS followed to set up this initiative.

QR Code 2.1

Example of combinatoric innovation in healthcare.

Risks for Failure

There has also been research into the factors that cause combinatoric alliances to fail. The most frequent reasons are change in management, change in priorities, slow/no results, cultural differences, weak commitment to the alliance, poor alliance management, poor communication, and changes in business environment.

Also, many people are comfortable in their current situation, which can result in a tendency to discourage innovation rather than encourage it. Just by making critical, energy-draining remarks, a person can negatively impact the enthusiasm of people and organizations for innovation. There are many such innovation-killer remarks (Iske, 2016a), and interestingly many of them suggest a fear of the unknown and of failure.

For example, "Can you guarantee that this will work?" is a perfect example of a question that should not be asked where innovation is concerned. As Einstein said, "If we knew what we are doing, we wouldn't call it research!" The word research in Einstein's statement could easily be replaced by the word innovation.

Other innovation killers related to fear of failure include, "That is impossible," "We have never tried this before," "You can never make this happen," "We will make a fool out of ourselves," "In our organization this will never work," "We have always managed without it," "You will never find a customer for this," and "We are too small for this."

Brilliant Failures

The importance of experimenting and daring to take risks to innovate, especially in these turbulent socioeconomic times, should not be underestimated. Progress and innovation go hand in hand with experimenting and taking risks, as Columbus found out long ago. It cost Dom Pérignon thousands of exploded bottles before he was able to bottle his champagne. And Viagra would never have been discovered if its manufacturer, Pfizer, hadn't persisted in looking for a new medicine for a completely different problem, that is, angina pectoris.

Healthcare systems may sometimes suffer from what can be called "corporate anorexia nervosa" and may create an unfavorable climate for enterprising people who want to explore the unknown, taking a chance that the result might not meet expectations.

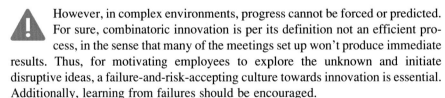 However, in complex environments, progress cannot be forced or predicted. For sure, combinatoric innovation is per its definition not an efficient process, in the sense that many of the meetings set up won't produce immediate results. Thus, for motivating employees to explore the unknown and initiate disruptive ideas, a failure-and-risk-accepting culture towards innovation is essential. Additionally, learning from failures should be encouraged.

Mediocrity, which is directly linked to fear of failure, just won't cut it. Michael Eisner, former CEO of the Walt Disney Company, is convinced that punishing failures always leads to mediocrity, because "mediocrity is what fearful people will always settle for." In other words, it is becoming increasingly important to have an open attitude to taking risks, experimenting, daring to fail, and learning from it.

The Institute of Brilliant Failures, which was founded in the Netherlands (QR Code 2.2), reinforces the culture of creating a failure-and-risk-accepting attitude towards innovation. The institute aims to reduce the fear in two ways: by increasing the appreciation of entrepreneurial activities and by stimulating learning from failed attempts. This is particularly relevant to combinatoric innovation, as the outcome of this process is by nature uncertain.

QR Code 2.2

Institute of brilliant failures.

The institute has seen the result of many failures. Often universal lessons are found within such failures: patterns or learned lessons that exceed a specific experience that can be applied in many other innovation projects. Based on these patterns, the Institute of Brilliant Failures has developed 16 archetypes that help people identify and learn from failures (Figure 2.5).

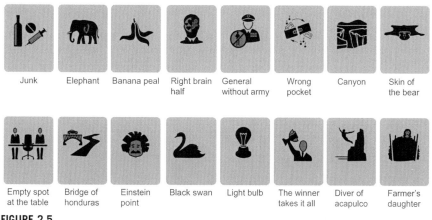

Junk — Elephant — Banana peel — Right brain half — General without army — Wrong pocket — Canyon — Skin of the bear

Empty spot at the table — Bridge of honduras — Einstein point — Black swan — Light bulb — The winner takes it all — Diver of acapulco — Farmer's daughter

FIGURE 2.5

Sixteen basic patterns (archetypes) of failure (Iske, 2016b).

The archetypes also function to classify. Failure can happen at (a combination of) four levels: system failure, organizational failure, team failure, and individual failure.

QR Code 2.2 provides a more detailed description of the archetypes.

Ideas Ready to Survive in a Complex World

Many innovative developments fail (brilliantly) because they cannot survive in a complex world. That is, something that works in a limited environment may be confronted with new circumstances and demands in a broader environment and may fail. In business development terms, one might say that a successful start-up will not automatically be successful in the next (scaled up) phase. There are essentially three phases:

- Proof of concept
- Proof of business
- Proof of success

At the point of transition between phases, it is important to consider certain aspects that might change or need to change. These include the team's skills (which could lead to changes in the team itself, as described in Chapters 19 and 21), the type of customers, and the model of financing and governance. Several brilliant failures stem from the inability to keep a concept alive in an increasingly complex context. The characteristics of each phase can be found in the book *Combinatoric Innovation* (Iske, 2016a).

When executing the goal of integrating new digital technology with pharmaceutical pathways, it is important to take these steps into account in order to develop a valuable product or service.

Chapter 3 discusses why proofing value-based innovation is important for the sustainability of future healthcare systems.

This means for circular pharmaceutical care:

- Pharmaceutical care providers should be equipped with the principles of innovation to prepare for upcoming disruptive innovations in the pharmaceutical care chain.
- Adhering to combinatoric innovation principles between current healthcare systems and (new) digital health providers will enhance the likelihood of successful innovation pathways towards circular pharmaceutical care.
- Vital conditions in which innovation can thrive need to be consciously facilitated in order to increase the likelihood of success and sustainability of digital innovation in pharmaceutical care.
- A failure-and-risk-accepting culture is crucial to stimulate innovation and learn from brilliant failures.

Value-based healthcare forestry

Claudia Rijcken

Price is what you pay. Value is what you get.
Warren Buffet

Not all forestry stakeholders agree that saving trees from harvesting is the best economic choice. In fact, a long-term saving approach may create opposition in a short-term, efficiency-driven society that prefers to cut the wood today and get immediate financial compensation. However, balancing short-term harvesting and long-term sustainable cropping strategy will result in higher and longer-lasting value; and as we have noted before, from both a health and geological point of view, doing so will ensure that we have the oxygen needed to warrant the survival of future generations. Thus, in this and other contexts, quantifying both short-term and long-term values is crucial.

In this chapter you will read about the principles of value-based healthcare and the Triple Aim concept, how to quantify the value of pharmaceutical interventions, and how this relates to the core values of the pharmaceutical care provider.

How to quantify a balanced approach to healthcare, in which the quality of future care, financial well-being, and the stability of governmental budgets are addressed, is a crucial question (refer to Chapter 1).

Current healthcare systems sometimes tend to focus on competing issues such as shifting costs, accumulating bargaining power, and restricting services rather than on creating true value for patients. This competition takes place more at the level of health plans, networks, and hospitals and unfortunately less where it matters most: in the diagnosis, treatment, and prevention of specific health conditions.

As Michael Porter indicated in 2006, the solution for keeping healthcare sustainable may be found in the implementation of value-based competition on outcomes (Porter, 2006).

Pharmaceutical Care in Digital Revolution. https://doi.org/10.1016/B978-0-12-817638-2.00003-1

In the value-based healthcare paradigm, healthcare providers are encouraged to proof the value of their interventions, as Porter described in this formula:

$$\text{Patient value} = \frac{\Delta \text{ Health Outcomes}}{\Delta \text{ Costs of Services}}$$

Any intervention that leads to a cost increase without better patient outcomes moves a system into an unsustainable, nonbeneficial situation and thus requires adjustment. Porter and Lee in 2013 defined six steps to transform healthcare organizations into value-driven ways of working; amongst these 6 steps, they considered rigorous measurement of value (outcomes and costs) as perhaps the single most important step to optimizing healthcare. When systematic measurement of results in healthcare took place, they found an improvement in the treatment results (Porter and Lee, 2013).

 Value-driven healthcare systems are characterized by the following measures:

- Focus on value for patients, not just on lowering costs.
- Drive for high-quality care that is most cost-effective.
- Focus on measuring value in the total patient pathway and beyond (broader societal value).
- Reduce variation by learning from failures and extrapolate best practices.
- Reward innovation that increases outcomes and value.
- Use technology as an enabler for the preceding characteristics.

Concerning the latter point, value-enhancing IT platforms are expected to be centered on patients and to use common data definitions and acquire holistic patient data that are accessible to all parties involved in care. These platforms will include expert systems for each professional attribution and will allow quick and easy analysis and extraction of data (Porter and Lee, 2013).

Measuring Outcomes

 The World Health Organization defines an outcome measure as a "change in the health of an individual, group of people, or population that is attributable to an intervention or series of interventions." Outcome measures (i.e., disease progression, mortality, readmission, patient experience, etc.) are the quality and cost targets healthcare organizations are trying to improve (for more detailed information see QR Code 3.1).

In addition to measuring differences in clinical parameters, outcomes can be measured by using, for example, the International Consortium for Health Outcomes Measurement (ICHOM), which offers of standardization of outcomes for a growing number of individual diseases (ICHOM, 2017).

Also, quality of life of health processes can be measured, for example, by Patient Reported Outcome Measures (PROMs) and Patient Reported Experience Measures (PREMs). PROMs measure a patient's health status or health-related quality of life

---

QR Code 3.1

WEF value of healthcare.

at a single point in time. PREMs are focused on measuring a patient's experience with healthcare processes. Both data can be tracked by surveys or by digital applications.

In addition to the standardized approaches to measuring patient outcomes, pharmaceutical care stakeholders can survey patients not only on direct outcomes but also on other determinants of health from a physical, mental, and societal perspective—for example, "what matters to patients" rather than "what is the matter with your disease?"

What People Value, Is Different for Everybody

Take for example an active hypertension patient, who is prescribed a beta blocker. Although the treatment choice may be completely according to clinical evidence and prevailing guidelines, the patient may decide not to take the pill. The adverse events of a beta blocker may be such that the patient feels hampered in active daily life, and thus the overall quality of life experience has deteriorated in the perspective of the patient. That negatively impacts therapeutic adherence and the outcome of a treatment.

In order to determine what patients value, a personalized holistic approach, potentially supported by digital data on lifestyle and life preferences, is recommended. Validated instruments like the global attainment scale can be used to monitor progress.

In the example case, an antihypertensive without fatigue adverse events could have been a better fit for treating this "specific" patient.

Taking this individual approach is essential once aiming a holistic value approach, where health status is just one parameter within a broader spectrum of aspects that determine positive health (IPH, 2018; Christensen et al., 2017).

In other words, because we know that every dollar invested in drugs has an approximate fourfold return in broader societal benefits, pharmaceutical care providers are recommended to put these broader determinants of health into the equation when moving to value-driven pharmaceutical care (WHO, 2014).

Triple Aim and Proving Value of Medicine

Value-based healthcare embraces the "Triple Aim" concept, which means that "any health-related" interventions should pursue and have a positive effect on (1) preventing disease, (2) providing better treatment, and (3) lowering overall healthcare costs (IHI, 2017).

In order to work according to the Triple Aim, the Institute for Healthcare Improvement (IHI) recommends a process that includes identification of target populations, definition of system aims and measures, development of a portfolio of project work that is sufficiently strong to move system-level results, and rapid testing and scale-up that is adapted to local needs and conditions (IHI, 2017). Some elements of this approach are embedded in the Digital by Design concept that we propose in Chapter 20.

QR Code 3.2

The value of medicines.

Health technology assessment (HTA) agencies all over the world are working on how to adequately define the value of medicines (see QR Code 3.2), the value of a life year, and how to regulate drug prices in a solidary way. Precision medicine tests, technologies, and therapeutics (see Chapter 16) are increasingly being adopted into clinical practice as evidence of their effectiveness grows; however, justification of their budget requires adequate measurement of outcomes and a growing need for regulatory reform to safeguard equitable access (Gronde et al., 2017).

A potential dilemma of the Triple Aim concept for pharmaceutical care professionals is reflected by the example that a proposed intervention may influence one of the three pillars positively but cause friction in another pillar. For example, clinical guidelines may conflict with economic arguments, and the latter may conflict with improving a patient's quality of life. This dilemma seems to occur more frequently in choices for innovative drugs, which, for example, may have a better tolerance profile but a higher budget impact. The professional standards that pharmaceutical care providers adhere to require a balanced judgment of the well-being of the patient versus societal economic arguments, which sometimes creates complex dilemmas that both physicians and pharmacists must deal with (more information in Chapter 18).

The Quantified Self to Measure Outcomes

The technologies mentioned in Part 2 of this book increase the possibilities for collecting remote patient data on outcomes, analyzing and visualizing results, and creating holistic pictures of patients and populations.

The movement towards gathering these kinds of personalized data and using them in big data analysis is generally referred as "the quantified me" or "the quantified-self", also known as "lifelogging". In brief, quantified-self delivers self-knowledge through self-tracking via technology.

The movement incorporates technology into the acquisition of data from person's daily inputs (e.g., food consumption, quality of surrounding air), states (e.g., mood, arousal, blood oxygen levels), and health status (mental, physical, and social).

Other examples of outcomes that can nowadays be continuously tracked are:

- self-monitoring and self-sensing devices that combine wearable sensors (e.g., EEG, ECG, and echography) and wearable computing;
- biometrics and biomarkers, which in 2019 are, for example, insulin, cholesterol, glucose and cortisol levels, DNA sequencing, microbiome testing, and so on;
- semantic data, for example, data on interactions with virtual personal assistants; and
- quality of life and other social and/or mental digital assessment scales.

This quantification approach makes it possible to measure outcomes (or ultimately value) of interventions in a very holistic and longitudinal way, and although governmental and commercial goals are often focused on short-term wins, longer term goals will become more interesting as prospective studies to proof effects of major reforms with better data are more feasible than ever.

Being quantified also means that less favorable lifestyle patterns are becoming more transparent and can be disclosed to a broader society. As humans may become advanced quantified selves in the future, global dialogues have started on how individuals can maintain autonomy (i.e., self-autonomy) in how their data is shared with others. Pharmaceutical care providers have an academic and professional background perfectly suited to support patients as they deal with this serious issue. To gain a better understanding of the moral and ethical considerations around this topic, see Chapter 18.

Driving Value as a Pharmaceutical Care Provider

With the aim to create as much health value as possible for patients, the world's pharmacy profession is moving from a product-oriented practice to a patient-centered practice.

In this respect, the primary contribution of the pharmaceutical care provider—beyond filling, dispensing, and counseling patients on how to take prescriptions—is a service best known as medication management, which is explained in depth in Chapter 6.

Studies have demonstrated positive value of pharmacist interventions on clinical outcomes, such as improved control of blood pressure, improved self-care activities for diabetes, and fewer drug-related adverse events. A reduction in the total cost for care has been suggested for some scenarios, such as lower treatment costs for patients with Type 2 diabetes (Hussein, 2012).

Also, instruments that measure medication-related burdens for patients are available, for example, the Medication-Related Burden Quality of Life (MRB-QoL) scale. With this type of measurement, the value of pharmaceutical care services can be visualized as well (Mohammed et al., 2017).

As indicated in Chapter 1, in many countries, recent reforms in payment indicate a shift to holding providers more responsible for outcomes and quality and for coordinated care to reduce variation and fill the gaps when patients move from one part of the system to another.

This shift offers opportunities for partnerships between, for example, general practitioners and pharmaceutical care providers, who on the one hand, have access to a broad set of patient data and, on the other hand, can harvest the advantage of a trusted, low-threshold, close relationship with patients, and thus are able to influence outcomes through both data and empathy.

This synergy is known to bring the highest value in healthcare systems and makes pharmaceutical care providers the optimal foresters for maintaining a sustainable balance in driving outcomes of drug intervention programs.

In the next Chapter 4, we will describe how new models for reimbursing these outcome-based activities look.

This means for circular pharmaceutical care:

- Value-based or value-driven healthcare principles support sustainable systems that embrace the Triple Aim concept: more prevention, better treatment, and lower costs.
- Value base healthcare focuses also on "what matters to patients" rather than "what is the matter with the disease"?
- In order to proof value, outcomes must be measured, preferably in a standardized way.
- Outcomes can, for example, relate to clinical results, disease measurement scales, quality of life, or broader societal benefits.
- Digitization of health has led to the quantified self, where broad personal health data are tracked.
- Balancing economic versus patient-related outcomes is a unique competency by which pharmaceutical care professionals can drive patient value.

Hunting grounds of outcome-based financing

4

Claudia Rijcken

Obstacles are those frightful things you see, when you take your eyes off your goal.
Henry Ford

The process of preserving and sustaining our forests and restricting mining activities in rainforests and sequoia woods is considered beneficial to mankind in general, but local foresters and loggers, who see their direct income from harvesting decreasing significantly, may see this as a loss.

However, incentive schemes can be adjusted to encourage the latter group to choose a balanced approach in their harvesting techniques and thus improve the sustainability, health, and productivity of forests, including preserving hunting grounds.

In this chapter you will read about the innovation of reimbursement schemes for pharmaceuticals, why outcome-based financing is considered a potential panacea, and how health digitization can augment the role of pharmaceutical care providers to drive these outcome-based agreements.

Similar to the advantage-versus-loss potentially felt by foresters, a healthcare revolution focused on sustainability may create winners and losers in the health provider space as well.

Groups that hunt for control in this future "value chain sustainability" can be placed in three general categories (The Economist, 2017):

- **Traditional innovators:** e.g., pharmaceutical firms, hospitals, and medical technology companies.
- **Incumbent players:** e.g., health insurance companies, pharmacy-benefit managers (which buy drugs in bulk), and all other payers in healthcare systems.
- **Technology insurgents:** e.g., the big four, Facebook, Google, Apple, and Amazon; and a host of eager entrepreneurs (like health-tech startups) that are aiming to disrupt healthcare.

From Activity-Based to Outcome-Based Financing

Players in the preceding categories have the same goal, that is, finding sustainable solutions that warrant accessibility to future drug innovations. They all tend to agree that the majority of innovative, specialty drugs referred to in Chapter 1 are not at all discretionary and cannot be dismissed as mere lifestyle improvement drugs, as many of these drugs represent significant medical innovations in their clinical realms. Thus, among other interventions, innovation in payment access schemes is a next step towards establishing sustainable future models.

> **Philips: From Products to Solutions**
> Traditionally, Philips was a company selling light bulbs.
>
> The company's sales model for many years was based on selling as many bulbs as possible. As the bulbs' quality grew better and were eventually replaced by long-lasting LED lights, the business model had to change.
>
> Philips had much more lighting expertise than just producing the bulb, thus their new business model is much more focused on integrated light solutions.
>
> Now when clients contract with Philips for a light-solution plan, the company is reimbursed for providing the clients with a customized, adjustable, continuous light solution. Philips is paid for the solution, rather than for only the product.

To optimize the cost-effective use of drugs and reward outcomes (refer to Chapter 3), payers increasingly demand "value-based" reimbursements; this means that if a drug doesn't perform as it is supposed to (i.e., according to outcomes in clinical trials), it will not be fully reimbursed. This is what we call performance-based or outcome-based financing (OBF).

The outcome-based or performance-based model takes a radically different approach to the structure of a health system by not funding the system by resources (i.e., personnel, budget, real estate). Instead this model gives organizational units the right to make decisions about their resources (i.e., autonomy), in order to reach set, predefined performance levels. In this new paradigm health systems may no longer be rewarded for providing patient interventions (i.e., activity-based interventions, delivery of drugs), instead they will be rewarded for providing effective solutions based on the outcomes explained in Chapter 3. This outcome-based approach happens in other industries as well, as shown in the Philips example.

The performance-based model is particularly marked in relation to drugs that are highly innovative and recently introduced, because societal risks are considered higher as real-world experience is less available, the outcomes are yet harder to predict (whether they resemble trial results) and the budget impact is often significant as compared to existing therapeutic options.

An important prerequisite for driving performance-based models is the availability of outcome data, as shown in Chapter 3. This is one of the biggest assets of the digital revolution; as in the days of the quantified self, much more health data are available. Medical records are digitized, interventions are digitally tracked, and all kinds of patient data are recorded by real-time sensors. These data give insurers and governments (let's call them "payers") better insight into which treatments and interventions worked and which didn't. Additionally, while connecting the different data sets and linking them with artificial intelligence (AI) software, all stakeholders are expected to better predict upfront what the outcome of treatments will be (also see Chapter 11).

To meet performance-based requirements of payers, physicians, manufacturers, and pharmaceutical care providers (PCPs) are requested, or even expected, to install mechanisms together with patients that prove actual outcomes of drug and care interventions.

Changing Models for Spending Control on Drugs

In order to be ready to move into outcome-based payment models, providers' business models are changing significantly.

For example, in the pharmaceutical industry, whereas in the past development, marketing and sales of a specific product were the core activities, today the optimal outcome for individual patients is becoming the core strategy, as shown in Table 4.1.

Table 4.1 Towards Proving Clinical Outcomes

Past	Future
Treating signs and symptoms For example, lowering cholesterol, opening up airways	**Proving relevant clinical outcomes** Fewer cardiovascular incidents, fewer COPD exacerbations
Offering products Drugs	**Offering solutions** Reduction of COPD via smart inhaler, drugs, and behavioral therapy
Negotiating price Transactional collaboration based on volume	**Partnering for better health** Collaboration based on best health outcomes

Many countries seek to control overall spending of drugs either directly or indirectly by controlling the price and access to specific drugs. Direct controls include spending or growth caps and payback schemes, not a drug's immediate performance. An example of indirect control is assigning dedicated separate budgets for, say, hepatitis or oncology. Other indirect controls focus on evidence-based assessment of the value of medicines, which then influences either price or patient access to the medicines or both.

Table 4.2 provides an overview of different payment schemes as they are currently implemented in different payer-provider relationships.

Table 4.2 Overview of Payment Schemes

More Outcomes/Performance Focus →		
Financial-Based Contracts	**Intermediate Outcomes**	**Final Outcomes/ Outcome-Based Financing (OBF)**
Price-volume (no. of units)	Intermediate patient outcome, which are a marker for disease state, e.g., LDL, CRP	Actual patient outcome, e.g., cancer survival or multiple sclerosis relapse
Capitation	No payment for nonresponders	System usage outcomes, e.g., avoided hospitalization/ER visits
Financial risk share	Reimbursement only with evidence development in real life	Experience of healthcare treatment, e.g., QoL improvement
Volume-based discount		Broader societal benefits, e.g., less sick days at work
Payment per channel		Health impact bonds, e.g., integrated societal impact
Free/discount treatment initiation		

Globally, innovative models are sometimes co-developed by the pharmaceutical industry and other relevant stakeholders such as physicians and patient associations. Figure 4.1 shows an overview of recent changes in spending control mechanisms in Europe; this overview indicates significant development of creative, innovative ideas for keeping access to drugs affordable and sustainable.

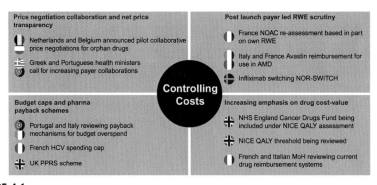

FIGURE 4.1

Changes in EU drug spending control mechanisms. Reproduced from Aitken (2016).

Real-World Evidence

As OBF schemes are becoming increasingly popular in many healthcare systems, there is a growing need to provide real-world evidence of the outcome of drugs. Real-world evidence is defined as data collected outside the clinical trial setting, including electronic health records, social media, and digital health devices.

Over the past decade many countries with outcome-based healthcare systems initiated registries to analyze the real-world experiences of people using medications. A registry is a collection of information about individuals, usually focused around a specific diagnosis or condition. Many registries collect information about people who have a specific disease or condition, while others seek participants with varying health statuses who are willing to participate in research about a particular disease. People provide information about themselves to these registries on a voluntary basis. Registries can be sponsored by a governmental agency, a nonprofit organization, a healthcare facility, or a private company.

Registries may make use of primary care data, hospital data, claims data, patient reported outcomes, and, increasingly, data from digital health devices. The most time-consuming work in these large databases is combining, formatting, cleaning, and processing data to prepare the data for analysis.

Advanced analytics techniques, with statistical methods or AI algorithms (as explained in Chapter 11), can be applied to the collected registry data to help organizations analyze much broader data sets as compared with past data. For example, upfront segmentation of patients based on RWE behavioral patterns and correlated risks of inadequate drug use can be considered, which in turn can help to develop better, more customized, and earlier intervention strategies.

Real-world evidence can be directly related to measuring the disease status or general health of a patient and may also look at benefits outside the direct healthcare environment. For example, spending on drugs may not only improve the health status of the patient but also decrease the need for care and improve work productivity.

Unfortunately, in many countries healthcare department and socioeconomic department budgets are yet completely separated, as profit-and-loss structures are organized in separate balances. Once spent in costs in healthcare result in benefits in work productivity, that real-world benefit should be considered as well when determining the real-world value of medicines.

In their assessment procedures for reimbursement, a number of European health technology authorities consider these broader societal benefits (BSBs) of drugs. Nevertheless, due to broad differences in the cost of living among different countries, it is rather complex to compare BSBs between countries and come to joint conclusions on a more holistic assessment of the economic value of drugs.

Broader Societal Benefits and Health Impact Bonds

In a value-based healthcare system, we need to look at both the direct advantages that medications have on the health of an individual or a population and the impact that drugs can have on people's ability to work or contribute to the economy and society.

There is a global trend in which employers are increasingly investing in the prevention of disease and the well-being of employees. Seventy-five percent of major US employers planned to offer telehealth services to employees in 2016, up from about 50% in 2015 (Gandhi et al., 2018). And that figure has been growing ever since.

> **BSB for Rheumatoid Arthritis (RA)**
>
> RA is a lifelong disease, with a variable pattern of symptoms and working ability of patients. Improved treatment possibilities have significantly optimized the prognosis.
>
> Benefits of adequate treatment are seen not only in less swollen joints and pain but also in productivity, for example, as more RA patients are able to continue working.
>
> The European Fit for Work initiative, which primarily looks at optimizing integrated living environments for patients with rheumatic arthritis, supports the broader societal view on the value of RA medication (The Work Foundation, 2018).

Although these figures are lower in Europe, the movement has started, and promoting high standards in working conditions, including in the area of health and well-being at work, is a key priority for the European Union (Eurofound, 2018).

In several countries there is as well a tendency towards building innovative health impact bonds (HIBs) (Brookings, 2017).

QR Code 4.1

HIB: a form of social impact bond.

HIBs are a type of social impact investment and can be defined as an investment that funds organizations addressing certain broader population-based health needs with the explicit expectation of measurable health and financial returns. Thus HIBs fall under the category of OBF models, directing the allocation of money to health programs that yield effective results (QR Code 4.1).

The difference between a HIB and a traditional OBF is the involvement of the private sector, which usually acts as an investor. This sector provides up-front financing to health service providers with the agreement to share the financial benefits once patient and/or population outcomes have been achieved. These outcomes may be, for example, lower health-related costs in a population, less time taken for sick leave, less need for care giving, and a higher quality of life, leading to healthier populations.

Pharmaceutical Care Providers as Drug Outcome Optimizers

The outcome-based payment schemes as previously described provide many opportunities for pharmaceutical care stakeholders. While the traditional activity-based model was focused on delivering products and care, evolving models are increasingly focused on incentivizing positive healthcare outcomes.

In the course of reading this book, you will see how digital health technology can augment the role of PCPs to deliver health solutions and patient outcomes as opposed to predominantly providing products. By thoroughly understanding the opportunities of this digital arena, by having access to broader health data sets, and by being able to use analytics, we may have the setup we need to make performance-based risk-sharing arrangements (PBRSA) in pharmaceutical care a reality.

 PCPs need to be highly involved in setting up these PBRSAs (which are often initiated by payers and pharmaceutical industries), as PCPs have the holistic insight of the individual patient and may positively influence drug outcomes by combining analytic insights with a human, low-threshold, and trusted approach.

As the earlier Philips example indicates (where Philips moved from selling light bulbs to warranting light solutions), we can anticipate that in future healthcare systems, the hunting grounds of drug budgets will be better balanced by PCPs being paid based on providing circular pharmaceutical care outcomes rather than on the number of prescriptions delivered.

In the next Chapter 5, we will take the perspective of patients on these developments.

This means for circular pharmaceutical care:

- Payment models in healthcare are shifting from activity-based to outcome-based schemes.
- Outcome-based reimbursement of drugs is increasingly possible due to better real-world insights.
- In addition to the value of medicines on health status, BSBs of drugs need to be considered as well when determining value and driving circular pharmaceutical care.
- Health impact bonds incentivize stakeholders to cross silos and jointly optimize the health of populations by igniting risk-benefit agreements for all collaborating partners.
- PCPs are essential partners in outcome-based payment models, as these providers can drive outcomes through strong, insightful analytics combined with low-threshold, trusted care relationship with patients.
- PCPs can be paid based on the provision of circular pharmaceutical care outcomes rather than the number of prescriptions delivered.

#PatientsIncluded™ botany

Claudia Rijcken

Diversity is the art of thinking independently together.
Malcom Forbes

In botany, a tree is a perennial plant with an elongated stem, or trunk, supporting branches and leaves in most species. Forests usually comprise multiple species of trees. Unless the needs of these individual species are understood, it is very difficult to maintain them in an appropriate way.

In healthcare systems, patients are metaphorical trees that produce the healthcare forest and determine its beauty and diversification. Only through recognition of the preferences and requirements of individual patients can systems within the forest of healthcare be equipped for the best possible circular approach.

In this chapter you will read about the emerging engagement of patients in healthcare system optimization, the principles of good care, the competencies for shared care partnerships, and the expectations for future pharmaceutical care.

Within this forest a growing number of engaged patients are daily researching, networking, and talking about health-related topics via the virtual world, accessing medical information that is freely available and shared. Increasingly, patients find themselves in the center of care.

Patient Centricity

Early patient engagement is an essential aspect in disease management, and patient centricity is a core element of the development of medicines and value-driven healthcare. In Chapters 3 and 4, we noted that health outcomes are highly dependent on active patient engagement and that there is a clear need for healthcare system providers to partner with patients in optimizing the adequate use of medicines, among other activities, to bring about better outcomes.

Pharmaceutical Care in Digital Revolution. https://doi.org/10.1016/B978-0-12-817638-2.00005-5

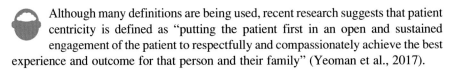 Although many definitions are being used, recent research suggests that patient centricity is defined as "putting the patient first in an open and sustained engagement of the patient to respectfully and compassionately achieve the best experience and outcome for that person and their family" (Yeoman et al., 2017).

This definition encompasses five clear themes: (1) achieving inclusiveness, (2) sharing goals that are patient- and family-centered, (3) empowering patients to take control of their own health, (4) working in a way that shows respect, compassion, and openness, and (5) working in partnership (Yeoman et al., 2017).

At first glance, the concept of patient centricity may seem easy to grasp; however, in today's society this concept cannot be taken for granted universally. Let us take a look in more detail.

Why Healthcare Systems Promote Active Patient Participation

Of the many forces that drive the goal of healthcare systems to actively engage with patients and consumers, we pick four to elaborate on as they seem the most relevant ones for the upcoming years.

- Consumerism to take autonomy on own healthcare
- Targeted information supply at individual literacy levels
- Care systems move from volume to value
- Regulatory interest in patient perspectives

Consumerism to Take Autonomy for Own Healthcare

As we indicate in Chapter 1, in many countries there exists dissatisfaction with current forms of healthcare systems, and more patients than ever are criticizing the healthcare industry's once-paternalistic approach. Therefore patients are increasingly taking charge of their own care and proactively communicating their needs, desires, and concerns to healthcare institutions.

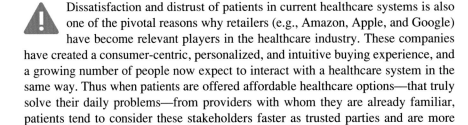 Dissatisfaction and distrust of patients in current healthcare systems is also one of the pivotal reasons why retailers (e.g., Amazon, Apple, and Google) have become relevant players in the healthcare industry. These companies have created a consumer-centric, personalized, and intuitive buying experience, and a growing number of people now expect to interact with a healthcare system in the same way. Thus when patients are offered affordable healthcare options—that truly solve their daily problems—from providers with whom they are already familiar, patients tend to consider these stakeholders faster as trusted parties and are more open to adopt their new services offered (Atluri et al., 2016).

Financially accountable, digital-savvy consumers therefore are soon expected to avail themselves to a wide range of digital health services from both traditional providers and new entrants in the healthcare industry. Many consumers want to create their own health-management ecosystems, act as stewards of their own care, and control not just where they access the care but also how and from whom they acquire it, as well as the price they have to pay.

Society is anticipating the evolution of consumerism largely through initiatives that disclose health information directly to patients. For example, those are institutions like MyTomorrows (whose goal is to disclose information that will ensure that patients with rare diseases and their physicians don't miss out on available treatment options), the Patient-Centered Outcomes Research Institute (which aims to improve the quality and relevance of the evidence available to help patients, caregivers, clinicians, employers, insurers, and policymakers make better informed health decisions), and Askapatient (see QR Code 5.1), which is an environment that gathers and discloses experiences of drug users, thus empowering other patients to take control of their health by being better informed through peers.

QR Code 5.1

Askapatient.

Targeted Information Supply at Individual Literacy Levels

In the movement to take charge of own health, access to tailored, understandable, and executable information to make informed decisions is essential. However, this is not so straightforward as it sounds; for example, having access to laboratory results is one thing, but interpreting the results as a layman and knowing how to adjust lifestyle or treatment accordingly is a different matter.

Offering optimal patient value is about supporting patients' holistic experiences and everything that goes into making those experiences as good as possible, including providing health information at an individual level of understanding. Thus many consumers and patients may not only look for how a medication works or what a certain disease comprises, they also may want to make completely informed and empowered healthcare decisions in order to reduce the likelihood of an inaccurate or delayed diagnosis, to lower the risk of hospitalization, and to maximize their quality of life. By becoming self-educated and gaining health literacy, they expect to optimize their own treatment pathways (Couch, 2018).

Herein lies a huge opportunity for pharmaceutical care providers. Digital pathways offer a variety of mediums that give patients access to health information in a personalized manner. Providing individualized written, visual, and digital information communication is possible nowadays and can be aligned with the personal preferences of patients. Part 2 of this book offers an extensive discussion about the different digital pathways that can be used to deliver information at the level consumers are seeking.

Prior to developing these information gateways, it is essential to involve both patient associations and individual patients. Thus together they can determine the highest priority areas for solving existing problems and also where most value can be created by implementing individualized support. All diseases are different, and preferences may be linked to the mobility of patient populations, the prognosis of a disease, age variations, treatment options, and so on. Involving patients as equal partners from the start, as opposed to near the end or at the point of redesign of a process, should be at the top of every health professional's mind and should be considered as "the new normal." (Engelen, 2018b).

Care Systems from Volume to Value

As we discuss in Chapter 3, precision medicine has been described as disruptive in its ability to drive down healthcare costs without compromising quality or outcomes, thus supporting the move from volume-driven to value-driven healthcare (Christensen, 2009).

Personalized medicine in this respect refers to an approach in which patients consider their genetic makeup with a focus on their preferences, beliefs, attitudes, knowledge, and social context. Conversely, *precision medicine* describes a model for healthcare delivery that relies heavily on data, analytics, and information. Precision medicine is an emerging model that aims to customize therapy to subpopulations of patients, categorized by shared molecular and cellular biomarkers, to improve patient outcomes. This model goes beyond genomics and has vast implications for a nation's research agenda and for its implementation and adoption into healthcare. To be successful precision medicine—and the ecosystem that supports it—must embrace patient-centeredness and engagement, digital health, genomics and other molecular technologies, data sharing, and data science (Ginsburg and Phillips, 2018).

The power of precision medicine is that it enables healthcare providers to choose the most effective treatment for an individual. Precision forecasting (e.g., which drug might provide the highest patient value) currently is not yet a common practice and cannot be easily drawn from only the results of clinical trials. Real-world outcomes may differ from those in clinical trial settings, mainly because populations in the real world are much more heterogenous as compared with populations in which medicines have been tested. Nevertheless, the current real-world health data offer a wealth of new opportunities once the data are synergized, for instance by combining clinical development data, patient experiences, and real-life digital health biomarkers.

As a result, using multi-criteria decision formulas that consider a broad set of data, third-party value assessment groups—such as the Institute for Clinical and Economic Review (ICER), the American Society for Clinical Oncology (ASCO), and the European Cardiology Society, as well as many national disease-specific scientific associations—increasingly publish in a structured approach their own balanced decisions about drug value.

Those insights, preferably created with patients included in the guideline setup, empower both providers and patients to make better informed decisions on treatments that best fit individual cases, thus fueling the goal of precision medicine within a circular care model.

Regulatory Interest in Patient Perspectives

The move from a volume model to a value model requires that regulatory authorities and health technology assessment bodies use a proactive patient-inclusive approach. For example, when pharmaceutical companies aim to market drugs for diseases of low prevalence (called orphan indications), costs to develop these drugs are often higher, as the risk of development failure may be increased and the return of investment distributed among a lower group of patients. Therefore, to increase the likelihood of development and reimbursement success, both pharmaceutical companies and regulators strive toward better and earlier integration of the experiences of people who endure low-frequency, but often very serious, illnesses.

As part of the Food and Drug Administration Safety and Innovation Act of 2012, the FDA set up a Patient-Focused Drug Development program to better engage with patients. As of 2018 the FDA had held 21 disease-specific meetings in the United States in which they ask patients for perspectives on their diseases, treatments, willingness to participate in clinical research, tolerance for risk, and digitalization perspectives on healthcare.

Also, the European Medicines Agency (EMA) has a structured approach to interaction with patients (EMA, 2016), collected in a framework based on the establishment of regular interactions within a network of European patient and consumer organizations. The framework aims at the following:

- Supporting the EMA to access real-life experiences of diseases and their management and to obtain information on the current use of drugs. This will contribute to understanding the value, as perceived by patients, of the scientific evidence provided during the evaluation process for the purposes of benefit/risk decision-making.
- Contributing to more efficient and targeted communication to patients and consumers, to support their role in the safe and rational use of drugs.
- Enhancing patients and consumer organizations' understanding of the role of the European Union's drug regulatory network.

What Do Patients Consider as Good Healthcare?

The importance of timely determination of whether expected outcomes of innovative treatments will meet patient expectations of good, and preferably easy, care has been explained. But what should we consider as the definition of good care?

Whereas there is considerable literature on this topic, here we want to focus on the findings within a 2018 project. One of the world's largest personalized health networks, PatientsLikeMe, fielded a six-question, online poll to a sample of its members, asking them what they consider as being "good care." A total of 2559 patients completed the poll, which asked a number of original multiple choice questions with a section for additional written responses (Delogne, 2018).

While opinions about care and provider performance varied across different disease conditions, in general patient groups agreed on the top factors that constitute "good" care:

- Active patient role in care
- Effective treatment selection
- Effective care delivery
- Focus on outcomes
- Doctor or provider competence
- Individualized and empathic care
- Collaborative care
- Effective staff communication
- Care accessibility and cost
- Office management of the respective care institute

The findings in this survey were pretty much in line with other research published in this field. Also, as in previous studies the "offer support in using digital health data and technology" has not been a dedicated item addressed.

Some of the 10 reflected topics can only be achieved by adequate use of available digital tools, thus one could state that adequate use of digital technology enables the different perceptions of what is good care.

Definitions of good care in the digital revolution may not be that different from those in the analog period, because digital technology is seen as a way to serve patients well just as human interactions do. Good care is the best possible outcome, and digital technology can be a vehicle for achieving that goal.

It is also crucial to realize that the more trust we place in future technology to deliver good care and support clinical decisions, the more studies and research we will need to validate such technology. Therefore we must continue to evaluate whether the goals of technology remain aligned with our human goals and whether they are consistent with the previously mentioned definitions of good care.

Shared Responsibility

To establish an environment in which good care can thrive, an increasing number of healthcare organizations have developed transparent communications on the shared responsibility of care providers and patients.

The way institutions provide healthcare can be found in their mission, vision, value, and process statements. Also, for many diseases, there are openly published regional, national, and international treatment guidelines (although not always at an appropriate literacy level). Additionally, institutional ambitions on private and secure data sharing, financial coverage, attitude, and expected professional behavior of providers are openly published in many healthcare environments. Thus patients are informed on what to expect from the healthcare provider and the healthcare process, and if a patient does not feel well-informed, a proactive attitude and hand-raising are expected in many healthcare systems.

Some healthcare institutions publish what they expect from a patient, which can be regarded as *psychological contract* between the healthcare system and the patient. An inspirational example is the UCLA hospital in Los Angeles, which transparently publishes its expectations to patients in public environment as (UCLA Health, 2017):

- To report to your physician, and other healthcare professionals caring for you, accurate and complete information to the best of your knowledge about present complaints, past illness, hospitalizations, medications, unexpected changes in condition and other matters relating to your health to be filed in your medical record, if applicable.
- To seek information about your health and what you are expected to do. Your healthcare provider may not know when you're confused or uncertain, or just want more information. If you don't understand the medical words they use, ask for a simpler explanation.
- The most effective plan is the one to which all participants agree and that is carried out exactly. It is your responsibility to tell your healthcare provider whether or not you can and want to follow the treatment plan recommended for you.
- To ask your healthcare provider for information about your health and healthcare. This includes following the instructions of other health team members, including nurses and physical therapists that are linked to this plan of care. The organization makes every effort to adapt a plan specific to your needs and limitations.
- To continue your care after you leave UCLA Health, including knowing when and where to get further treatment and what you need to do at home to help with your care.
- To accept the consequences of your own decisions and actions, if you choose to refuse treatment or not to comply with the care, treatment, and service plan offered by your healthcare provider.

It is interesting that many of the responsibility statements publicly available from hospitals and other healthcare providers do not yet make specific statements about the responsibility to transfer relevant quantified-self data (although this may be included in "sharing all knowledge about your health available"). Patients are not obliged to share these digital data, however, as data may be crucial for adequate treatment, actively reminding patients about this asset may help produce a favorable outcome of the proposed care.

Therefore adding a statement about the potential use of such data, specifying that they may contain important health information required to optimize the outcome of the chosen treatment, might be considered, such as the following:

- *To discuss with your healthcare provider the option to transfer relevant digital health data (e.g., mobile apps, wearables, home robotics), as they may contain important information for your treatment plan.*

Patients Getting Acquainted with Digital Health Technology

In general the rate of global adoption of digital health technology largely relates to a population's health and technology literacy. In situations where there is no awareness of why a healthy lifestyle is important, technology will not be the primary answer to stimulating consciousness on the necessity of maintaining fitness and well-being. And if health literacy exists but interest in or access to technology is limited, the adoption rate of digital health tools is still at risk.

Health technology industries are anticipating these factors by increasing integration of health monitoring tools with low-threshold devices like watches and other wearable devices that do not need to be actively operated. In a global study comprising 160 patient groups, Deloitte showed that 65% of the respondents used smartphones, of which 70% used their phone to manage their disease and about 50% did so regularly (Tailor et al., 2017). Chapter 7 provides more information on factors that impact the adoption of digital health technologies.

In a 2015 study the rate of patient engagement with digital health technologies was found to increase by 60% or more when physicians used apps and online portals to facilitate ongoing communication with patients. Thus the expanding digital environment is opening avenues for providers to improve communication with patients and remotely monitor disease status. Therefore, technology has the potential to bridge the still existing gap between patients and the healthcare ecosystem (Wicklund, 2015).

A recent survey of 2301 US health consumers also suggests that consumers become more accepting of machines—ranging from artificial intelligence (AI), to virtual clinicians, and home-based diagnostics—and those machines have a significantly greater role in their overall medical care. For example, one in five respondents (19%) said they have already used AI-powered healthcare services, and most said they are likely to use AI-enabled clinical services, such as home-based diagnostics, virtual health assistants, and virtual nurses, that monitor health conditions, medications, and vital signs at home (Accenture, 2018).

We cannot include all the available information on patients' adoption of digital healthcare in this book, but one commonality is obvious: it is the focus on simplifying and solving basic patient needs that drives adoption in healthcare, not the novelty or degree of innovation of the tools. Based on the fact that in 2018 there were about one billion chronically ill patients worldwide, it is clear that digital innovations are or are expected to become vital tools enabling patients to play an informed role in their healthcare, which is one of the strongest prerequisites for making value-driven healthcare systems work.

Some Examples Where Patients are Making a (Digital) Difference

An interesting example of where patients are voluntarily sharing health data that can be used to improve the health of specific populations is DigitalMe. The goal of this platform is to stretch the limits of breakthrough technologies to find new answers to existing and upcoming healthcare questions.

It is an initiative of the platform PatientsLikeMe (a health data sharing platform), which combines multiple sources of patient health data, pulling together experiential, environmental, biological, and medical information to create a digital version of the participating patient. The platform has a business model of selling data to pharmaceutical companies and others, which contributors to the platform agree to up front (QR Code 5.2).

QR Code 5.2

DigitalMe.

Based on the a patient's disease-specific data, what the platform is seeing across conditions, and what the platform learns from the data, it will choose from the most advanced scientific resources available, such as machine learning to examine RNA and DNA, proteins, antibodies, microbiome, and metabolites.

Ultimately, the platform aims to make it possible for a patient to try an intervention first in the digital version of himself (called an avatar or digital twin) and see how it works before deciding with a healthcare provider to continue the treatment. Needless to say, adverse events and contraindications will be much better modeled upfront than is done in current practices.

Orcha and myhealthapps.net are other examples of where patients can contribute their own or find the health experience and knowledge of others.

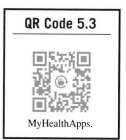

QR Code 5.3

MyHealthApps.

The site myhealthapps.net brings together information about healthcare apps that have been tried and tested by patients. Each app is reviewed by healthcare communities from all over the world, including empowered consumers, patients, care providers, patient groups, charities, and other not-for-profit organizations. It is a community-based platform that endeavors to disclose information in a more user-friendly way than general app stores do and that adds experiences that contributors had when they used a particular app (QR Code 5.3).

The website gives consumers, patients, and care providers a quick-and-easy way to find trusted apps that can make a difference in a patient's health or that can support caregivers. Although the platform is not fully matured yet, it provides a good example of how patients can take power into their own hands and build a knowledge base worldwide (see also Chapter 9).

Orcha is a leading provider of health-and-care app reviews and of the assessment of digital activation solutions. Orcha is part of the NHS England National Innovation Accelerator program and supports many NHS (National Health Service) and local government organizations to drive the uptake of digital health among their populations. Orcha's aim is to help remove the barriers that currently inhibit the true potential of digital health solutions and prevent the widespread adoption of great products and services by patients, health and care professionals, and health and care systems.

What Patients Can Expect from Pharmaceutical Care

Pharmacists in many countries around the world are praised for their professional service and their accessibility. Next to being trusted advisors, the waiting time for pharmaceutical services pales in comparison with the waiting time many patients experience in a doctor's office. Although many doctors are praised for their good services, there is a growing demand for care, and if patients cannot get a timely appointment with their doctor and their condition deteriorates, they often turn to more expensive care providers such as emergency rooms or other hospital facilities. Often, pharmaceutical care is regarded as the highly educated, professional intermediary that may prevent the need for emergency care and that can provide support for disease-related questions.

Also, for example, research has shown that US patients perceive their pharmacists as one of the most trusted care providers. The pharmacists' high rating is due mainly to the fact that they are regarded as clinically trained medication experts, who—at a low threshold—adequately and quickly answer patients' questions and offer solid advice about their drug profile as well as their disease (Gallup, 2016).

Pharmaceutical care providers strive to understand how patients think about their health and illnesses. Patients' personal perceptions of their health tells something about their ideas, feelings, and expectations about illnesses and their motives for why and how they see medication as a value in impacting their health. By talking with patients, pharmaceutical care providers often know the patients pretty much as good as their doctors to, especially in rural areas. Thus pharmacists know what matters most to patients and can align advice about treatment with the personalized situation that a patient may be in.

Unfortunately, pharmaceutical care is in many countries still a relatively untapped resource. Once pharmacists have access to key individual health information (preferably specific data from both first- and second-line care), they, together with physicians, are able to offer quick support to patients who need urgent advice, or need unplanned care, or even need help when their doctor's office is closed or busy.

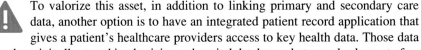 To valorize this asset, in addition to linking primary and secondary care data, another option is to have an integrated patient record application that gives a patient's healthcare providers access to key health data. Those data may be originally stored in physician or hospital databases, but can also be part of an online or mobile personal health dossier. Patients (or their representatives) may grant pharmaceutical care providers access to certain medical data, if local regulations allow. Conversely, physicians should have access to pharmaceutical care data, for instance, on adherence, adverse events, or other drug-related facts such as those acquired from digital health devices that a patient is using (you can find more on the topic of Personal Health Applications in Part 2 of this book).

The level of trust that patients have for sharing their health data with pharmaceutical care providers will grow as the providers continue to positively adapt to the changing nature of healthcare delivery. These changes include, for example, setting up more coordinated care with other healthcare providers, analyzing and using shared health data, and ensuring understanding of the data with the aim to drive better health outcomes.

Not Just a Shop or Department

Although there is great variability among regions and countries, sometimes hospital pharmacies are criticized as being invisible in direct patient care, and community pharmacies are often seen as being just a shop, with drugs dispensed at the back of the facility and employees focusing on earning money by selling over-the-counter medications. In those settings, it seems to be difficult for many people to position the pharmacist as the healthcare professional, with a five-to-six-year postgraduate education, who is able to drive the highest patient value and outcome.

Also, in the digital epoch that we are approaching, new logistic entrants are claiming to be better capable of the pure drug "distribution and shopping" concept as compared with traditional pharmacy models.

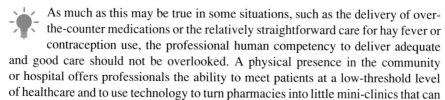 As much as this may be true in some situations, such as the delivery of over-the-counter medications or the relatively straightforward care for hay fever or contraception use, the professional human competency to deliver adequate and good care should not be overlooked. A physical presence in the community or hospital offers professionals the ability to meet patients at a low-threshold level of healthcare and to use technology to turn pharmacies into little mini-clinics that can consult on all kinds of health and wellness concerns (Engelen, 2018a).

Additionally, in the digital epoch where blended care approaches will thrive, certain pharmaceutical interventions will require a trusted face-to-face interaction or a direct drug delivery within minutes to hours. Examples from daily practice that continue to require human support include accompanying patients with complex polypharmacy interaction profiles; dealing with difficult innovative drug administration schemes in hospitals (e.g., in oncological situations); consulting with patients on ethical questions, for instance, euthanasia; or urgent recall situations with polluted drugs like the valsartan recall in 2018 (EMA, 2018).

In some of the patient surveys done in past years, overall outcomes have revealed that those patients living longer with multiple morbidities prefer to see pharmaceutical care providers especially visible, actively promoting tools around health promotion and screening, supporting efficient medication management of long-term conditions, enabling easy and accessible drug monitoring, educating the public about timely and innovative (digital) tools that are easy to integrate into patients' daily lives.

However, more extensive client-satisfaction surveys are required to gain a deeper understanding about how our metaphorical trees, that is, patients, can be optimally nurtured in the future pharmaceutical forest.

In Chapter 6 we discuss how pharmaceutical care providers view their role and responsibilities in this endeavor.

This means for circular pharmaceutical care:

- A growing number of patients play a responsible role in their own health, which is a strong prerequisite for making value-driven healthcare systems work.
- Many forces drive increasing engagement of patients in healthcare system optimization, with some of the important drivers being consumerism, information supply, value-driven healthcare, and regulatory patient interests.
- A number of factors determine the experience of "good care" delivery, in which a dedicated description of the impact of digital health data sharing.
- Actively depicting both institutional responsibilities and patient responsibilities in a healthcare environment can help to ensure that the patient's voice is really heard.
- Patients' preferences about the format (digital) of future pharmaceutical care need to be further researched.

Scenery of pharmaceutical care

6

Claudia Rijcken

There are only two ways to live your life: as though nothing is a miracle, or as though everything is a miracle.
Albert Einstein

Our forests have long been considered as sacred sites, the place where the spirits of nature and the spirits of our ancestors live. Forests help to purify the air we breathe; they provide edible plants and animals for food and the materials we need to build our homes, furniture, and numerous other items we depend on. It is important that we remain grateful for our wealth of forests and that we act responsibly in our care of them so that future generations can experience their richness, too.

In this chapter you will read about the principles of pharmaceutical care and medication management, the concepts and causes of inadequate drug use and nonadherence, and the personalized opportunities that digital pharmaceutical care provides to optimize the value of drugs.

Likewise, pharmaceutical care can be a rich and gratifying experience, as it can help improve a patient's health and quality of life. To benefit from the options in our metaphorical forest of drug treatments, we must treasure the values of good pharmaceutical care, just as we treasure our natural forests.

Pharmaceutical care (PC) is a philosophy of practice in which the patient is the primary beneficiary of the pharmacist's actions.

Pharmaceutical Care

Pharmaceutical care is defined as a professional patient care practice, which, when provided as an organized service, is experienced, documented, evaluated, and paid for as a medication management service (Cipolle et al., 2012). Pharmaceutical care can also be defined as the pharmacist's contribution to the care of individuals in order to optimize medicines use and improve health outcomes (PCNE, 2013). The goal of pharmaceutical care is to optimize the patient's health-related

Pharmaceutical Care in Digital Revolution. https://doi.org/10.1016/B978-0-12-817638-2.00006-7

quality of life and to achieve positive clinical outcomes, within realistic economic costs (APhA, 1995–2018).

The practice was developed to meet the standards of and to be consistent with the professional practices of the fields of medicine, nursing, dentistry, and veterinary medicine. As a professional practice, pharmaceutical care is guided by a philosophy, a purpose, and values in its resolution of specific problems. This mandates a strong commitment to using the profession's knowledge for the good and well-being of others, which implies a clear ethical component (turn to Chapter 18 for more on this topic).

Pharmaceutical care providers are professionals, as they became competent in their role through solid academic training; they maintain their skills through continuing professional development and commit to behaving ethically to protect the interests of the individual in the context of societal needs.

Pharmaceutical care focuses on the functions, knowledge, responsibilities, and skills as well as the attitudes, behaviors, commitments, concerns, and ethics that a pharmacist is required to fulfill, as previously defined. Above all, the provision of people- or patient-centric drug therapy has the goal to drive optimal outcomes towards patients' health and quality of life.

To understand what drives the patient, it is necessary to understand what patients value most (refer also to Chapter 5). Clinical intervention is more than the competent application of pharmaceutical knowledge to the resolution of health problems. It is also the value-laden context in which the provider deals with the process of decision making, judgment, and justification of choices made (Cipolle et al., 2012).

The pharmaceutical care process can take place in a hospital setting (hospital pharmacists), in the transition phase from hospital to home care (e.g., elderly wards), and in an outpatient, homecare setting.

The patient care process parallels the practice management activities conducted by pharmacists and ensures personnel support, document management, a supply chain, good distribution and manufacturing practices, and so on (Figure 6.1).

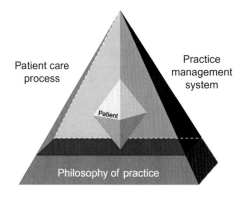

FIGURE 6.1

Components of patient-centered pharmacy practice (Cipolle et al., 2012).

Although not all have equal accountability for patient-oriented programs, pharmacists with a pharmaceutical care focus can be found in clinics and hospitals, in community pharmacies, in the pharmaceutical industry, and in pharmaceutical wholesale companies. They may also work in policy-making organizations, health insurance companies, research laboratories, governmental agencies, and may be involved in academic and post-academic education and research.

Digital Pharmaceutical Care

A patient's medication experience can be described as the sum of all the events the patient has in his lifetime that involve drug therapy. These combined experiences reveal how the patient values his health, how he makes personal decisions about medications, and his beliefs and habits around adhering to proposed healthcare interventions.

Increasingly, components of those experiences are built by and recorded in digital ecosystems. The technologies discussed in Part 2 of this book, combined with data on social media and on geographic, demographic, and cultural environments, and so on, form a patient's medication footprint, which pharmaceutical care providers need to understand. To gather all the insight required to personalize care pathways, it's crucial that the healthcare provider is part of that digital ecosystem.

Historically, pharmaceutical care was provided predominantly in a face-to-face manner; however, over time it has gradually shifted towards a format that includes digital environments, which we discuss in detail in Part 2 of this book. Based on the situation, pharmaceutical care can (and will) be given remotely; it should also consider multiple sources of digital health data and be augmented by analytics more so than in the past.

 Therefore, Digital Pharmaceutical Care (DPC) can be defined as responsible digital provision of pharmaceutical care for the purpose of achieving definite outcomes that improve a patient's quality of life.

In many cases it is up to the professional whether pharmaceutical care can be provided in a full digital manner or whether (additional) human interaction is required. A blended care approach may be a feasible option for most patients: *digital if possible and human where required* for patients' well-being.

Whereas the professional's choice is largely led by the patient's preference, considerations like the complexity of dosage regimens, native versus refill medication, and historical experience on adherence may be taken into consideration when deciding whether to provide care digitally or in person. Pharmaceutical care professionals have a responsibility to support adequate understanding about the use of medications as well as the use of the digital technology, as we further elaborate on in the course of this book.

Independent of the mode in which it is provided, pharmaceutical care must consist of a number of activities that ensure a structured and solid approach, as discussed in the following section.

Five Essential Domains of Pharmaceutical Care: The Role of Pharmacists

The American Pharmacists Association defined five domains for pharmaceutical care providers (PCPs), mainly pharmacists, which determine adequate pharmaceutical care (APhA, 1995–2018):

 A. Establish and maintain professional relationship with patients

 B. Maintain adequate collection and recording of health data

 C. Review health data and provide adequate PC proposal

 D. Ensure patient alignment and facilitate execution of PC plan

 E. Ensure circular management of PC plan

Although the outcome of either digital or human provision of pharmaceutical care should be focused on achieving optimal patient outcomes, digitization of healthcare interventions will have an impact on the execution of those domains. In Chapters 9–15 we take these five domains through an iterative process to explain how each type of technology is expected to change the paradigm of the domains.

First, let us take a deep-dive into the basic expectations of each of these five domains, where we focus primarily on the role of the pharmacist as the pharmaceutical care provider, while realizing that a number of other stakeholders support this process as well (pharmacy technicians, physicians, etc.) (APhA, 1995–2018):

 A. A professional relationship must be established and maintained.

Interaction between the pharmacist and the patient must occur to ensure that a relationship based upon caring, trust, open communication, cooperation, and mutual decision making is established and maintained. In this relationship, as in the Hippocratic Oath, the pharmacist holds the patient's welfare paramount, maintains an appropriate attitude of caring for the patient's welfare, and uses all of her professional knowledge and skills on the patient's behalf. As part of the relationship (as we note in Chapter 5), the patient gives consent to supply personal information and preferences and participates in the therapeutic plan. The pharmacist develops mechanisms to ensure that the patient has access to pharmaceutical care at all times.

B. **Patient-specific medical information must be collected, organized, recorded, and maintained.**

Subjective and objective information regarding the patient's general health and activity status, past medical history, medication history, social history, diet and exercise history, history of present illness, and economic situation (financial and insured status) must be collected. In general, this is done by the physician and the pharmacist, and ideally a connective data set is shared by the two.

Sources of information in addition to the patient's perspective may include, but are not limited to, Quantified Self data, medical charts and reports, pharmacist-conducted health/physical assessment, the patient's family or caregiver, the insurer, and other healthcare providers, including physicians, nurses, mid-level practitioners, and other pharmacists.

Since it will form the basis for decisions regarding the development and subsequent modification of the pharmaceutical care plan, the information must be timely, accurate, and complete, and it must be organized and recorded to ensure that it is easily retrievable and is updated as necessary and appropriate.

In addition to the preceding data sources, it is imperative to consider data regarding patients' beliefs, concerns, and expectations (BCE) for medication use, as they carry great weight in determining how patients regard their medication intervention. Also, discussing and recording what matters most to patients in other domains that determine a "good life" should be taken into account in order to develop a plan that is as personalized as possible. Two concepts that propagate the idea that to improve health a holistic approach to individual values is needed are the Positive Health approach and the Whole-Person approach. They are relatively new concepts within healthcare that consider six domains of what determines good life: physical functioning, mental well-being, meaningfulness, quality of life, participation, and daily functioning (IPH, 2018).

These approaches focus on supporting people in defining how to live a truly meaningful life, more than on recovering from a disease (which is not always possible). Taking data from an IPH measurement tool into account will enable pharmaceutical care providers to make a more holistic treatment plan with a higher likelihood of the patient's acceptation and adherence by the patient.

Patient information must be collected and maintained in a confidential and privacy-compliant manner (one can find more information on this topic in Chapters 17 and 18).

C. **Patient-specific medical information must be evaluated and a pharmaceutical care plan developed mutually with the patient.**

Based on a thorough understanding of the patient's beliefs and his condition or disease and its treatment, the pharmacist must, with the patient and with the patient's other healthcare providers if necessary, develop a value-driven, outcomes-oriented pharmaceutical care plan.

The Five Steps of Medication Management

- Service needs to be delivered directly to a specific patient.
- Service includes assessment of specific patient's medication-related needs. A personalized care plan is developed.
- Care must be comprehensive because medications impact all other medications and all medical conditions.
- Work of pharmacists and medication therapy practitioners are to be coordinated with other care team members.
- Service is expected to add unique value to the care of the patient.

(Taskforce PCPCC, 2012; De Gier et al., 2013)

The plan may have various components that address each of the patient's diseases or conditions. In designing the plan, the pharmacist must carefully consider the psychosocial aspects of the disease as well as the potential relationship between the cost and complexity of therapy and patient adherence.

As one of the patient's advocates, the pharmacist assures the coordination of pharmaceutical care with the patient's other healthcare providers and the patient. In addition, the pharmacist strives to achieve medication literacy by explaining at the patient's level of understanding the various pros and cons of the options relative to drug therapy and instances where one option may be more beneficial based on the pharmacist's professional judgment.

The pharmaceutical care plan must be documented in the patient's pharmacy record and communicated to the patient's other healthcare providers as necessary.

 D. The pharmacist assures that the patient has all supplies, information and knowledge necessary to carry out the pharmaceutical care plan.

The pharmaceutical care provider must assume ultimate responsibility for assuring that the patient has been able to obtain, and is appropriately using, any drugs and related products or equipment called for in the pharmaceutical care plan.

The pharmacist also assures that the patient maintains a thorough understanding of the disease and the therapy and medications prescribed in the plan.

 E. The pharmacist reviews, monitors, and modifies the pharmaceutical care plan as necessary, in alignment with the physician and in close collaboration with the patient and healthcare team.

The pharmaceutical care provider takes a circular approach towards the service provided, which means feeding patient's information on response, tolerability, and beliefs into a continuation or adaptation of the care plan, with a focus on achieving best patient outcomes possible.

From Hospital or Community to Home Pharmaceutical Care

Provided infrastructure and technology allows, in a growing number of countries an increasing number of patients are being treated with complex therapies in intermediate care facilities or in their own homes. For example, the Mercy Virtual Hospital is transforming healthcare by creating new care models fully supported by telehealth teams and technology. Patients no longer have to physically seek out care or entirely reorient their lives to gain access to specialists. Virtual technology brings care to them (Mercy-Virtual, 2018). We tend to call this care "hammock healthcare."

There are a number of reasons for the shift towards homecare:

- Most patients prefer to stay at home, if possible.
- The number of elderly people in the population are overtaking the capacity of hospital beds.
- Hospital treatment timelines have reduced significantly in past years (think, e.g., about a hip replacement, which used to be a seven-to-ten day hospitalization and now is almost an outpatient intervention).
- There are lower costs projections when treating patients at home.

Consequently, PC provision is expected to increasingly extend beyond the traditional pharmacy establishments, which emphasizes the need for different types of pharmacists and other care providers to collaborate and exchange data in an integrated care environment to ensure continuity of PC, optimize strategies, and reduce where possible harm from medication (WHO, 2017).

Integrated Care

With the patient's well-being at the center of decision making, it is vital to have one environment where all data are accessible to relevant care providers. Ideally, this is an environment managed by the patients themselves, where they authorize care providers to see, use, and review data as needed. This environment is referred to differently in various countries, for example, Personally Controlled Electronic Health Record, My Health Record, or a Personal Health Application (PHA), which we use in the remainder of this book. The PHA should always be accessible via a centralized cloud or a decentralized type of technology, as we discuss in Chapter 8.

In general, information on the patient is currently stored in an electronic health record (EHR).

In many countries there is a big challenge to connect siloed healthcare applications with this electronic health dossier, as shown in Figure 6.2.

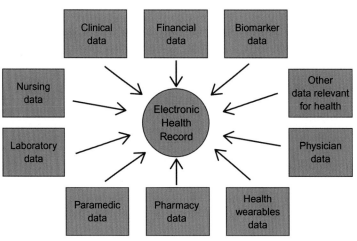

FIGURE 6.2

Electronic health record.

Technology may be a strong driver towards this connectivity, but it is currently lagging, as many different healthcare applications exist but many of the systems are not (yet) compatible.

The Internet of Things (IoT) will enable interoperability, machine-to-machine communication, information exchange, and data movement that makes healthcare service delivery effective. One can find more information on establishing integrated data systems with standardization of interoperability in Chapter 8.

An important responsibility of PHA system owners is to establish a systematic approach to warrant literacy for patients, as medical and pharmaceutical transparency that is not understood may inadvertently create stress for patients and caregivers. When patients have access to health data and cannot understand their relevance, questions may arise and explanation should be given. Providing this transparency can be handled by making literacy a crucial part of the design phase (e.g., add explanatory text fields to the PHA) and offering a virtual personal assistant that explains to the patient how to interpret data in the PHA, before concerns are raised by the patient, which would create more work for providers and more discomfort for the patient.

 Maintaining the balance between having as much patient transparency as possible and avoiding unnecessary worries and questions makes achieving PHA literacy a complex matter.

Preventing Inadequate Drug Use

The objective of reducing avoidable harm due to medication and inadequate drug use has received global attention in recent years.

Avoidable Harm Due to Medication

In March 2017 the World Health Organization (WHO) launched a global initiative to reduce severe, avoidable medication-associated harm in all countries by 50% over the next 5 years.

Medication errors injure approximately 1.3 million people annually in the United States alone. Although low- and middle-income countries are estimated to have rates of medication-related adverse events similar to those in high-income countries, the impact is about twice as high in terms of the number of years of healthy life lost. Many countries lack good data, which now will be gathered as part of the WHO initiative.

Globally, the costs associated with medication errors (not including indirect costs related to nonadherence) have been estimated at $42 billion annually or about 0.5% of total global health expenditure (WHO, 2017).

Inadequate Drug Use

In principle, inadequate drug use can be placed in four main categories (Cipolle et al., 2004). Table 6.1 depicts a number of situations that lead to inadequate drug use.

Table 6.1 Categorization of Inadequate Drug Use

Indication	Effectiveness	Safety	Adherence
Drug therapy unnecessary: - No medical indication - Duplicated therapy - Nondrug therapy indicated - Treating avoidable ADR - Dose set too high in clinical trials - Unnecessary dose escalation or combinations	**Requires different drug product:** - More effective drug available - Condition refractory to drug - Dosage form inappropriate - Not effective for condition - Dosage too low	**Adverse drug reaction:** - Undesirable effect - Unsafe drug for patient - Dose changed too quickly - Allergic reaction - Contraindications present	**Drug not taken according to directions:** - Directions not understood - Patient prefers not to take - Patient forgets to take - Drug product too expensive - Cannot swallow/administer - Drug product not available More reasons reflected below in text
Additional drug therapy required, but not provided: - Untreated condition - Preventative/prophylactic - Synergistic/potentiating	**Wrong dose:** - Frequency inappropriate - Duration inappropriate - Drug interaction - Dose set too high in clinical trials		

Adapted from Cipolle et al. (2004).

Depending on a specific problem in adequacy of drug use of a patient, digital health technology may offer solutions to limit the occurrence of situations described in Table 6.1. Those technologies are described in Part 2 of this book, and referrals will be made to the topics in the preceding table to address potential benefits to reduce avoidable harm.

Adherence, Its Relevance and Taxonomy

 Medication adherence is the process by which patients take their medication in accordance with the mutually agreed upon care plan.

As the healthcare community adopts the concepts of patient centeredness and activation, it is moving away from the previously more frequently used term *compliance*, which implies a certain patient passivity in following the prescriber's recommendations.

Another term often heard in relation to adherence is *persistence*, which refers to the length of time from initiation to discontinuation of therapy as compared to the initial treatment goals.

Medication nonadherence is an important public health consideration, strongly affecting health outcomes and overall healthcare costs. It is widespread and varies by disease, patient characteristics, and insurance coverage, with nonadherence rates ranging from 25% to 50% (Iuga and McGuire, 2014).

Chronic conditions such as diabetes, hypertension, and asthma can be effectively managed with low-cost medications. Unfortunately, around 50% of people taking pills for these conditions fall out of adherence (Heldenbrand et al., 2016). And of that 50%, half will stop taking their pills within the first year (Neura, 2017).

Classification System for Nonadherence Using the Theoretical Domains Framework (TDF)

Successful interventions in medication adherence ideally target current modifiable determinants and are tailored to the unmodifiable determinants.

Potential interventions and patient determinants from published literature on medication adherence can be categorized in 11 domains according to the Theoretical Domains Framework (TDF) (Lawton et al., 2016):

Knowledge	Skills	Social/professional role and identity
Beliefs about capabilities	Beliefs about consequences	Intentions
Memory, Attention and decision processes	Environmental context and resources	Social influences
Emotion	Behavioral regulation	

Those categories are useful to consider as both modifiable and unmodifiable determinants need to be assessed at inclusion of intervention studies to identify patients most in need of an adherence intervention (Alleman et al., 2016).

Medication nonadherence places a significant financial burden on healthcare systems. Although some literature suggest that healthcare costs attributed to nonadherence are as much as $300 billion each year in the United States and about $125 billion each year in Europe, (no global data are available), current research assessing the economic impact of medication nonadherence is limited and of varying quality, failing to provide transferable data sufficient to influence health policies. Differences in methods make comparison among studies challenging, and an accurate estimation of the true magnitude of the cost is still impossible (Cutler et al., 2018) (QR Code 6.1).

Multiple studies and meta-analyses show that more than 700 different factors are associated with adherence as reflected in Table 6.1 (Kardas et al., 2013).

To classify all these factors, various concepts have developed globally, for example, the ABC taxonomy or the depicted example of the TDF framework. The latter one focuses predominantly on categorization of nonadherence factors.

 The first one, the ABC taxonomy, is an initiative of the European Union (EU) to standardize adherence-related terminology for clinical and research use (Vrijens et al., 2012).

The taxonomy conceptualizes adherence to medications based on principles of behavioral and pharmacological science, as a response to a 2003 WHO call for action to address the disease burden associated with poor medication adherence (WHO, 2003).

The ABC taxonomy (Figure 6.3) defines the overarching concept of "medication adherence" as the process by which patients take their medication as prescribed, and then subdivides it into the following three essential elements, thus capturing the sequence of events that must happen for a patient to experience the optimal benefit from the prescribed treatment regimen.

QR Code 6.1

An explanation of adherence.

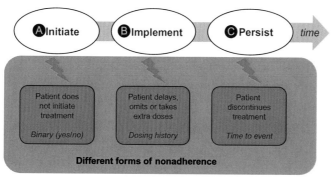

FIGURE 6.3

Taxonomy of medication adherence (Vrijens et al., 2012).

The three adherence process steps can be described as follows:

- **Initiation:** When the patient takes the first dose of a prescribed medication. This is typically a binary event (patients either start taking their medication or not in a given time period).
- **Implementation:** The extent to which a patient's actual dosing corresponds to the prescribed dosing regimen from initiation until the last dose is taken. This is a longitudinal description of patient behavior over time, that is, their dosing history.
- **Persistence:** The time elapsed from initiation until eventual treatment is discontinued (i.e., time to event); after discontinuation a period of nonpersistence may follow until the end of the prescribing period.

This taxonomy can be helpful in implementing digital solutions that link to the typical adherence problem related to a certain phase of the treatment. Digital solutions may enable monitoring and quantification of adherence patterns and may enable patients to reduce the likelihood that nonadherence stimuli will occur.

Measuring Adherence

A key process in the management of adherence consists of monitoring and supporting a patient's adherence to proposed treatments and interventions.

Pharmaceutical care stakeholders have a key responsibility to drive adherence in a positive direction, as this is one of the primary elements of the joint pharmaceutical care plan.

Adherence patterns can be measured indirectly or directly. Table 6.2 gives an overview of systematic calculation of adherence rates.

As reflected in Table 6.2, a frequently used indirect metric can be derived from refill data on prescriptions, which most pharmacies now collect in automated systems called electronic pharmacy records (EPRs). The refill rate divides the number of days pharmacy medication was picked up within a certain time period by the number of medications prescribed by the physician.

Table 6.2 Methods to Measure Adherence

Methods	Data Source	Definition
Indirect measurements used in research and administrative settings		
MPR[a]	Pharmacy claims	= (total days supplied)/(number of days between the first and last refills)
PDC[a]	Pharmacy claims	= (total days supplied)/(number of days in refill interval)
Indirect measurements used in patient care settings		
Self-report	Patient	Patient recalls medications taken in response to care team query
Questionnaire	Provider	Use of validated tool for adherence markers
Pill counting	Provider	Staff member reviews patient supply for doses remaining
Dose counting device	Device	Device includes electronic or manual counter that tracks doses released
Electronic-prescribing	PBM interface	Reports transmitted from a pharmacy benefit manager to provider usually via EMR link
Direct measurement		
Direct observation	Provider	Patient receives and takes medication at health care facility
Drug levels and markers	Laboratory	Patient blood or urine sample tested

[a]*Generally not used in direct patient care.*
Abbreviations: MPR, *medication possession ratio;* PDC, *proportion of days covered;* PBM, *pharmacy benefit manager;* EMR, *electronic medical records.*
From Iuga and McGuire (2014).

Other indirect adherence metrics, reflected in Table 6.2, that have been used for decades in pharmaceutical care research are the medication possession ratio (MPR) and the proportion of days covered (PDC), both referring to measuring continuous medication availability (CMA). A more recent way to measure CMA is found in the AdhereR example box.

AdhereR

AdhereR is an add-on package for the widely used free statistical software R developed for the estimation of adherence based on electronic healthcare data (EHD) (Dima and Dediu, 2017).

AdhereR implements a set of functions consistent with current adherence guidelines, definitions, and operationalizations. It is open source, runs on any platform on which R runs (including MS Windows, macOS, and various others); and its source code is openly available in a public GitHub repository.

Researchers and clinicians can use AdhereR to visualize patient medication histories and calculate medication availability and persistence in a flexible, transparent, and reproducible way. Users can choose among different options depending on their needs, perform sensitivity analyses with alternative options, and share their analysis code.

Being written in R and hosted on GitHub, AdhereR allows independent development and testing of new functionalities by different teams, which will be incorporated regularly in new AdhereR releases.

An MPR of 80% is often used as the cutoff between adherence and nonadherence based on its ability to predict hospitalizations across selected high-prevalence chronic diseases; however, although it is frequently used, this percentage is not based on sound arguments.

Technology to Support Adherence

In past decades, many (digital) applications have been developed that help patients remember to be more adherent and to adapt their lifestyle towards adequate use of drugs.

 For example, improving adherence can be achieved through:

- better understanding of a patient's beliefs, concerns, and expectations;
- better education;
- value-based insurance plans;
- use of patient incentives;
- adoption of medication adherence systems, including hardware-based medication adherence systems (e.g., smart pill bottles, smart caps, automated pill dispensers, electronic trays, smart cabinets, smart medical watches, smart medical alarms, wearable health sensors, packaging systems, and robotics); and
- software applications (e.g., mobile apps, sensor-enabled software solutions, mobile medication management applications, patient portals, health programs, web portals, voice-user-interfaces, and others) (Dangi, 2017).

To choose the technology that fits the needs of an individual patient, it is crucial to identify which measures are best suited for each stage of medication adherence (using the ABC taxonomy), as shown in Table 6.3.

Table 6.3 Overview of Assessment Methods of Adherence

	Time		
	A. Initiate	**B. Implement**	**C. Persist**
Direct measurement tools	Institutional sampling after prescription	Institutional sampling/home sampling by digital devices	Institutional sampling/home sampling by digital devices
Self-reporting	Survey/digital tools/phone calls	Survey/digital tools/phone calls	Survey/digital tools/phone calls
Pill counts	Dispensing tools/digital counting	Dispensing tools/digital counting	Dispensing tools/digital counting
Prescription and refill databases	Link physicians with pharmacy database	Combined database analysis	Combined database analysis
Electronic monitoring	Hardware and software solutions including initial support	Hardware and software solutions including behavioral support	Hardware and software solutions, including behavioral support

Adapted from Heidbuchl and Vrijens (2015).

Once a method is selected, it is important to realize that a tool can create a certain bias, and this should be considered when analyzing the data. For instance, home sampling may be forgotten, patients may be "white-coat" adherent, or self-reporting may have a desirability and recall bias.

Some tools, such as SMS reminders and behavioral apps, have changed the needle to the positive side in certain settings (Comstock, 2016; Mack, 2017; Vrijens et al., 2014), whereas others could not yet make a significant difference (Choudhry et al., 2017).

Individualized Goal Setting

It is clear that the adherence landscape is full of choices when it comes to finding a vehicle that best meets the expectations of an individual patient and that delivers the lowest level of bias.

Please refer also to Chapters 3 and 4, where the importance of considering holistic individual life preferences regarding "what matters most to patients" from a physical, mental, and societal perspective are described. Common sense tells us that patients will engage most readily in adherence goals, directed towards beliefs, concerns, and expectations that are important to them. The consensus among experts in the adherence community is that successful interventions need to target individual reasons for nonadherence and require tailoring to patient characteristics. Thus only personalized multifaceted interventions show positive effects at a population level.

 Therefore, pharmaceutical care providers ideally understand, for example, how an individual rates being healthy, being able to maintain a social life, fulfilling all work environment obligations, as well high-risk sports.

Through ongoing dialogue between the patient and the pharmaceutical care provider, negotiations of shared goals that are not only realistic but also well aligned to the patient's priorities for drug adherence will lead to increased satisfaction with the overall outcome of the intervention.

Goal attainment scaling (GAS) is a technique that can be used, for example, as a mathematical supportive technique for quantifying the achievement of goals set. GAS outlines the process of setting goals appropriately so that the achievement of each goal can be measured on a 5-point scale ranging from −2 to +2, and then explains a method for quantifying the outcome in a single aggregated goal attainment score (Turner-Stokes, 2009).

The goal attainment scaling process can further facilitate pharmaceutical care by helping to identify patients' priorities and by providing a systematic method for measuring and achieving outcomes that are important to the patients.

As we move into the era of the longitudinal quantified self and an integrated personal health application, it will become easier to understand and track individual health benefits obtained from adequate pharmaceutical care adherence interventions and then recalculate them in in terms of cost benefits.

This transparency is crucial as it will not only reinforce the value of pharmaceutical care support but also deliver a rationale for appropriately reimbursing adherence tools.

Return of Investment of an Adherence Program

The majority of direct costs attributed to medication nonadherence result from avoidable hospitalization. Due to the progression of controllable diseases, additional direct costs are incurred through (1) increased use of services at physician offices, emergency rooms, and urgent care and treatment facilities such as nursing homes, hospice facilities, and dialysis centers, (2) avoidable pharmacy costs related to intensified therapy as comorbid conditions develop, and (3) diagnostic testing that could be avoided by controlling the primary illness (Iuga and McGuire, 2014).

Indirect costs include factors such as loss of the caregiver's productivity and loss of the patient's autonomy.

Strategies to enhance drug adherence need to consider the impact on overall healthcare costs, weighing potentially increased drug expenditures against savings from improved outcomes and a better quality of life.

 Quantifying the benefits of investing in adequate drug use programs is rather complex, mainly for the following reasons:

- **Lack of standard approach:** this lack is due, for example, to different ways of reporting costs within and between countries.
- **Bias effect or "healthy-user" effect:** the type of patients who voluntarily enroll in adherence studies may not be representative of the general population.
- **Time preference trade-off:** stakeholders may not be willing to trade short-term increases in medication costs and complementary goods or services for long-term savings or health gains.
- **Time to attain return of investment (ROI) differs across stakeholders:** this is definitely an issue for pharmacists, who are often paid on a population-based level and will see benefits of adherence interventions only after a certain amount of time (less hospitalization, less deterioration). Patients may even receive a later ROI (depending on the progression rate of a condition), as well as the payers, who may see lower healthcare costs only after a significant amount of time due to better treatment of patients. This variability of return and the relative short-term focus of many systems may discourage healthcare system partners from making investments (Cognizant, 2016).

In conclusion, the scenery in the forest of pharmaceutical care is one of many picturesque vistas, but the scenes from past decades will not be the same as the ones in the coming years. Part 2 describes the technologies that will restructure this scenery.

This means for circular pharmaceutical care:

- Pharmaceutical care providers are value-driven healthcare team members and the gatekeepers for reducing avoidable harm due to medication and for the optimization of medication outcomes.
- DPC can be defined as responsible digital provision of pharmaceutical care for the purpose of achieving definite outcomes that improve a patient's quality of life.
- Optimal pharmaceutical care is facilitated once the patient's perspective and all patient data are collected in a Personal Health Application, a digital environment that puts all health-related data in one dossier that is owned and managed by the patient or a patient representative.
- Personal Health Applications should entail a system to warrant literacy for patients, as nonunderstood medical and pharmaceutical transparency may cause avoidable stress for patients and caregivers.
- Depending on the specificity of individual adherence challenges, digital health technology may offer personalized solutions to optimize medication management.
- The choice for a particular digital health technology support tool for pharmaceutical care should depend on individual beliefs, concerns, and expectations of the patient as well as the treatment phase.
- In digital pharmaceutical care, professionals have a responsibility to support adequate use of medication as well as the use of digital technology.
- Strategies to enhance drug adherence should consider the impact on overall healthcare costs, weighing potentially increased drug expenditures against savings from improved outcomes and better quality of life.

What: Digital advances to innovate pharmaceutical care journeys

Abiotic digital health technologies

Claudia Rijcken

Technology is neither good nor bad; nor is it neutral.
Melvin Kranzberg

As noted in this book's introduction, forests have two main components: biotic and abiotic ones. Biotic components are the living things in the ecosystem, such as trees, plants, animals, insects, fungi, and bacteria. Abiotic factors are the nonliving things in the ecosystem, such as light, water, minerals, heat, and rocks, which influence the size and composition of the living parts of the forests. We can apply this perspective metaphorically to healthcare systems, with the biotic factors being doctors, nurses, and pharmacists and the abiotic factors being, for instance, money, healthcare machines, and digital technology. It is the balance between these factors that determines the success of both ecosystems.

In this chapter you will read about the classification of digital health, considerations for adoption, economic benefits, and potential hurdles. We also consider the impact of persuasive techniques and serious gaming on uptake of digital health technology.

Let's start with a hypothetical example of patient Jeanny, reflecting how digital health is changing treatment paradigms.

Jeanny had not felt well for the past several weeks, and she could not fully grasp what was going on. Although she used to be in top physical shape, for days she had been sweating while sleeping, she had been feeling very tired for weeks, and she had lost some weight, even though she had stopped dieting some time ago. Okay, her daily job had been rather stressful for a number of months, and she did not have sufficient time to relax and do sports-related activities, but could that explain the decline in health she was experiencing?

Also, her smart health trackers and home equipment reflected issues. Her number of daily steps had decreased, her sleep-tracking mattress was emitting stress signals, the microchip in the toilet was detecting elevated lab markers in her urine, the smart scale measured ongoing weight loss, and her digital mirror reflected an unhealthy pale look with large, dark circles under her eyes. Then suddenly she received a digital

Pharmaceutical Care in Digital Revolution. https://doi.org/10.1016/B978-0-12-817638-2.00007-9

invitation to run a triage chatbot and subsequently see her doctor face to face. Probably this invitation was raised based on ongoing health data that some years ago Jeanny had decided to share with her healthcare team.

Although she thought her malaise might just be the result of her stressful job and many side activities, according to the data collected by the sensors, the symptoms could also point to an underlying malignant process, which she and her doctor now might be able to catch in its earliest stage and thus prevent a further deteriorating illness that could have a lifelong effect. On the other hand, her condition might be such that it could be easily treated in a homecare situation, allowing her to receive the care she needed from her comfortable hammock.

This example is no longer the stuff of science fiction. It is fast becoming "science fact." It is to a certain extent already possible, and it is expected to become a full reality in the upcoming years.

Technology is shifting power away from traditional healthcare providers and placing it more and more in the hands of consumers (patients), payers, and emerging digital entrants. Moreover, when individuals integrate smart technology into their living environment, they are able to monitor their disease and intervene more effectively.

People like Jeanny are now better informed, more connected, and increasingly engaged in keeping fit as long as possible (as we also note in Chapter 5). They prefer to receive their care at home as long as possible, and avoid having to visit their doctor's office or go to hospitals and other healthcare facilities.

As of 2018, mobile phones are a thousand times more capable than they were only 10 years ago, and they will become at least a thousand times more powerful over the next 10 years. Together with the sensors in their homes and on and within their bodies, Jeanny and many others will feel reassured that potential health issues will be identified in a timely way and that they will get the best outcomes from care and experience a better quality of life, even when ill.

Millennials are currently known to be the largest group to seek out alternative modes of healthcare delivery (Ebri, 2018) and like Jeanny, they are the earliest adopters of a broad range of digital health innovations.

Digital Health

When technology meets medicine, it is generally referred to as telehealth, telemedicine, e-health, or digital health.

The World Health Organization (WHO) describes telemedicine as follows: *The delivery of healthcare services, where distance is a critical factor, by all healthcare professionals using information and communication technologies for the exchange of valid information for diagnosis, treatment and prevention of disease and injuries, research and evaluations, and for the continuing education of healthcare providers, all in the interests of advancing the health of individual as their communities* (WHO, 2010). QR code 7.1 visualizes the definition further.

Telehealth, or as we call it in the remainder of this book, digital health, has to a certain extent become in the eyes of many a panacea for the democratization of healthcare (bringing it into people's homes and environment), as well as an opportunity to fight the challenges caused by an aging society, the epidemic of noncommunicable and chronic diseases, and the dramatically rising costs of healthcare, as we describe in Chapter 1.

QR Code 7.1

What is telehealth?

Booming Digital Health Environment

Digital health is expected to grow significantly in many countries in the upcoming years.

Figure 7.1 gives an overview of the digital health technologies and timelines, which are expected to disrupt the way healthcare systems are organized and how patients are treated.

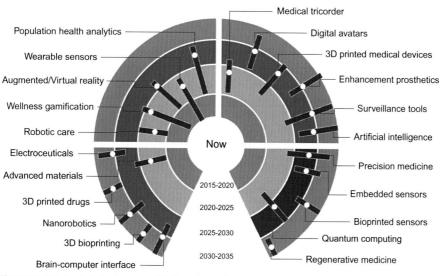

*Bars represents horizon for technology commercialization and maturation

FIGURE 7.1

Digital health technologies time frame through 2035 (Sullivan, 2016).

The digital health market in the United States is expected to grow approximately 27.5% with a value of about $9.5 billion in 2021 (PRnewswire, 2016). Also, the European digital health market is expected to grow significantly with a value of $13 billion in 2019 and beyond (Mordorintelligence, 2017).

Chapters 9–16 describe in detail the digital health technologies that the authors assume will have the most impact on future pharmaceutical care.

Digital Health Classification by Type of Data Transfer

There are many classification systems for digital health. One involves the classification in two categories that are based on the type of data transmissions (Badowski and Michienzi, 2017):

1. Store-and-forward technology, which involves the transmission of packages of data.
2. Real-time interactive services, involves direct (virtual) interaction.

Both categories are relevant for pharmaceutical care providers.

With regard to the first category, in many countries electronic pharmacy records (EPRs) are already linked to laboratories that, for example, transfer renal or liver function data into EPRs. The same is applicable in some countries where data such as genomic data on poor or fast metabolization of drugs are transmitted into EPRs, as essential information to better predict responses on medication and the occurrence of adverse events.

The second category of real-time virtual interaction is being adopted gradually by pharmaceutical care stakeholders. For example, data from health trackers, virtual personal assistants (VPAs), and digital therapeutics can be connected to electronic medical records (EMRs) and EPRs, allowing for a better understanding of response to treatment and to personalized follow-ups. Interconnectivity and the possibilities for secure data transfer are potential hurdles to adoption of these innovations, as we describe later in this part of the book.

WHO Classification of Digital Health Interventions

The WHO offers a classification of digital health interventions (DHIs) that categorizes the different ways in which digital and mobile technologies are being used to support health system needs. Historically, the diverse communities working in digital health—including government stakeholders, technologists, clinicians, implementers, network operators, researchers, and donors—have lacked a mutually understandable language with which to assess and articulate functionality. A shared and standardized vocabulary was recognized as necessary to identify gaps and duplication, evaluate effectiveness, and facilitate alignment across different digital health implementations. The classification framework aims to promote an accessible and bridging language for health program planners to articulate functionalities of digital health implementations and facilitates the dialogue between public health practitioners and a technology-oriented audience (WHO, 2018).

 The WHO DHIs categories are organized into the following overarching groupings based on the targeted primary user:

- **Interventions for clients:** clients are members of the public who are potential or current users of health services, including health promotion activities. Caregivers of clients receiving health services are also included in this group.

- **Interventions for healthcare providers:** healthcare providers are members of the health workforce who deliver health services.
- **Interventions for health system or resource managers:** health system and resource managers are involved in the administration and oversight of public health systems. Interventions within this category reflect managerial functions related to supply chain management, health financing, and human resource management.
- **Interventions for data services:** this consists of crosscutting functionality to support a wide range of activities related to data collection, management, use, and exchange.

Details of the content of the classification can be found in QR Code 7.2.

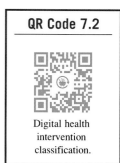

QR Code 7.2

Digital health intervention classification.

Health Technology at Different Stages of the Patient Pathway

Digital health technology can be used in different stages of a treatment pathway. From a patient's perspective (which may differ from a physician's point of view), an example of classification of tools within this pathway may look as shown in Figure 7.2.

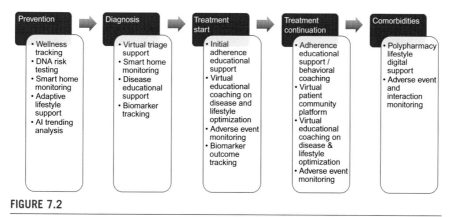

FIGURE 7.2

Examples of digital health in different patient pathway stages.

The choice of a particular technology in the initial phase of a patient pathway can seriously impact treatment in a later stage. For example, if virtual triage or digital disease education is done in an inappropriate way or results in suboptimal care, that might lower a patient's trust in digital supportive technology at a later stage, resulting in technology adversity or nonadherence later in the disease. Conversely, positive experiences in an early stage may result in better virtual expectations during the remainder of the treatment.

Additionally, once a certain technological platform or device is chosen to support the patient at the start of treatment and the patient becomes familiar with a certain platform and interconnectivity, switching to another platform or device may be increasingly complex and hard to achieve. The necessity of the Bring Your own Health Device strategy is explained in Chapter 10.

As pharmacists traditionally perform their role in close proximity to society and because pharmacy is one of the most trusted professions globally, it is considered as a low-threshold environment for professional care; thus a pharmaceutical care provider may take on additional responsibilities in future care systems.

Technology Adoption

In general, the adoption rate of digital technology varies among countries, as shown in Figure 7.3.

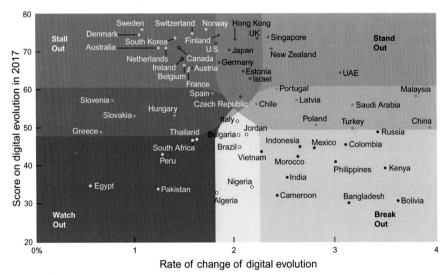

FIGURE 7.3

How countries scored across four drivers on the Digital Evolution Index. 100% on Y-axis is maximum (Fletscher School, TUFTS University 2017).

Healthcare in general has always been a technology-receptive area, embracing the development of diagnostic support tools such as X-ray, MRI, ECG, and so on. In the pharmaceutical care environment, since the beginning of the third revolution (around 1969), drug development, production, and distribution have been increasingly infused by technological advances like genetic profiling, robotics, and EPRs.

For two decades, digital advances in patient interaction have been adopted by healthcare sectors. With the global digital developments in and around 2000, many healthcare providers became aware of the need to offer online information about their services via their own website.

Around the same time, providers began to use social media to reach a greater number of customers and also offered support through interactive health services on Facebook and Twitter, for example.

Subsequently, providers' digital priorities changed again towards having their own health apps, which put the healthcare provider directly in the pocket of the patient.

Since 2018 more healthcare providers have been considering use of voice-user interfaces (VUIs) like chatbots, which take health and pharmacy records, clinical assessments, and other data to be processed by algorithms into supportive machines, thus helping both patients and providers.

The Promise of Smartphones

In the digital revolution, the adoption of mobile technology has been extremely fast, and it is estimated that there were about 4.3 billion mobile phone users in 2016, representing 58.7% of the global population. Mobile phones gradually are being replaced by smartphones, which are mobile phones with a touchscreen and a connection to the internet, that can perform a range of similar functions like a computer.

North America is expected to be the worldwide leader in adoption, with 78.7% of mobile phone users toting smartphones in 2016. Western Europe will not be too far behind at 71.7%. By 2020 the share of smartphone users is forecasted to reach 87.1% and 82.7% of mobile phone users in those regions, respectively (eMarketer, 2016).

The services smartphones offer are improving, and recent studies confirm that millennials check their phones about 150 times a day, and 73% of millennials say technology has given them a better work—life balance; for example, it has contributed to a better understanding of work projects and has helped them develop better friendships outside the workplace. Interesting fact is that in another test group comprising of about 8000 respondents globally, only 47% of older generations said tech has given them a better work–life balance or improved relationships (Accel+Qualtrics, 2017).

Nevertheless, as Figure 7.4 shows, US research indicates that baby boomers and generation X have also adopted mobile technology quickly.

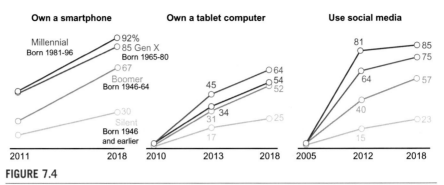

FIGURE 7.4

Adoption rate of mobile technology in the United States. Reproduced from Pew Research Center (2018).

The frequent connectivity via the smartphone makes it the ideal device for monitoring, checking, coaching, guiding, and supporting health topics. In Chapter 8 we discuss how the smartphone can become the home of an entire Personal Health Application (PHA). Also, many biosensors are now either integrated in or connected to smartphones, making the device suitable to track health parameters through, for example, ECGs, ultrasounds, and biomarkers. Applications like triage chatbots are increasingly "standard" on mobile phones, and are further explained in Chapter 12.

Even with these positive opportunities offered by mobile phones, many predict that the smartphone is only an intermediate vehicle and that within a decade augmented reality via glasses, body-worn solutions, and implanted neural laces will be our future, thus creating a cyborg-like, human-machine fusion called "transhumans." That may be the end of machines that we carry with us passively and the beginning of something that fuses our bodies directly to digital information. Yet, this vision also raises a number of ethical questions, which are discussed in Chapter 18.

Challenges of Health Technology Adoption

Many futurists and visionaries considered digital health technology as fast transformers of healthcare; for example, Fortune predicted in 2016 that wearables would enter the market and become speedy substitutes for costlier medical therapies. These wearables combined with behavioral apps were expected to offer less invasive but highly effective treatments for diseases. Business models in healthcare were expected to change fast based on the medical value wearables were expected to create, as they had done in the wellness, entertainment, and education sections for which many had been developed (Fortune, 2016).

Recent research by RockHealth involving 4000 US respondents shows a clear upward trend of consumers taking control of their healthcare via the use of digital tools like telemedicine, wearables, and online provider reviews. The percentage of respondents adopting at least one digital health tool increased from 80% in 2015 to 87% in 2017. Value drivers for adoption were empowerment for managing one's own health, open information, enablement of health data ownership, improved access to care, and a decrease in healthcare costs (Rockhealth, 2018).

Although the adoption of wearables and other digital health tools is definitely in an upward phase, the fast transformation of healthcare systems into one that uses predominantly digital pathways is not yet a reality in most countries.

 There may be a number of underlying reasons for this situation, such as the following:

- As addressed in the Foreword of this book as well as in the principle of **"first do no harm"** is one of the primary precepts of bioethics that all healthcare professions are taught in school, and it is a fundamental principle throughout the world. As long as digital innovation is in the early phases and its safety has not been proven sufficiently, healthcare professionals may regard its use as a risk for patients, which hinders adoption.
- Use of digital health in general will **require a different approach** to care delivery. Systems as well as cultures will have to adapt and engage informed patients while encouraging care providers to relinquish some control in exchange for useful real-time data.
- Those who market and develop new digital health technologies may yet underestimate the **distance between designing a wellness-like product** that appears to be associated with a healthy lifestyle and disease monitoring, versus **a tool that has also the capacity of providing scientific evidence** to support underlying health claims.
- **Pharmacists, doctors, and patients are not always involved** in the development of digital tools that are supposed to influence interventions set up by or for them. Thus not involving key stakeholders may lead to innovations that (initially) do not adequately meet customer needs.
- Digital healthcare has posed a variety **of data validation, privacy, security, and reimbursement challenges** as is explained in detail in the remainder of this book.
- **Connectivity** of different digital health solutions is yet suboptimal. Much of the data from wearables and apps available since 2018 have only limited ability to connect with existing electronic health software, thus an integrated outlook for circular pharmaceutical care is not yet achievable.
- **Amara's law** may be a potential rationale for slower adoption as well: people often overestimate the speed at which innovations will be

implemented, but underestimate how these innovations will ultimately have a very significant impact on changes in long-term healthcare systems.
- The healthcare sector as a whole also may have **insufficiently focused on truly meaningful problems**. The question, "What healthcare or patient challenges need to be solved?" in some cases has become, "How can technology solve a healthcare problem?" This may sound like a subtle distinction, but the result is a glut of mobile technologies searching for a medical purpose and not meeting the future needs of healthcare systems.
- **Governmental priority** is variable among countries. A great European example in this respect is Estonia, where since 2008 the government has developed a strong digital (health) policy and has repeatedly focused on the right questions and prioritized the right solutions for enabling fast adoption and has modeled frameworks so that they are quickly integrated into systems.

In Estonia doctors can access patients' electronic records, no matter where they are and can make better informed treatment decisions. Each person in Estonia who has visited a doctor has an online e-health record, which contains his medical case notes, test results, digital prescriptions, and X-rays, as well as a full log file tracking access to the data. Patients own their health data, and hospitals have made their data available online since 2008. Today over 95% of the data generated by hospitals and doctors have been digitized, and blockchain technology is used for assuring the integrity of stored EMRs as well as system access logs.

Because of its focus on digitization in healthcare as well as in other sectors, Estonia has been referred to as the "most advanced digital society in the world" (e-Estonia, 2017).

Despite all the challenges to adopting digital health solutions in an adequate way, there is a strong, ongoing proliferation of applications. In order to stimulate adoption and retention, persuasive health technology techniques may be needed.

Persuasive Health Technology to Drive Adoption

 Persuasive health technology is broadly defined as technology that is designed to change attitudes or behaviors of consumers through persuasion and social influence, but not through coercion.

Persuasive technologies are used regularly in sales, diplomacy, politics, religion, military training, public health, and management, and may potentially be used in any area of human-human or human-computer interaction. Examples of ways these technologies influence behavior include specific push-messages, question-and-answer techniques, and guidance signals.

Providers may utilize digital persuasive techniques and social influence strategies to increase user engagement, including, for example, gamification activities through competitions and challenges, publication of visible feedback on performance utilizing social influence principles, and reinforcement in the form of virtual rewards for achievements (Fogg, 2003; Eyal, 2014).

Extrapolating these techniques to healthcare does make sense, as successfully changing a patient's health habits is exceptionally difficult, even though doing so may provide huge health benefits in preventive healthcare, treatment adherence, disease management, and so on.

Past behavior is said to be the key enemy to forming new habits (not only those related to health), and research suggests that old habits die hard, as can be seen in the example of Google. Even when we change our routines, neural pathways remain etched in our brains, ready to be reactivated when we lose focus (Duhigg, 2012).

Old Habits Die Hard

Google users have switched marginally to the Bing searching platform, which is a perfect alternative to the better known Google, although Google is not liked by everyone.

Apparently, internet searches on Google occur so frequently that it has been able to position itself as the one and only solution in many users' minds, making it very difficult for new platforms to enter the market successfully.

Google identifies users through tracking technology, and it automatically improves users' search results based on their past behavior in order to deliver more accurate and personalized experiences, thus reinforcing the users' preference for the search engine.

Nevertheless, in 2018 Google was penalized for "serious illegal behavior" in its attempt to secure the dominance of its search engine on mobile phones.

For new behaviors to really take hold, they must occur often. That is why technology uses the principle of creating hooks to stimulate the occurrence of new habits.

Persuasive "hooks" can be defined as experiences that connect a user's problems to a supplier's solution with enough frequency to form a habit. The more often users run through these hooks, the more likely they are to form habits, most often linked to the supplier behind a product.

The hook always begins with an internal or external trigger that motivates a person to find the technology. In this respect, often the external trigger raises the interest of the user (the app sends a message, for example, on the risks of obesity and cardiovascular disease), whereas the action mostly follows only when the internal trigger is profound enough to drive activity (can I use digital tools in my app to help me lose weight).

The user then carries out a particular kind of activity (e.g., performs an exercise) and subsequently gets a reward, which can be tokens, applause, or perhaps even a reduction in health insurance fees. The next phase starts with discomfort when the exercise is not done and no reward is received and, for example, push messages are received with narratives about people who felt much more healthy at BMI 21 after successfully using the losing-weight app.

Such situations will motivate many people to perform the activity again, obtain a reward for positive behavior, and feel good. This is how the hook is created, and this is how the new habit, after a number of reiterations, is slowly formed.

In nonhealthcare environments, companies with habit-forming services usually link the services to users' daily routines and emotions. Many marketing companies, large or startups, are now trying to change behavior profoundly by guiding users through a series of experiences, that is, through hooks, as previously described.

 Some interesting fiction depicting what hooks can do to society can be found in the books *Zero* by Marc Elsberg and *The Circle* by Dave Eggers, which has been transformed into a movie plot as well (Elsberg, 2014; The Circle, 2017).

In terms of improving adequate use of medication in general and medication adherence in particular, the principles behind creating appropriate digital persuasive hooks combined with human pharmaceutical support can be strongly augmented.

Creating Hooks to Improve Adequate Use of Drugs

Being adherent to the use of a prescription drug is a fundamental habit, but one that for many is not easy to do (refer also to Chapter 6). Thus pharmaceutical care providers have a clear professional responsibility to support optimization of adherence behavior.

 To change nonadherent behavior, it is crucial that the external trigger for adherence is transformed into an intrinsic motivation. This means that patients need to be honestly convinced to use drugs in order to care for or cure their disease, or at least to alleviate the symptoms towards the best possible acceptable level. It is recommended that pharmaceutical care providers determine what a patient sees as personally relevant outcomes of treatment and to consider a holistic perspective of determinants influencing health (see Chapter 3 for more information).

Once an intrinsic motivation has been sparked, persuasive technology may call for a personalized action to use the medication, which ideally should be rewarded by something that the individual finds relevant and that makes the adherence activity attractive enough to prompt future action. This is where the GAS score of Chapter 3 and the IPH principles of Chapter 4 have relevance: when the pharmacist knows what matters most to the patient, the intrinsic motivation may be easier to spark. A blended care approach of digital as well as human coaching most often produces the greatest chance for success.

Also, all programs, digital or blended, that strive to change habits of patients, must at least have the principles of behavior change interventions (BCIs) integrated in them. A plethora of frameworks of behavior change interventions exists, but there is no gold standard yet. Therefore, before developing a digital tool that has the goal of changing behavior, it makes sense to analyze which BCI framework could best support the tool's goal and thus further increase the likelihood of a successful innovation.

Serious Gaming to Change Habits

Gamification may also be considered as a suitable technique for achieving behavioral changes. Gamification triggers the brain's reward pathways and can be designed to promote positive action and reinforcement for the correct adherent behavior.

Serious gaming can be defined as the use of game principles for the purposes of learning, skill acquisition, and training. Serious gaming, as reflected in QR Code 7.3, has shown in patient care to improve patients' cognitive abilities, rehabilitate disabled patients, promote healthy behavior, educate patients, enhance disease self-management, and attract participation in medical research.

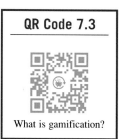

QR Code 7.3

What is gamification?

Serious games are expected to be increasingly prescribed as autonomous treatment regimens for patients. At the time of this writing, the company Akili Interactive (which is described in Chapter 15) is filing for FDA approval to market AKL-T01, a video game specifically designed to treat pediatric ADHD. This is one of the first games to be seriously considered as a legitimate treatment option for pediatric ADHD (Graafland, 2014).

A couple of other examples of serious gaming apps in the cognition improvement area are Lumosity and Elevate, which in 2018 had already acquired millions of users striving to maintain or even improve their cognitive skills on a regular basis. Users are updated on improvements (or decline) after running the game and can gain access to new levels (the reward) by continuing to play the game. Based on the data acquired in this way, the apps can even signal improvement or deterioration and potentially underlying disease conditions.

Another interesting example may be the Mango Health App, an adherence support app that allows the user to earn points every time medication is taken properly and healthy habits are maintained according to data input. Points earned unlock the chance to win gift cards, and charitable donations in raffles are held frequently.

A critical comment is that commercial models and the varying scientific reasoning behind some health-related games may negatively affect their potential for use and may require a thorough investigation before they can be recommended as being appropriate in pharmaceutical care. Future regulation and certification by authorities will provide the games' level of quality and indicate their ease of use.

The ability to use the data that the games gather and to analyze behavior patterns for continuous improvement of both the app and disease management are expected to be game-changers in healthcare.

Economic Benefits of Digital Health

The main benefits associated with digital health are often positioned as being improved personalized access to healthcare, ameliorated health insights, and reduction of healthcare-related costs.

Due to digital healthcare, patients may also experience a better quality of life, as they are treated in a more personalized and often geographically convenient way; and with digital health's strong focus on prevention, people are protected as long as possible from deterioration or perhaps even from getting sick at all.

 This can result in broader societal benefits, as we describe in Chapter 3; for example, people may need less sick leave time and may have the ability to work or live autonomously longer.

Digital health adoption as such will create additional benefits for healthcare systems as implementation may (or should) lead to more cost-efficient care, predominantly in home-situated environments. Thus the need to maintain large, expensive hospitals and care institutions may gradually decrease as well.

Additionally, the digital health epoch creates more opportunities for new entrants in the care arena, startups as well as big corporations, who see the attractiveness of a suboptimal system that can benefit from digital optimization.

Research on Digital Health Cost-Effectiveness

Structured analysis on the costs, benefits, and added value of digital health innovations is needed to form the basis for developing new business models in healthcare and to facilitate payment systems to support the most promising services. In the absence of solid evidence, key decision makers in government and paying authorities may doubt the effectiveness of digital innovations which, in turn, limits investment in and adoption of such models.

Fortunately, a significant amount of vital research is being done in this area. The scope of this book is too broad to provide a detailed discussion on this research; instead, here we look at a number of representative recent examples.

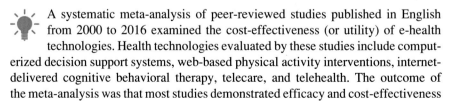 A systematic meta-analysis of peer-reviewed studies published in English from 2000 to 2016 examined the cost-effectiveness (or utility) of e-health technologies. Health technologies evaluated by these studies include computerized decision support systems, web-based physical activity interventions, internet-delivered cognitive behavioral therapy, telecare, and telehealth. The outcome of the meta-analysis was that most studies demonstrated efficacy and cost-effectiveness

of the intervention using a randomized control trial and statistical modeling, respectively. However, the quality of the evidence so far was considered limited, and further research is warranted to clearly demonstrate the long-term cost-effectiveness of e-health technologies from the healthcare system and societal perspectives (Sanyal et al., 2018).

Telemonitoring is becoming increasingly important for the management of patients with chronic conditions, especially in countries with large distances such as, for example, Australia. Recent research tested 100 patients and 137 controls; the 100 patients were supplied with a telehealth vital signs monitor and were remotely managed by a trained clinical care coordinator, while control patients continued to receive usual care. At-home telemonitoring of chronically ill patients showed a statistically robust positive impact increasing over time on healthcare expenditure, number of admissions to hospital, and LOS as well as a reduction in mortality (Celler et al., 2017).

As an example of the financial benefits that further implementation of healthcare digitalization could bring, according to McKinsey research and analysis, technologies that make it possible to deliver primary care in the United States less expensively would save $175 billion to $220 billion a year if they were to have widespread use.

Although consumers are likely to be (and should be) the primary beneficiaries of the savings, payers like the government, managed care organizations, and insurers will capture some of that money as well. In addition, the McKinsey research shows that increased automation and self-service in the United States are expected to lower overall administrative costs by an additional $24 billion to $48 billion annually through productivity gains (Atluri et al., 2016).

Research by the European Commission estimated a 2:1 return on e-health investment. When benefits were given a euro value, the average breakeven point for the 10 e-health initiatives studied was five years.

The authors forecasted that on average these solutions could reduce the health expenditures of most European countries by 0.31% GDP or 5% less spent on health by the taxpayer. A more conservative assumption connected only with telehealth usage as e-prescriptions, ICT systems, and fraud control could lower the expenditures to about 0.13% GDP, which saves about 2% on the health budget (or makes these funds available for other treatments) (Boni, 2017).

Thus, in summary, the abiotic vegetation of digital technology in healthcare thrives in a luxuriant way. The synergy with the human vegetation shows great promises, provided that research underscores the benefits of the different new technologies and adoption hurdles are mitigated.

Proving the advantages of digital health adoption requires a strong data environment, which is the topic of Chapter 8.

This means for circular pharmaceutical care:

- Digital telehealth technologies will further mature towards 2024, offering possibilities for care in every stage of the patient pathway, whereas smartphones still seem to be the ideal devices to provide digital pharmaceutical care.
- Adoption of digital health tools by care providers still faces a significant number of rate-limiting hurdles.
- Persuasive technology and serious gaming are techniques that may positively stimulate adoption and retention of digital health tools.
- To integrate digital health technology effectively into current healthcare systems, further systematic research on the (broader) economic benefits is crucial.

Data outback of an internet of (pharma) things

8

Claudia Rijcken

It is a capital mistake to theorize, before one has data.
Arthur Conan Doyle

The Outback is characterized by a unique combination of factors, such as its low human population density, its impressive natural environment, and its low-intensity land use. Biotic and abiotic materials are meticulously intertwined into what is called one of the largest remaining intact natural areas on Earth. This fascinating intertwinement has some resemblance to what is becoming the largest manmade network of biotic and abiotic materials: the Internet of Things (IoT).

> *In this chapter you will read about data in the Internet of Health and how to turn them into value, the use of digital biomarkers, the blooming future of integrated personal health records, the need for FAIR data, and the interoperability of healthcare applications, facilitated by HL7-FHIR.*

The IoT can be defined as a structure of interrelated mechanical and digital devices, objects, animals, or people, each featuring unique identifiers and the ability to transfer their respective data over a digital network without requiring human-to-human or human-to-computer interaction.

A "thing" in the IoT is always assigned an Internet Protocol (IP) address and can be, for instance, a pet with a biochip transponder, a light bulb with a WIFI connector, a person with a heart monitor implant, or an automobile with built-in sensors to alert the driver when the tire pressure is low. Figure 8.1 shows how the principle of the IoT works.

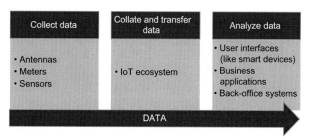

FIGURE 8.1

How the IoT works.

Pharmaceutical Care in Digital Revolution. https://doi.org/10.1016/B978-0-12-817638-2.00008-0

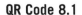

Internet of Things
explained.

Identification of every "thing" is closely tied to IoT governance, security, and privacy (see Chapter 17 for more information on compliance). Different forms of identification are key components of multiple layers of the IoT, from those embedded in the user's device to those enabling data routing and discovery (QR Code 8.1).

Rather than using the term IoT, some prefer to talk about the "internet of everyone and everything" (IoEE), as the IoEE connects all separate nodes into one cohesive whole. It's not just about allowing devices to talk to each other, it's also about allowing everything (people and devices) to talk about each other (Iske, 2016a).

As such, IoT connectivity has created radically different paradigms of infrastructures in our society; for example, it enabled the development of smart cities, of smart metering, disruptive e-commerce, and far-reaching home automation, which has large implications for healthcare as well.

IoT Explosion

Market research by the International Data Corporation (IDC) in 2017 projected that an average person's interaction with connected devices, anywhere in the world, would increase from about 200 times per capita per day in 2015 to nearly 4800 times per day in 2025—basically one interaction every 18 seconds (IDC, 2018).

It is difficult to estimate how many connected "things" are linked to the preceding figure, as estimates are most often based on active devices but may ignore those that are dormant, retired or the identifier provisions for future devices.

At the high end of the scale, Intel projected that the use of internet-enabled devices would grow from 2 billion in 2006 to 200 billion by 2020, which equates to nearly 26 smart devices for each human on Earth. A little more conservative, IHS Markit said the number of connected devices will be 75.4 billion in 2025 and 125 billion by 2030.

Other companies have tempered their numbers, taking smartphones, tablets, and computers out of the equation. Gartner estimated 20.8 billion connected items will be in use by 2020, with IDC coming in at 28.1 billion and BI Intelligence at 24 billion.

Internet of Health

The healthcare industry has been somewhat slower than other industries to adopt Internet of Things technologies. Nevertheless, the Internet of Health (IoH), or Internet of Medical Things (IoMT), is expected to help monitor, inform, and notify not only caregivers, but will also give healthcare providers actual data that will enable them to identify health problems before they become critical or to allow for earlier invention. The Internet of Health refers to the connected system of medical devices and applications that collect data that is then provided to healthcare IT systems through online computer networks. In early 2018 there were 3.7 million medical devices in use around the world; these devices are connected to and monitor various parts of the body to inform healthcare decisions (Marr, 2018a).

Figure 8.2 depicts the scope of the device types that are integrated into the Internet of Health (IoH).

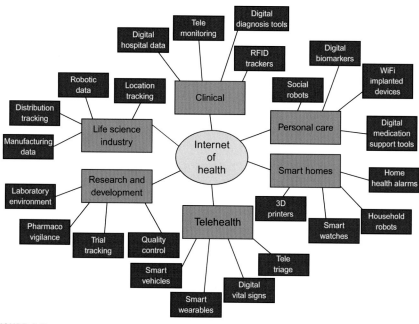

FIGURE 8.2

The Internet of Health (Adapted from Romeo and Corey, 2017).

The explosive growth in medical monitoring applications is predominantly driven by

- broad adoption of wearable tools and medical products, for example, smart watches, bracelets, and clothing;
- new types of measurements for the advancement of medical treatments;
- reduction in size and cost of devices and proliferation of device types; and
- availability of semiconductors and MEMS (micro-electromechanical systems) technologies.

These monitoring devices create a data-sea on digital biomarkers, which are defined as consumer-generated physiological and behavioral measures, collected through connected digital tools that can be used to explain, influence, and predict health-related outcomes.

Health-related outcomes can vary from reporting disease states to predicting drug responses to influencing fitness behaviors. In general, patient-reported measures (e.g., survey data), genetic information, and data collected through traditional medical devices and equipment may be stored digitally, but are not digitally measured or truly dependent on software, and thus are not regarded as digital biomarkers (Wang et al., 2018).

Ultimately, the digital health monitoring platforms (as described in Chapter 7) may replace a large swath of activities that now take place physically in various healthcare facilities. Connectivity and interoperability will allow for better connected, more efficient care in a better-informed stakeholder landscape.

Internet of Pharma Things

IoT technology and pharmacy automation will also shift the focus of tomorrow's pharmaceutical care providers. Many pharmacies around the world already use electronic pharmacy record (EPR) databases, often connected with information systems of general practitioners and hospitals, that is, electronic medical records (EMRs).

A number of EPR platforms also provide connectivity to supply chain automated solutions to achieve good distribution of medications, for instance, by connecting radio frequency identification (RFID) data (on medication), production data, and distribution data (e.g., from robotic medication dispensing systems). In addition to generating a lot of interesting data, the latter solutions help reduce counterfeit medication and recall situations. In the coming years, these platforms may be further augmented by digital health data, derived from the devices mentioned in subsequent chapters in this book.

Through connectivity of these different data sources, the Internet of Pharma Things (IoPT) will grow into a powerful medium that enables in-depth data analysis, stratification, and precision medicine.

For instance, it will help optimize and monitor adherence (which we address in Chapter 6), thus resulting in one the largest areas of improvement in the adequate use of drugs.

Figure 8.3 illustrates how IoPT connectivity can empower pharmaceutical care providers through better data on precise medication adherence.

Successful IoPT platforms like the concept shown in Figure 8.3 will incorporate continuous feedback loops that, through monitoring, measurement, and scale, can facilitate dashboards that support circular pharmaceutical care.

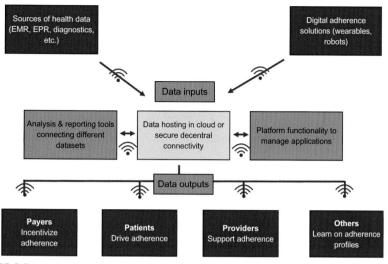

FIGURE 8.3

Internet of Pharma Things: An example of adherence.

IoPT platforms will give the various stakeholders an action perspective, contributing to better and well-informed decision making. In addition to being medication experts and excellent communicators, tomorrows' pharmaceutical care providers are envisioned to be data analytic translators, who, based on dashboards derived from data as shown in Figure 8.3, can respond in real time to emergencies and provide risk-based analysis of patients' profiles. The essential competencies required to perform in these changing roles are discussed in Chapter 19.

Data in the Internet of Things

IDC forecasts that by 2025 with the rise in connected devices, the global data sphere will grow to 163 zettabytes (10^{21}). The astounding growth comes from both the number of devices generating data and the number of sensors in each device. As just an example how much data are generated in normal life, a car like a Ford GT for instance, carries 50 sensors and 28 microprocessors and is capable of generating up to 100 GB of data per hour (IDC, 2018).

Thus the amount of data we produce every day is truly mind-boggling. At our current rate, 2.5 exabytes (10^{18}) of data are created each day, and the pace will accelerate with the growth of the IoT. Over the past 2 years alone, 90% of the world's data was generated (Marr, 2018b).

The enormous amount of data generated are often referred to as big data, which are data sets that are so big and complex that traditional data-processing application software is not capable of structuring them appropriately.

The challenge here is to turn big data into "smart data." Processing and organizing big data has become complex, as countless sources are involved, and many of these sources use different methods of data collection, including various sensors, automated reports, historical trend analysis, and so on.

 Big data comprises five dimensions

- **Volume** refers to the huge amounts of data currently being collected.
- **Velocity** refers to how fast data can be produced and processed (speed of connection, e.g., 4G or 5G technology, as well as maturity of applications).
- **Variety** refers to the different content of data sets, whether structured, semistructured, or unstructured.
- **Veracity** refers to the uncertainty of data (related, e.g., to biases, noise, abnormalities, ambiguities, and latency).
- **Value** refers to the ability to convert the data into meaningful value.

How the balance between these big data dimensions in a particular business area like pharmaceutical care is defined depends on whether the available and relevant data can be absorbed, processed, and examined within a time frame that meets a particular business's requirement.

For instance, if data on a patient's wearables are considered to be essential to track medication responses, the value of the data is highly dependent on whether ongoing data can be obtained; the speed at which the data is transferred into, for example, an EPR environment; whether the wearables collect fixed data (like heart rates) or spoken information; and whether the data are collected by a regulatory-approved, safe, and secure health device.

Data in the Health Ecosystem

As previously discussed, the healthcare industry is generating a vast amount data that is driven by a wide range of medical and healthcare functions, including data from wearable devices, clinical records, health-and-wellness apps, medical images, genomic data, clinical decision support tools, disease surveillance, and public health management. The global digital healthcare data were estimated in 2014 to be 500 petabytes (10^{15}) in 2012 and are expected to reach 25 exabytes (10^{18}) in 2020 (Madsen, 2014).

Again, estimates differ according to definitions and to ongoing insights; according to a Stanford Medicine Stanford white paper in 2017, 153 exabytes (10^{18}) of health data were produced in 2013, and an estimated 2314 exabytes (10^{18}) will be generated in 2020, translating to an overall rate of increase of at least 48% annually (Stanford, 2017).

In general, an EMR is meant to contain medical and clinical data gathered in a healthcare provider's office. An EPR contains pharmaceutical data gathered in a pharmaceutical care providers' space.

Electronic health records (EHRs) go beyond the data collected in an individual provider's office and include a more comprehensive patient history, connecting different providers (e.g., EMRs and EPRs) and other data sources (e.g., digital health data or diagnostics). When building an EHR, it is vital to address the mechanics of creating a health record and concepts such as a single logical health record and managing patient demographics and externally generated (including patient-originated) health data. Data may be captured using standardized code sets or nomenclature (which is crucial for using the data in further digital derivates), depending on the nature of the data, or captured as unstructured data, like open fields or even speech.

With the patient's well-being at the center of decision making, an EHR is ideally an ecosystem where all data are accessible for relevant care providers and the environment is managed by the patient, with the patient able to authorize care providers to see, use, and review data as required. In Chapter 6, we refer to this environment as a Personal Health Application (PHA). PHAs can be developed on autonomous platforms but also within existing environments, like the Apple example in QR Code 8.2.

> **QR Code 8.2**
>
>
>
> Example of a personal health application.

A single record for each patient should always be identified and maintained, as this is needed for legal purposes, as well as to organize care unambiguously for all stakeholders. By connecting all different health data from the unique patient with the unique identifier, a so-called Single Point of Truth (SPoT) on the patients' health information is created. This SPoT can than be used by all stakeholders in the health ecosystem as a joint knowledge position to organize a well-aligned and optimized individual health management plan for the patient. There is still an ongoing dialogue about whether this SPoT should reside in one place (e.g., one server) or can be created by getting access to the constituting data and be generated and maintained at various locations.

By connecting EHRs, PHAs, EPRs, and data such as behavioral, claims, and socioeconomic data, we will be able to create a 360-degree, "digital-twin" overview of patient profiles, compare them with other populations, and make hyper-personalized care plans that extend beyond the canned information that is linked to current rather siloed systems.

Exogenic data like socioeconomic environment, psychological profile, exercise patterns, metabolism, literacy level, and so on can further help in determining the care needs of an individual. Once connected to a genetic profile—which companies like Helix and 23andme have offered customers since 2016—a personal health dossier can be constructed that provides a complete and holistic overview of a person's life, well-being, health risks, and opportunities.

HL7-FHIR and the Interoperability of Healthcare Applications

As of 2019 many healthcare applications are not yet standardized and interoperable, so health research and patient data are yet still redundantly collected and not shared, or are collected by different methods and formats that are not interchangeable. Thus, the Single Point of Truth on individual health information cannot yet be created.

A large part of this is derived from the fact that medical data and information are not yet optimally standardized.

Many standardization initiatives have been introduced in past decades to resolve this problem, such as the Clinical Data Interchange Standards Consortium (CDISC), the International Statistical Classification of Diseases and Related Health Problems (ICD) and Health Level Seven (HL7). All coding and classification systems have the aim to develop and incorporate industry standards that improve the way different healthcare computer systems share data, have uniform interpretations, and allow for consolidated analysis. Also, coding systems are used for reimbursement and resource allocation in some health systems.

HL7 is an international community of healthcare subject matter experts and information scientists who created a framework (and related standards) for the exchange, integration, sharing, and retrieval of electronic health information, to increase the effectiveness and efficiency of healthcare information delivery. HL7 collaborates with other standards development organizations and national and international sanctioning bodies (e.g., ANSI and ISO), in both the healthcare and information infrastructure domains to promote the use of supportive and compatible standards (HL7, 2018).

HL7 developed (as a follow-up on HL7-V3 standards) the Fast Healthcare Interoperability Resources (FHIR) structure, which is a standard describing data formats, elements, and an application programming interface (API) for exchanging EHRs. FHIR facilitates real-time exchange of data using web technology. FHIR can construct and deconstruct CDA documents from various data sources and systems (HL7-FHIR, 2018).

With FHIR as the standard format for cloud EHRs, patient-facing mobile applications and wearables, telemedicine platforms, analytics platforms, and care coordination systems, interoperability of healthcare applications has come to a new phase, by solving many problems associated with healthcare domain complexity, data modeling, medical data storage, and custom integrations with legacy systems that resulted in long development cycles and high costs.

One of the latest efforts in 2018 towards interoperability is the Argonaut Project, which is a private sector initiative to advance industry adoption of modern, open interoperability standards. The purpose of the Argonaut Project is to rapidly develop a first-generation FHIR-based API and Core Data Services specification to enable expanded information sharing for EHRs and other health information technology based on internet standards and architectural patterns and styles (Argonaut, 2018).

FAIR Data Exchange

One of the other grand challenges of data-intensive science is to facilitate knowledge discovery by—in an open structure—assisting humans and machines in their discovery of, access to, integration and analysis of task-appropriate scientific data and their associated algorithms and workflows. The aim of having open health data exchange may be twofold: on the one hand, facilitating transparency of the health sector effectiveness, and on the other hand, providing a valuable resource that can drive science, innovation, and outcome measurement.

To develop valuable and reliable AI applications, organizations often need access to massive training data sets (see also Chapter 11). Making predictive models requires enormous data sets, which is why tech giants like Facebook, Amazon, Microsoft, and Apple (FAMGA) and China's Baidu, Alibaba, and Tencent (BAT) are leaders in the field of AI. But for many other companies, obtaining these large data sets can be challenging.

Emerging blockchain companies have dived into this problem, by re-imagining internet services and access to decentralized data, proposing a way to create data marketplaces that democratize access to AI training data. These marketplaces would coordinate users offering their data with projects in need of it—and because the exchanges are on a blockchain, there's no middleman handling files, ensuring that the shared data stays secure. More information on blockchains can be found in Chapter 14.

Because not all data being shared are curated, often it is not the lack of appropriate technology that creates the hurdle for developing smart AI tools; the reason more often is that digital objects did not receive the careful attention they deserved.

Therefore, in order to make data reusable and feasible for research, it is recommended to ensure that data comply as much as possible to the FAIR principles (Wilkinson et al., 2016), which are as follows:

- Findable
- Accessible
- Interoperable
- Reusable

As of 2018, although in many healthcare institutions the goal for large data integration exists, the key challenges for using and connecting health data sets are to

- ensure that personal data are confidential and protected;
- guarantee high quality and FAIR data;
- maintain control mechanisms for access;
- warrant data are used in an integral way; and
- make data usable for all.

Turning Health Data Into Knowledge

Connecting different data sets creates infrastructures that are set up for better dissemination of knowledge by making research data publicly available so that many research groups throughout the world can start working on them.

However, to use the information to make well-informed decisions, data must be turned into knowledge. This requires standardization of information models as previously described, but also an approach for modeling of knowledge and knowledge-based processes. In these models a consistent and systematic way is needed to deal with semantics, files, processes, and information modeling. Only with this structured approach, can a SPoT for health data be created.

An interesting example in this respect is Health-RI in the Netherlands, whose goal is to bundle and connect a wide range of resources, including biobanks, IT technologies, facilities, and data collections, into one large-scale research infrastructure (Health-RI, 2017).

> The ICT backbone of Health-RI is largely built as a "life science and health workflow & data exchange," which supports seamless access, interoperability, reuse, and trust of data among all the resources contained within the infrastructure. Highly specialized reasoning algorithms help process data as part of migrating research workflows, making it possible to go beyond observation, theory, and simulation into exploration-driven science by mining new insights from vastly diverse data sets.

The Health-RI approach may eventually give pharmaceutical care providers access to data that will help produce more effective treatment evaluations.

Imagine the possibilities if a Health-RI-type initiative is ultimately linked to broader health-wellness-socioeconomic data sets, in which case even more extensive integrated research will be possible, such as calculating the actual societal benefits of drugs, as described in Chapter 3.

Considerations for Future IoT Uptake

While IoT devices clearly offer new benefits for healthcare provider organizations, adoption is lagging compared to other industries. Healthcare system stakeholders still have several key concerns pertaining to the IoT, such as missing standards, inadequate security, difficult interoperability and compatibility, and the high cost to interlink all devices.

The siloed ecosystem of many healthcare systems throughout the world does not make adoption of IoT devices easy, as most healthcare providers have their own goals and their own roles to play and systems are not set up to create a fully uniform approach (e.g., in some countries, systems purposely adopt a free market strategy, which results in different providers competing for the same pot of software development money and thus potentially developing different ecosystems for the same purpose).

To achieve alignment in all the health optimization initiatives, just getting them connected is not enough. The connectivity needs to do something more; it needs to add true value to the healthcare chain (the fifth "V" in the five dimensions). If patients see the PHA as the holy grail to getting the best possible care and policymakers are convinced that this is the way to reduce waste and harm in the system, then these factors may drive the pressure required to really achieve interoperability.

Privacy and Security

In general, privacy and data protection and information security are complementary requirements for IoT services. In particular, information security is regarded as preserving the confidentiality, integrity, and availability (CIA) of information.

General information security requirements should apply for IoT; however, since IoT is more of a vision than a concrete technology, it is still difficult to properly define all the requirements. More information on the background of privacy and security with a focus on the healthcare industry can be found in Chapter 17 and the Appendix.

To conclude, one has to admit that the largest manmade "outback" is, to say the least, an impressive "thing" and will be followed closely in the coming years. Provided that mankind ensures the proper conditions, the IoT will be a synergistic breeding ground for all the digital health technologies described in Chapters 9–16.

 This means for circular pharmaceutical care:

- The IoT can be defined as a structure of interrelated mechanical and digital devices, objects, animals and/or people.
- Data as such are only as valuable as the way they are used; therefore the challenge is to transform big data into smart data.
- Data has five dimensions, Volume, Veracity, Velocity, Variety, and Value, and in principle they must be Findable, Attributable, Interoperable, and Reusable.
- Health data are tracked in many scattered databases, such as EHRs, pharmacy and paramedic databases, and decentralized digital tools.
- Connecting all these different health data sets may result in the Integrated PHA, which is a 24/7—accessible integrated secure environment with all personal health data from all providers, managed by the patient.
- A crucial factor for developing PHAs is standardization in data recording and facilitation of interoperability of healthcare applications, for instance, by adoption of HL7-FHIR standards.
- Digital biomarker data are defined as consumer-generated physiological and behavioral data, collected through connected digital tools.

The jungle of health apps

9

Claudia Rijcken

My powers are extraordinary. Only my application brings me success.
Isaac Newton

A jungle is covered with dense vegetation dominated by trees that tend to grow in a chaotic way, making it difficult to trudge through the landscape. "It's a jungle out there," people say, and their point is clear. They mean that the outside world is dense, diverse, and sometimes dangerous. With more than a quarter million healthcare apps available in different app stores globally, finding the right one for your purposes might be like trudging through a jungle.

In this chapter you will read about healthcare apps and their use in the pharmaceutical ecosystem as well as how to decide which ones are relevant, safe, and secure for pharmaceutical care and how to build a sustainable future for health apps.

As of 2018 it is estimated that at least 300,000 health-related smartphone apps are globally available for download, with about 200 new health apps added every day. General wellness apps account for the majority of apps available to consumers. Nevertheless, apps focused on optimizing specific health conditions form a rapidly growing sector. An increasing number of health apps have an evidence-based background, allowing the apps to be adopted as treatment options in clinical guidelines (Parkinson, 2018).

Technology

 A mobile app is a computer program designed to run on a mobile device such as a smartphone or tablet computer. The term "app" is a short version of the term "software application."

Over the past decade an entire industry has emerged to support the use of mobile health technology. In 2017 more than 84,000 app developers around the world

Pharmaceutical Care in Digital Revolution. https://doi.org/10.1016/B978-0-12-817638-2.00009-2

created apps, of which an estimated 3.6 billion health apps were downloaded (mostly Android software). Most users of apps utilize 20 or fewer health-related apps. Health insurance companies are expected to be the main drivers for the future use of health-related applications (Research2Guidance, 2017).

Categories of Health Apps

Health apps can have many different objectives, scopes, and functions. Here are a few examples (categorization adjusted from Atluri et al. (2016)):

- **Quantified self and wellness** apps that help patients improve their lifestyle via behavioral tools (refer to Chapter 7).
- Apps that **support patient self-service** of healthcare (e.g., apps that provide disease and treatment information or apps that run self-triage; see Chapters 11 and 12 for more on these applications).
- Apps that **improve clinical transparency** and support an individualized, holistic health view (like the Personal Health Application discussed in Chapter 6).
- Apps that have a **disease and/or deterioration prevention** scope.
- Apps that support **transparency** on healthcare processes and expenses and make insurance flows easier.
- **Healthcare information apps** that disseminate research and professional knowledge in an easy and accessible way.
- **Digital therapeutic apps** that act as a classified healthcare intervention.

Ideally, apps are developed to integrate seamlessly with patients' mobile devices and to comply with the international interoperability standards, as described in Chapter 8.

Impact on Core Responsibilities in Pharmaceutical Care

The extensive variety of health-related apps is forecasted to make a huge impact on the way pharmaceutical care providers execute their responsibilities.

While the consistent advancement of medical research makes pharmaceutical care providers perennial students by default, due to the volume of material that mobile phones can support, the providers no longer have the burden of lugging heavy books.

Moreover, customer health applications allow both patients and providers (once data are shared) to view a health profile within a narrative context of sorts, creating a more holistic health profile "story."

Here is the general impact that health apps are expected to have on the five domains of pharmaceutical care provision (refer to Chapter 6 for a more detailed discussion):

A. **Professional relationship between PCPs and patients:** Increasingly, information and communication flows via digital applications

B. **Adequate collection and recording of health data:** Apps allow for better insight of individual, 24/7 remotely obtained health data

C. **Review health data and provide adequate PC proposal:** This involves a broader health data spectrum for pharmaceutical care planning, one that specifies how to use health app data to optimize outcomes

D. **Patient alignment and facilitate execution of PC plan:** Use shared app data to augment human pharmaceutical support

E. **Circular management of PC plan:** Use optimized remote monitoring, with a focus on prevention and easier adjustment of the PC plan based on individual patient outcomes, retrieved via apps

Implementation in Daily Practice

As we describe in Chapter 7, due to the establishment of websites and social media, an increasing number of healthcare providers now recognize opportunities to deliver patient services via mobile applications.

Additionally, within the labor sector, providers are also increasing their use of professional support tools that are delivered via mobile applications.

In the following sections, we talk about a number of applications that are particularly relevant for pharmaceutical care providers.

For Professional Support: Medical and Pharmaceutical Reference Apps

Medical and pharmaceutical reference apps promote evidence-based medicine by offering low-threshold access to a broad scientific knowledge base, ideally on mobile platforms directly integrated into the daily workflow. In the case of pharmacists, there are an increasing number of online and mobile apps that provide clinical drug information, for example, monographies, patient leaflets, and other drug-related information. Apps like Lexicomp, iPharmacy, and Micromedex make retrieving clinical and drug information easier, as they provide the latest updates on safety and efficacy and are easy-to-use reference applications that are always available right in your pocket.

With all these mobile applications, some people believe that over the next few years physical pharmaceutical libraries will become a thing of the past.

> Some apps also support pharmaceutical decision making, such as Epocrates, an app that enables a review of drug prescribing and safety information for thousands of brand, generic, and OTC drugs. The information includes, for example, dosing advice, black box warnings, safety monitoring advice, pharmacological features, and so on.

Logistic Prescription Management Support Apps for Providers and Patients

Many health apps are now available to support smooth prescription management for both the pharmacist and the patient; for example, they offer automatic prescription refills, refill reminders, and direct connection with insurance companies for reimbursement.

Whether it is uploading a copy of your prescription, ordering medicines via WhatsApp, or getting a price reduction when ordering a drug via the pharmacy's app, these digital applications can lower the threshold so that medications are ordered in a timely way and support is personalized, and sometimes the apps being used can be utilized in conjunction with other wellness applications.

Ideally, the data in these types of health apps link directly into the electronic pharmacy record (EPR), which improves the quality and completeness of the individual data environment of the EPR software. For instance, once an app links directly into an insurance environment, the administrative burden is reduced for both the patient and the provider (as data don't have to be manually digested for claims individually submitted). Thus during drug distribution pharmacists can focus on providing optimal care instead of bureaucratic administrative work.

Chapter 12 discusses the emerging growth of voice-user interface apps and how some of these apps already nowadays can support to administer pharmaceutical narratives in an efficient way. These apps automatically convert speech to text and thus record either dialogues or professional narratives directly into the EPR, which automatically augments the patient's record without all the data having to be entered by hand.

Disease Management Apps

The potential benefits of health apps seem particularly compelling for managing chronic conditions such as COPD, heart failure, diabetes, and hypertension, from which in 2030 about half the global population is expected to suffer. Using a disease management app, patients regularly monitor their vital signs (generally, blood pressure, blood glucose, and weight) and other specific symptoms and also their adherence to taking medications on time. Use of such apps results in an earlier awareness of health issues and less need of a physician's support.

Also, in complex manageable, multifactor diseases, like oncological and orphan disorders, structured guidance in disease-specific apps may provide relief in both logistics and the knowledge level of patients, care givers, and providers.

The technology for these chronic disease management (CDM) apps is impressive, and many supportive apps for each part of the patient pathway (as described in Chapter 7) have been developed. Often, country-level overviews of the top-rated apps in specific disease areas are available.

A Wealth of Adherence Improvement Apps

Only two and a half decades ago, when the mobile phone was introduced, the pharmaceutical sector sent reminder SMSs (Session Manager Subsystems) to improve adherence to drug treatment profiles. In practice, those reminder services might have been valuable for individual patients or certain disease areas, but in general research shows mixed outcomes when such services are used as stand-alone interventions (Tao et al., 2015; Kenyon et al., 2018; Kashgary et al., 2017).

With the availability of smart 4G mobile platforms, intuitive apps now empower patients to self-manage their medication regimens and appointment schedules from their mobile and tablet devices. When connected to cloud-based platforms, these technologies allow healthcare providers to communicate with patients to clarify their understanding of conditions, complex drug regimens, and potential side effects; likewise, patients can more easily connect with healthcare providers about questions, suggestions, and so on.

On the other hand, when setting up a digital adherence improvement program, we know that it is preferable to build a connected adherence ecosystem that is a multifaceted combination of a digital tracking and alerting device, a behavioral modification app, and a connected (human) healthcare environment (Choudhry et al., 2017).

Figure 9.1 shows what an ideal integrated adherence environment looks like.

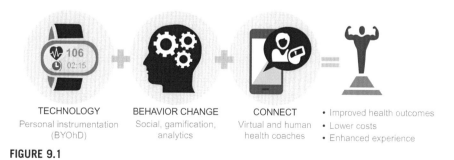

TECHNOLOGY	BEHAVIOR CHANGE	CONNECT	
Personal instrumentation (BYOhD)	Social, gamification, analytics	Virtual and human health coaches	• Improved health outcomes • Lower costs • Enhanced experience

FIGURE 9.1

Optimal digital adherence environment (Cognizant, 2016).

Over the past decade numerous applications and devices to improve drug adherence have been developed by both big corporate organizations and startups. These smart solutions make adherence support easier, and they also often link the data directly into electronic pharmacy records to allow for timely and appropriate ordering of refills, checking on contraindications, and making the management of chronic conditions much less complex.

The adherence apps take a variety of different approaches to improve adherence to adequate drug use and address both intentional and unintentional nonadherence (refer to Chapter 6 for classification of adherence problems).

Some examples of action profiles of adherence apps are

- preferred adherence pattern built into a serious game (refer to Chapter 7 for more info on gamification);
- exchange of visual information on color and form of drug to be taken via virtual pillboxes to reduce confusion (see also QR Code 9.1);
- calendar-based alarm notifications via mobile device apps as well as health wearables and virtual personal assistants (see Chapter 12);
- avatars (as well as robots) that support adequate drug intake; and
- remote quality of life measurement after dose intake.

QR Code 9.1

Example of adherence innovation.

As noted, different applications can be used in parallel in a multifaceted approach and may create synergy in outcomes.

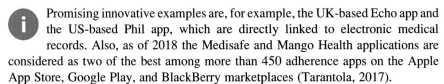 Promising innovative examples are, for example, the UK-based Echo app and the US-based Phil app, which are directly linked to electronic medical records. Also, as of 2018 the Medisafe and Mango Health applications are considered as two of the best among more than 450 adherence apps on the Apple App Store, Google Play, and BlackBerry marketplaces (Tarantola, 2017).

Considerations

In the fertile jungle of health applications, it is easy to get lost, as the example box of the dilemma of pharmacists reflects. Nevertheless, pharmaceutical care providers can play

App Dilemmas of Pharmacists

Suppose a community pharmacy has about 10000 patients registered. Hypothetically, the number of diseases covered by these patients may be about 130.

Now assume that all these individual patients have different apps to manage their disease and all these apps are requested to be linked to or integrated within the pharmacy information system in order to allow health data synergy, as described previously.

The dilemma occurs: Is it the pharmacist who is responsible to make sure the app data are reliable and securely stored? And would they need to check timely updates of the app? Who is responsible for organizing connectivity and compatibility?

And what if the cohort of COPD patients in this pharmacy want to use 10 different refill-ordering apps or 15 different COPD medication support apps?

What knowledge level does a pharmacist need in regard to all these apps?

an essential role in selecting and offering the digital services that really matter to patients. Providers may decide to build their own apps (that meet all the requirements) or choose the best one available (certified and warranted) via one of the many online providers. Following are a couple of important considerations to increase the likelihood a health app's data will have real value in the pharmaceutical care process.

Responsibility for Connecting and Working With Health Apps

Pharmaceutical care providers are confronted with prescription drugs from many different companies regardless of whether they are active in a hospital or in a retail pharmacy. Often, due to nonharmonization of apps, a new app connected to an individual product is introduced nearly every time a new drug is dispensed, frequently with different levels of connectivity with the individual patients' devices as well as with prevailing pharmacy software.

In addition, patients may be enthusiastic about the health apps they are using and request that their data are linked to the electronic pharmacy records, as described in the example box.

 This brings a number of questions that the pharmaceutical care provider needs to consider:

- Does the app **comply with privacy, quality, and security** regulations, as referred to in Chapter 17, and is the **informed consent** process transparent for both the patient and the provider?
- Does the app gather data that are **FAIR** for researching and augmenting electronic pharmacy records (as indicated in Chapter 8)?
- Is the app **interoperable** with the pharmacy information system; for example, is data transfer HL7-FHIR-standardized?

Those seem to be questions that can be answered only with an awareness of the content of the app, of the technological conditions a specific app should meet, of the health app's validation, the potential availability of alternatives, and so on.

The following sections and subsequent chapters will help provide some of the answers, but in general, a systematic approach to adopting and advising on the merits of health apps will face further development needs in the upcoming years.

Simplification Efforts Ongoing

To deal with the challenges healthcare providers are facing with the growing variety of digital applications, more than 25 big pharma companies joined forces in 2017 to create a single sign-on login for doctors and healthcare providers to access online pharmaceutical content (QR Code 9.2).

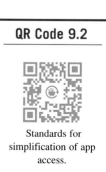

QR Code 9.2

Standards for simplification of app access.

The goal of the group is to create two industry standards, one for identification and authentication and the other for consent and communication preferences. In 2019, the identification and authentication standard to enable single sign-on for HCPs has already been established, you can find more information via QR code 9.2 (Alignbiopharma, 2017).

QR Code 9.3

Example of an app reviewing platform.

Assessing the Quality of a Health App

As of 2019 a number of health app reviewing platforms target either healthcare professionals, or patients, or both. These platforms aim to review and assess available health apps and rate their feasibility for use (QR Code 9.3).

Some platforms focus on one aspect or (disease) area and use subjective review input from patients and healthcare providers. Others strive for a multifaceted robust examination of quantifiable evidence and data.

Elements that are considered in app review processes are

- rationale for why an app was developed and whether it aims to improve patient outcomes;
- compliance with global and local standards and regulation on privacy, quality, and security (see Chapter 17 for more information);
- functionality with regard to the purpose;
- evidence base and transparency of their algorithms; and
- level of user friendliness and ease of integration in a disease management program.

Inspirational Examples of App Review Platforms

The global list of review platforms and medical app checklists is to extensive to include in this chapter, but here are some inspirational examples:

- Orcha: www.orcha.co.uk (UK, provider of health and care app reviews and assessments).
- myhealthapps.net: http://myhealthapps.net (US, apps reviewed and recommended by global healthcare communities).
- NHS Apps Library: https://apps.beta.nhs.uk (UK, apps have passed a review to prove their safety and compliance with data protection rules).
- iMedicalApps: www.imedicalapps.com (US, a platform that provides reviews, research, and commentary by health professionals).
- Health Navigator: www.healthnavigator.org.nz/app-library (NZ, peer-reviewed recommendations by medical experts).
- Practical Apps: https://practicalapps.ca (CND, family physicians reviewing apps for primary care peers).
- Xcertia: http://www.xcertia.org (US, to develop and disseminate mHealth app guidelines).

In addition to evaluating content on the online review platforms, before making recommendations to patients, healthcare providers are advised to perform a thorough, structured approach to determining which health app is most appropriate for a given patient, as follows (Boudreax et al., 2014):

- Review scientific literature, if available.
- Search app clearinghouse websites on potential certification details.
- Search app stores on availability.
- Evaluate app descriptions, user ratings, and review platforms.
- Conduct a social media query within profession and, if available, patient networks.
- Pilot the app within your own environment.
- Elicit user feedback from patients.

Certification of Healthcare Apps

Only a limited number of health apps, often used in clinical programs or as digital therapeutics (see Chapter 15), are certified and validated at time of writing of this book. This process includes clinical trials and is often considered expensive and time-consuming. Most apps do not yet (have to) follow the entire regulatory process. Many countries now have regulations that specify how apps must be registered and whether they need to have a CE mark or certification. If the app meets the definition of a medical device, specific regulations are in place, as explained in Chapter 17.

The FDA revised its guidance on regulating health apps and apps that can function as medical devices in February 2015. The FDA is taking a tailored, risk-based approach that focuses on the small subset of mobile apps that meets the regulatory definition of "device" and that are intended to be used as an accessory to a regulated medical device or that transform a mobile platform into a regulated medical device (FDA, 2016). The new EU Medical Device Regulations of 2020 will provide strong guidance on whether a health app classifies as a medical device class II, III, or even IV.

In 2017 the FDA announced that it had chosen nine companies out of more than 100 for its Software Precertification (Pre-Cert) program, which will essentially "pre-certify" health-focused apps and possibly health devices offered by these companies.

This means that a PreCert company provides the FDA with the steps to create, test, and update the health apps offered. According to a set of standards, the FDA grants the company a PreCert certificate and will make periodic audits to ensure that all steps in the quality management are obeyed. The primary goal of this program is to support the development of a regulatory model that assesses the safety and effectiveness of software technologies without inhibiting patients' quick access to these technologies (FDA, 2017).

⚠ An additional complexity is how a healthcare provider monitors the maintenance and use of an app after it has been recommended and patients use it. As we discuss in Chapter 6, digital pharmaceutical care implies that the provider is responsible for adequate use of drugs as well as the tools to accomplish this use. That begs the question: who is responsible or even liable if errors occur during usage or, for example, updating of the health app is ignored, which means that the app can no longer be used in a secure and quality-warranted way (with the possibility of pharmaceutical emergencies being missed)? Responsibility probably should rest jointly with the app manufacturer, the healthcare provider, and the end user. Such questions require that new legal frameworks be developed in the coming years, most probably based on real-life dilemmas that require immediate solutions.

Much more information on the regulation of digital health technology can be found in Chapter 17 and the Appendix.

Are Apps as Effective as They Promise?

Although many apps promise to support patients and improve outcomes, a significant number of versions still seem to have basic technological flaws. In 2015, after evaluating more than 400 apps and user-testing 100 of the best-rated ones, researchers noted that nearly 25% of the top-scoring adherence apps could not mitigate a basic nonadherence function (like issuing a medication reminder), could not be installed by a student healthcare professional, or had other barriers to appropriate use (e.g., compatibility issues) (Heldenbrand et al., 2016).

A report by the American Journal of Preventive Medicine sketches an even clearer picture of certain apps' developmental needs. The researchers looked at medication adherence apps and the way they applied established health behavioral change techniques (BCT) to drive adherence change (see Chapter 6 for more information on this topic). BCT is an evidence-based list of ways to change people's behavior that has been used to test fitness and dieting apps. The study coded 166 apps using the Behavior Change Technique Taxonomy (v1) for the presence or absence of established behavior change techniques. Of the possible 96 different behavioral techniques that could have been used in the apps, only 12 appeared, which means that established behavior change techniques used in medication adherence apps are currently limited; therefore medication adherence apps may not yet have benefited fully from advances in the theory and practice of health behavioral change (Morrisey et al., 2016).

Recent research also found that the overall low quality of the evidence on the effectiveness of health apps greatly limits their prescribability. Twenty-three RCTs evaluating 22 available apps that mostly addressed diabetes, mental health, and obesity were meta-analyzed. Most trials were pilots with a small sample size and of short duration. Risk of bias within the included reviews and trials was considered high. Eleven of the 23 trials showed a meaningful effect on health or surrogate outcomes attributable to apps. In general, the conclusion of this research was that there is a strong need to have more apps evaluated by more robust RCTs that report between-group differences before becoming prescribable (Byambasuren et al., 2018).

Reimbursement of Apps

It is obvious that health apps have not yet lived up to their full potential, which relates not only to efficacy but also to the reimbursement systems in which they exist. Digital health apps are difficult to sell directly to patients; thus the leading buyers are providers (health systems or primary care practices) or payers (self-insured employers or health insurers). Yet payers worry that patients will not use these apps as regularly as required to manage their disease effectively and so outcomes may be suboptimal.

 To succeed under these circumstances, developers of health apps need to first consider who the primary (that is, paying) customers of their technologies will be (Huckman and Stern, 2018). They may then develop an approach to ensure that a customer's willingness to adopt an app also translates into sustained use of the app and relevant clinical outcomes. Moreover, as long as many healthcare systems face a predominant fee-for-service reimbursement system that pays substantially more for seeing a patient in person than for managing care electronically and remotely, adoption of remote app technology may be hindered as well.

In conclusion, we can say that the jungle of apps is becoming more passable, but there are still sufficient challenges in this dense environment. For now, there is a vision of a race between the tech giants, in which each tries to come up with the ultimate app, a single program that everyone will find incredibly easy to use and that will do everything we want it to do.

In the next Chapter 10, one can read how data from wearables are converted to useable information in apps.

This means for circular pharmaceutical care:

- Health apps can have different objectives, scopes, and functions, such as supporting the quantifying self, disease self-management, clinical transparency, holistic health overview, disease prevention, disease insight, financial transparency, and provision of professional background knowledge.
- Before recommending a health app to patients, a care provider is advised to use a structured approach and assess the privacy, quality, security, and feasibility level of the app.
- Globally, an increasing number of reviewing platforms offer insights in the validation of health apps.
- Authorities are continuing to develop regulations to certify app software as medical devices, with a focus on thorough investigations and clear deliverables in the upcoming years.
- More research is required to determine the true cost-effectiveness of health apps and thus make them more feasible for adequate reimbursement.

QR Code Animation

Health Apps.

An animation—kindly adopted by the Albert Schweitzer Hospital Dordrecht, the Netherlands—on the topic of Health Apps can be found on www.pharmacare.ai.

Rainforests of wearables and insideables

10

Claudia Rijcken

Attention is the scarce resource in this Quantified Self space.
J. Paul Neeley

Rainforests are characterized by millions upon millions of species of plants, insects, and microorganisms, many of them still undiscovered in tropical rainforests. Research of this flora and fauna has given us many solutions for previously unsolved medical problems, and with more research, the forests will continue to do so.

In this chapter you will read about how the quantified self is becoming a reality with digital bio-marker data due to wearables and insideables, how this broad range of health parameters can augment pharmaceutical care, and the vital conditions required to integrate these digital assets successfully in pharmaceutical care.

In many ways, the unexplored opportunities of rainforests are like the world of wearables and insideables, a world that is experiencing rapid and monumental development with the potential to offer mankind a wealth of longitudinal, real-world data that may change forever the way we approach healthcare and well-being.

Technology

Wearables are smart electronic devices with micro-controllers that can be worn on the body, in clothing, in accessories, and even in tattoos. In the health ecosystem, they can track a number of parameters that reflect personal health and well-being and thus provide better understanding of health outcomes and what drives optimization.

It is expected that by 2021 one billion wearables will be connected to the Internet of Things (IoT) (Statista, 2018).

The first wearables were sports bracelets and fitness trackers, which essentially were a sort of advanced pedometer. The bracelets allowed individuals to track things like number of steps taken, distance traveled, calories burned, and sleep patterns.

Pharmaceutical Care in Digital Revolution. https://doi.org/10.1016/B978-0-12-817638-2.00010-9

The integration of these assessments within a smartwatch opened up opportunities for improved user experience, and many more features have been added, including GPS linking, detection of a rapid heart rate, and ECG trackers.

However, wearables have advanced far beyond wellness tracking. Figure 10.1 exemplifies the broad range of assessments that are currently available and that help to map a true quantified self.

As explained in Chapter 3, the concept of quantified self is characterized by the use of technology to acquire data on various aspects of a person's daily life, including those related to input (food consumption, quality of surrounding air), state (mood, arousal, blood oxygen levels), and health, whether mental, physical, or social. Moreover, these data are often tracked via wearables or home robotics.

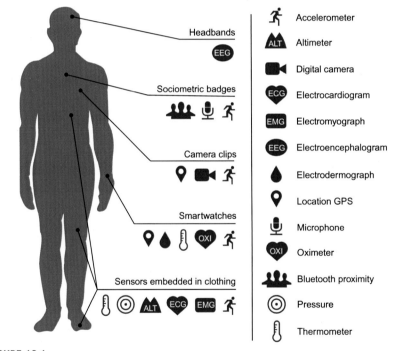

FIGURE 10.1

Overview of wearables (Piwek et al., 2016).

Medical wearables collect body-metric-derived digital biomarkers (for definition, see Chapter 8). These devices are connected to and monitor various parts of the body in order to inform healthcare decisions; as such the devices can help prevent disease and can monitor specific diseases, particularly chronic diseases such as Parkinson's, dementia, COPD, cancer, and heart failure; and they can also monitor pain management. The efficacy of medical grade devices is being intensively studied, as they must undergo thorough clinical research and meet strict regulatory requirements, which we address in Chapter 17 (Snyder et al., 2018).

Examples of innovative wearables are orthopedic wearables that determine walking patterns, earbuds that measure temperature, and a smart ovulation tracking bracelet that provides real-time detection of a woman's 5.3-day fertile period; also rehabilitation gloves to reduce joint stiffness due to rheumatoid arthritis, headbands to enhance the effectiveness of meditation, and devices that measure stress levels via the skin pores on our fingertips.

Here are some of the concrete benefits derived from using health wearables:

- **Personal health management:** Individuals can continuously monitor different fitness, health, and wellness characteristics to develop the quantified self and to track progress toward health goals or to signal deviations before becoming ill.
- **Disease management:** Those with health conditions that need to be closely monitored can use a wearable device to remotely track essential health indicators and quantify complications, deterioration, or improvements.
- **Holistic health data sharing:** Data from wearable devices can be easily shared with healthcare providers and thus give physicians, pharmacists, or disease team stakeholders a more detailed understanding of a disease's status.
- **Behavioral change:** Better insight in combination with a motivational app may empower people to change and sustain habits according to their personal goals.
- **Social engagement:** People can connect their data to social media sites or patients' networks, and thereby increase the understanding and motivation of others in working toward their goals.

Insideables and Digestables

Insideables are considered the next phase after external wearables. These electronic devices can be implanted in the body, or digested and integrated into the body, or attached under the skin. They perform a diagnostic task or monitor one or more bodily functions.

Digestible interventions include, for example, the use of smart pills or nanoparticles, which upon digestion send an electronic signal demonstrating when a patient took medication. Those insideables can, among other things, monitor the biologic availability of a drug, measure levels of blood parameters like glucose, or send an alert in the case of food allergies (QR Code 10.1).

QR Code 10.1

Example of an insideable.

Digital Pills

The first drug with an ingestible sensor was Proteus Health's Abilify Mycite, which was approved by the FDA in 2017.

As soon as the pills are digested, the ingestible sensor send a simple signal (derived from a very small current activated by stomach fluids) to a patch worn on the patient's torso.

This patch sends the information encrypted via Bluetooth to a mobile app that analyses the data and is able to alert healthcare providers and caregivers when adherence expectations are not met.

Another interesting innovation is AngelMed Guardian, which received FDA approval in 2018. It is an implantable cardiac device designed to rapidly detect ST-segment changes—ST shifts—that may signify major cardiac events, such as coronary artery occlusions caused by life-threatening plaque ruptures.

Once an ST-segment shift is detected by the AI algorithm that identifies it as an abnormality, and even if the patient has no symptoms yet, the system alerts patients to seek medical care by delivering a series of vibratory, auditory, and visual warnings (AngelMed Guardian System, 2018).

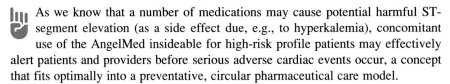 As we know that a number of medications may cause potential harmful ST-segment elevation (as a side effect due, e.g., to hyperkalemia), concomitant use of the AngelMed insideable for high-risk profile patients may effectively alert patients and providers before serious adverse cardiac events occur, a concept that fits optimally into a preventative, circular pharmaceutical care model.

Virtual Personal Assistants and Wearables

Another promising development is the connection between the dynamic data flow of wearables and the use of virtual personal assistants (VPAs, described in Chapter 12), which will enable algorithms to continuously interpret the wearable's collected data and translate it into personalized (spoken) advice.

This technology grew significantly in last years, is still in its infancy, however, as voice interaction with VPAs is expected to become standard on consumer devices and wearables, its functionality will become more personalized, opening up new opportunities for healthcare services. Some services will come straight from the next generation of AI features and could include alerts to health professionals and designated caregivers, as well as predictive algorithms to help prevent or manage lifestyle diseases such as Type 2 diabetes and hypertension.

Gartner estimates that by 2020 no-touch interfaces will account for about 15% of personal health-related devices and wearables. A more natural interface delivered with voice, movement, and gesture will increase ease of use and help bring devices into mainstream healthcare use (Gartner, 2018).

Impact on Core Responsibilities in Pharmaceutical Care

Using data from wearables and insideables provides insight on the results of their use and the safety and efficacy of medication and gives pharmaceutical care providers the opportunity to assess more real-world data that are representative of patients' responses to medication and general quality of life.

Here is the general impact that wearables and insideables are expected to have on the five domains of pharmaceutical care provision (refer to Chapter 6 for a more detailed discussion):

 A. **Professional relationship between PCPs and patients:** Enhances insight due to real-time patient data of wearables

 B. **Adequate collection and recording of health data:** Provides broader set of remote, real-time data to be considered in electronic pharmacy records

 C. **Review of health data and provision of adequate PC proposal:** Makes available a broader set of health data to measure outcomes for pharmaceutical planning that includes a suitable digital monitoring proposal

 D. **Patient alignment and facilitate execution of PC plan:** Provides informed consent on wearable data that can augment a care plan and support personalized care

 E. **Circular management of PC plan:** Offers optimized possibilities through the results obtained by remote monitoring and more appropriate adjustment of the plan based on individual real-time data

Implementation in Daily Practice

As with health apps, wearable and insideable devices are meaningless without the applicable use of the data collected. Use of dynamic APIs and powerful artificial intelligence, health metrics from multiple wearable devices, connected in a personal health application with, among others, hospital and pharmacy data, could provide valuable insight into the health and disease status of patients. Individual data can also be compared against anonymous averages of millions of people with the same characteristics (e.g., age, gender, and genetic predispositions), thus creating the possibility for a clinical benchmark.

Because more people are tracking different data with regard to their health, many healthcare providers and organizations are seeking how to best leverage wearable data to help guide and augment their clinical care practices.

Pharmaceutical Care Providers as Consultants on Use of Health Wearables

In a landscape filled with hundreds of health wearables, it is difficult to determine which ones meet the requirement to strategically augment a pharmaceutical care plan and provide reliable, specific, and sensitive data. With patient stratification being central to emerging concepts such as precision medicine and population health management, providers need a better understanding of the wide range of regulated and clinically vetted wearable technologies that can seamlessly capture reliable vital signs and selectively package the wearables most critical for management of specific diseases.

There are still limited databases or oversights that depict and compare health wearables and provide a structured review, as is increasingly available for health apps (refer to Chapter 9).

Healthcare providers need a platform that compares health wearables, as shown in Figure 10.2, and that can help them enable care providers and patients to select the most appropriate devices to augment clinical and pharmaceutical care plans.

A future health wearables comparison platform would show most important features and may give relative scores on the following domains:

Features	*User experience*	*Potential disease support*
Accuracy	*Health benefits*	*Medical classification*
Validity	*Trials*	*Certification status*
Quality assurance	*Maintenance*	*Security*
Privacy	*Price*	*Reimbursement*
Interoperability		

FIGURE 10.2

Key features of a wearable comparison platform.

Specific requirements for the privacy, quality, and security compliance level for wearables are discussed in detail in Chapter 17.

Manufacturers of wearables, academia, and digital health training centers may even consider developing an educational literacy roadmap for healthcare providers who want to work with innovative wearables and insideables, something that in many countries in not available in regular medical training programs or in postacademic medical educational settings.

Wearables That Empower Pharmaceutical Care Providers' Work

An upcoming group of wearables does not focus on tracking health data but on easing a healthcare provider's workload. They are in general AI-powered devices that, among other things, help providers handle paperwork by updating a patient's EHR, for example, by listening to a provider's conversation with a patient. The device can even come up with an action plan based on the knowledge it collects about the provider's preferences and pharmaceutical practice guidelines. More information on these applications can be found in Chapter 12.

Also, body-worn cameras powered by AI technology (e.g., augmented reality glasses; see Chapter 13) may augment the future role of pharmaceutical healthcare providers, which will enhance triage and communication skills with real-time facial and body recognition and allow predictive alerting of events that deviate from the desired health situation.

Although these supportive tools are definitely in their infancy, they may offer pharmacists an opportunity augment the dialogue with patients about their pharmaceutical care and reduce the administrative burden as spoken data can be directly transferred into the EPRs. This will increase the time that pharmacists can spend with their patients and reduce the amount of time they spend in front of a computer, thereby providing the opportunity to enrich the quality of the human pharmaceutical support interaction.

Considerations

The threshold to track health data has lowered over time as smart watches, bracelets, and rings have become more affordable. At the same time, as reflected above, the features and possibilities of health wearables are fast expanding and more people are using the devices, which is increasing the collection of valuable data.

Retentive Wearables Use: Bring Your Own health Device

Many patients may have more than a decade of experience with wearable devices that are connected to their smartphones and other digital applications and that add value to their life. A younger cohort of adopters, most of whom fall into the 25–34 age range, are usually focused on fitness and wellness wearables, whereas adopters between 55 and 64 are more focused on improving their overall health and extending their lives.

Studies found that the attrition rates for fitness devices are rather high; that is, users report increased physical activity after purchasing a sensor, but the longer they own it, the less they use it. Nearly one third of all users cease tracking activity 6 months after purchasing a device. Qualitative analyses of the reasons for this behavior include forgetting to wear the device, discomfort during exercise, lack of aesthetic appeal, and loss of interest. In some cases users report they have met their fitness goals and no longer rely on the device (Fox et al., 2017).

Previous studies about patients' use of medical wearables show that leveraging peer support to encourage activity and other healthful habits achieves more favorable health outcomes than self-motivation (Fox et al., 2017).

Persuasive technology tactics, as described in Chapter 7, may improve users' motivation to stay connected. Also, including the end user's preferences and goals early in the design of a device can optimize retention of use. Moreover, the value of virtual disease management for the prevention of disease or worsening of the disease is an important factor for retaining medical wearable use.

Once experiences have been positive and retention is achieved, people are often hesitant to switch to a different wearable platform. Therefore, prior to proposing wearable data tracking as part of the pharmaceutical care plan, healthcare providers may need to assess which wearable device the patient already uses and whether it can be used to connect to the EPR. This is called a Bring Your Own health Device (BYOhD) strategy.

Provided the used devices meet the clinical needs and comply with regulatory requirements on data privacy and security, this BYOhD approach may provide the flexibility needed to capture patient data across different systems and channels, in which case the patient will not have to deal with additional technology that might not be compatible with other devices or with a double add-on situation (Cognizant, 2016).

As we describe in Chapter 8, the growing tendency of wearables to offer interoperability by using HL7-FHIR standards is expected to give a boost to the integration of different digital health devices and will allow the PCP to connect wearables data more easily to a pharmacy information system.

From this perspective, it is counterintuitive "to force" patients to use a new or additional wearable device or app, as part of a "packaged medical intervention" proposed, for instance, by drug manufacturers, payers, or healthcare providers. Although these "beyond-the-pill" concepts may be valuable to support better outcomes, think for example of polypharmacy patients who would get a (potentially free) health tracker for each medication they need to use. A patient would need extra arms after a certain point in time. Also, switching patients between different devices and letting patients use various platforms could create confusion and is labor-intensive and thus jeopardizes optimal treatment outcomes.

Therefore, in a "beyond-the-pill concept" working with the device that the patient is already used to, often has the highest likelihood of adoption and successful, sustainable data tracking.

Is a Wearable the Best Solution?

Proving the added value of wearables is an area that still needs substantial, systematic research. Although some studies have already shown beneficial outcomes (Snyder et al., 2018), other research is less positive on the actual advantage of using wearables. A recent meta-analysis published in *Nature* evaluated a set of randomized controlled trials (RCTs) that assessed the effects of using wearable biosensors (e.g., activity trackers) for remote patient monitoring on clinical outcomes. It revealed no statistically significant impact of remote patient monitoring on six reported clinical outcomes, leading to the conclusion that there are still substantial gaps in the evidence base that should be considered before implementation of remote patient monitoring in a clinical setting (Noah et al., 2018).

 Thus, before asking the question whether using a wearable technology can augment a pharmaceutical care plan, it is advised to make a systematic analysis of the potential added value of the wearable:

- In which phase of the patient journey, as described in Chapter 6, could digital biomarker data help optimize treatment outcomes?
- Can these digital biomarker data be tracked reliably by wearables or insideables?
- Which kinds of digital biomarker data of the patient are already tracked?
- Is it possible to use these existing data from a validity, accuracy, interoperability, safety, quality, security, and privacy point of view?
- How are data going to be analyzed to prove that the wearable augments the pharmaceutical care plan?

Medically certified wearables and insideables that in principle must undergo regulatory approval are further explained in Chapter 15.

Digital Health Compliance of Wearables

Using health wearables in a new strategy and in a BYOhD strategy requires a strong governance approach to ensure that the device complies with the global and local medical device regulations.

Also, when wearables data are included in a formal pharmaceutical care program, the device must be appropriately maintained and the related responsibilities must be considered. For example, adequate documentation of informed patient consent, who owns the data, how and which data will be consolidated, how the data are processed, how privacy and security is warranted, and how updates of the devices are tracked are rudimental for the development of safely connected IoT environments with medical wearables.

Worth Reading the Provisions

Given the very strict privacy and security regulations globally, all professional wearable companies have transparent statements on which features they track, how patients can grant sharing of their data and with whom, how the data are processed, how users can have their data removed, and whether any data are shared and with whom. Also, criteria for the quality and maintenance (like ISO) is worth reading up front in order to determine the professional level of the manufacturer.

More information on the digital health compliance aspects is given in Chapter 17.

Reliability of Digital Biomarker Data

Once new technology is part of a formal pharmaceutical care plan, patients as well as providers should be able to rely on the tracked health data as the gospel truth. However, as with many innovations, the limits and capabilities of new technology may not be completely mapped, and medical grade accuracy may still be under research.

Noninvasive devices that are intended for general wellness use hardly ever undergo strict certification, whereas medical wearables with a clear clinical purpose, both in the United States and Europe, are subject to medical device classification and regulation.

Looking at the data from the perspective of their purpose is essential; for example, a mainstream heart-rate tracking wristband used to measure moderate exercise in a totally healthy patient is less expected to sensitively alert minor deviations from normal heart-rates as compared to wearables used to determine the boundaries of an intensive interval training for a patient with arrhythmia (in the latter case, one would expect the highest level of accurate detection of abnormalities).

 Thus accuracy, specificity, and sensitivity, in relation to the risk posed once the wearable gives inadequate data, is crucial to consider.

It is to be expected that more guidance and regulation for healthcare providers will become available in years to come, as more patients (potentially stimulated by payers, driving measurable value-based outcomes) request to have their wearable data added to their Personal Health Application (PHA).

Resistance to Using Wearables or Insideables

Society is already used to insideables without smart technology; for example cochlear implants and artificial hips and even smart devices like pacemakers are well accepted. However, what if the new knee has a WIFI connection and can be remotely followed to monitor its effectiveness, disclosing as well data on the owner's walking patterns? Or what if the adherence tool alerts that a patient decides one day not take the beta blocker because he has a full day tomorrow and doesn't want to be burdened by things like tiredness, which often happens with beta-blockers?

Moreover, while many people use fitness trackers, a number of other people have a certain resistance to engaging with technology. The fear of being alerted when medical issues appear, technology adversity, the burden of having to charge the device and aesthetic shortcomings, the knowledge that false positive alerts (as well as false negatives) may pop up, and the big-brother-is-watching-you culture are all reasons why patients may not be willing to track or share their health status.

 Although insurance companies' incentive programs may stimulate, even with financial benefits, the use of wearables or insideables to improve health conditions and treatment outcomes, a patient has and will have the right to refuse wearing digital technology and sharing data (as further explained in Chapter 18).

In summary, there is a clear need to further explore and develop the beauty of the rainforest of wearables, but as with the Amazon Rainforest, it is recommended to do this with a proper amount of balance to assure digital biomarker data from wearables and insideables can truly augment the pharmaceutical care plan.

In Chapter 11 we discuss how wearables' digital biomarker data are processed to deliver insight into relevant patient outcomes.

This means for circular pharmaceutical care:

- Wearable technology or wearables are smart electronic devices (with micro-controllers) that can be worn on the body, in clothing, in accessories, and even tattoos.
- Insideables are the next phase after external wearables; these devices are implanted in the body, or are digested and integrated into the body, or attached under the skin.
- Most wearables do not understand the data they track and cannot account for the differing health needs of an individual. Data have to be analyzed in an application that can offer actionable health information.
- Health care providers would benefit from a structured platform that gives an overview of the characteristics of wearables and insideables to enable care providers and patients to select well-informed and appropriate devices to augment clinical and pharmaceutical care plans.
- A Bring-Your-Own-health-Device strategy may increase the likelihood of retentive wearables use and may be the most customer-friendly way to collect health data for a pharmaceutical care plan.
- Tracked health data cannot yet be considered as the gospel truth. Depending on the purpose, medical grade device certification should clarify whether data are reliable, accurate, sensitive and specific enough to augment clinical decision making
- A patient has and will have the right to refuse wearing digital technology and sharing data.

An animation—kindly adopted by EFPIA—on the topic of Wearables can be found on www.pharmacare.ai.

Wearables.

Sequoias of artificial intelligence

11

Claudia Rijcken

AI is likely to be the best or the worst thing happening to humanity.
Stephen Hawking

Sequoias, a genus of redwood coniferous trees, are the oldest and tallest trees in the world. Their appearance is overwhelming, and their influence on the Sierra Nevada landscape in North America has been significant. At least metaphorically this influence resembles the impact many people think artificial intelligence (AI) will have on society in general and on the healthcare sector in particular.

In this chapter you will read about how artificial intelligence is changing healthcare paradigms and the conditions under which algorithms augment pharmaceutical practice and thus drive apothecary intelligence.

With the data explosion, the availability of more than 300,000 health apps, and the ever-growing information flow on the internet, there is a bright light on the horizon (QR Code 11.1).

Actually, global tech giants are in a race to become the first to come up with the ultimate app. This app is envisioned as being a single, fully integrated, AI-driven program that will be incredibly easy for anyone to use and that can do everything it is asked to do, and thus act like a personal virtual assistant (similar to the chatbots described in Chapter 12).

This vision is not as farfetched as it might sound, as our world is increasingly dependent on artificial intelligence, which is becoming the backbone of the major providers' big-data analytic strategy. For example, a survey done by the World Economic Forum's Global Agenda Council on the future of software and society reported that people expect artificial intelligent machines to be part of a company's board of directors by 2026 (WEF, 2015). Therefore let us have a look at what this technology comprises.

QR Code 11.1

What is artificial intelligence?

Pharmaceutical Care in Digital Revolution. https://doi.org/10.1016/B978-0-12-817638-2.00011-0

Technology

 Artificial intelligence (AI), which is often called machine intelligence, is intelligence demonstrated by machines, in contrast to the intelligence displayed by humans. AI research is defined as the study of "intelligent agents," which is any device that can perceive its environment and maximize achievement of its goals. Colloquially, the term "artificial intelligence" is applied when a machine mimics "cognitive" functions that humans associate with other human minds, such as learning, anticipation, or problem solving (Wikipedia, 2018a) (QR Code 11.2).

As shown in Figure 11.1, AI is built to solve questions that include planning, reasoning, knowledge, natural language processing, perception, and the ability to move, manipulate, or omit objects. Methods used draw on statistical methods, computer science, mathematics, cognitive behavioral techniques, psychology, linguistics, and philosophy.

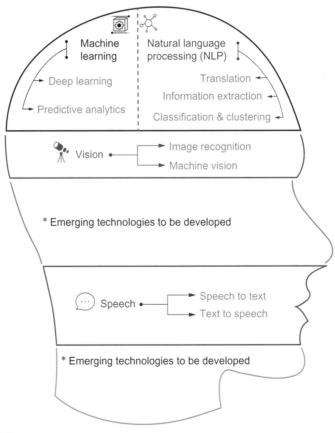

FIGURE 11.1

Domains of artificial intelligence.

Algorithms are the basis of AI, and they can be defined as a process or set of rules to be followed by computers in calculations or other problem-solving operations to generate answers to a prespecified problem.

The Promise of Machine Learning

Since the 1970s algorithms have "taught" machines how to read documents and answer questions based on their content, but the machines' capabilities were limited at that time by their computational power and the amount of data available to feed the machines.

With more and more content becoming available digitally and online and with super-fast processors being available, systems now have increasing access to a large pool of natural language data combined with broad data sets, which gives the systems a deeper and more widespread understanding of many topics (QR Code 11.3).

 Machine learning (ML) is defined as a subset of artificial intelligence in the field of computer science that often uses statistical techniques to give computers the ability to "learn" (i.e., progressively improve performance on a specific task) with data, without being explicitly programmed (Wikipedia, 2018c).

ML in general uses an algorithmic approach that takes both structured and unstructured historical data through a mathematically driven process to generate a model that recognizes patterns and contextual meaning. ML can be used in both supervised and unsupervised ways, as exemplified in Figure 11.2.

QR Code 11.3

Impact of machine learning.

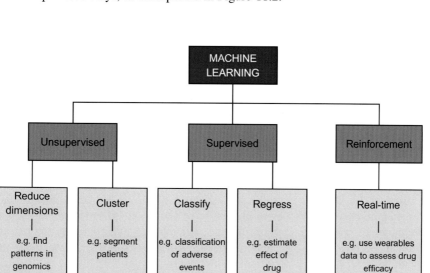

FIGURE 11.2

Different forms of machine learning.

The majority of current AI models are trained through "supervised learning." This means that humans must label and categorize the underlying data, which could be a sizable and error-prone task. Unsupervised or semisupervised approaches reduce the need for large, labeled data sets, as the AI system can group unsorted information according to similarities and differences even though no categories are provided.

Unsupervised learning algorithms are able to execute more complex processing tasks than supervised learning systems. However, unsupervised learning is sometimes more unpredictable than the other model. While an unsupervised learning AI system might, for example, figure out on its own how to sort black and white cats from Dalmatian dogs, it might also add unforeseen and undesired categories (like stracciatella yogurt pictures), creating chaos instead of order.

Reinforcement learning is an example of an unsupervised technique that was used to train AlphaGo, the AI system that defeated the world champion of the board game Go. The technique allows algorithms to learn tasks simply through trial and error. Goals can be implicitly induced by rewarding some types of behavior and punishing others. In pharmaceutical care, this is a potential technique in which the AI system can learn about the factors that determine patients' adherence profiles and how to deal with them to improve adequate drug use.

While AI capabilities have developed dramatically over time, most instances of AI that we encounter today is of the class "Narrow AI" or "Specialized AI." That is, it can handle only a narrow task of capabilities, such as identifying cats and dogs in an image *or* (not *and*, like with humans) identifying a bone fracture in an image. But give a dog-identifying AI an image with the word "dog" written on it, most AIs will not know what to do with that input. Thus, with all the progress on specialized applications of AI, we are still some distance from creating a system on a level with the learning ability of a human baby.

Stream-Mining in Continuous Data Flows

Regarding dynamic data streams, there is an interesting form of AI called stream-mining that is potentially relevant for pharmaceutical stakeholders. In streammining, AI is programmed over a constant flow of data in a system where individual data do not have to be stored. This capability is valuable in healthcare, for example, in intensive care or in home-monitoring situations, where a variety of technologies provide an endless flow of patient health data, but only the outliers need to be picked up by care providers and acted on. For example, with this technology stratification of patients with the highest risk for adverse events from medication can be done continuously once personal data are shared with pharmaceutical care providers.

AI Technology in Our Current Era

The effects of AI implementation on society in general have been spectacular. Since its development in the 1950, AI now has proven to be capable of matching or surpassing some of the most impressive intellectual feats of humans, including in healthcare, as shown, for example, in QR Code 11.4. The big promise of machine learning is the possibility of exponential learning, as trend analysis and scalability of learnings can be done much faster.

QR Code 11.4

AI in healthcare.

AI has defeated human world champions in chess; in the world's most complex game, Go; and in poker games. It is already superior to the average person in multiple aspects of recognizing faces, videos, or words from speech. And it is also developed as a successful opponent in debating competitions.

AI-enhanced IT systems are used in business to automate increasingly complex tasks that humans used to perform. These include, for example, chatbots that mimic customer service agents and enable new sales channels, loan officers' IT systems that approve and arrange loans, self-driving cars, or security guard systems that automatically check IDs, which is being used extensively at airports. AI is used increasingly in healthcare to automate structured scientific reasoning, accelerate innovation to find new treatments, and find correlations in previously considered large data sets.

Once all these competencies are combined, a computer is said to have superintelligence, which refers to an intellect that greatly outperforms the best human minds across many cognitive domains (Bostrom, 2014).

If computers were to become smarter than the world's entire population, that would prompt what is called a "singularity moment." There are various opinions about the exact time this might happen, and these opinions range from a number of years to a number of decades. Mathematician Vernor Vinge predicts it will occur by 2023, and futurist Ray Kurzweil says by 2045 (Ross, 2016). Recent research suggests there is a 50% chance that AI will outperform humans in all tasks in 45 years and will automate all human jobs in 120 years, with Asian respondents expecting these dates to occur much sooner than North Americans do (Grace et al., 2018).

The potential is there: different from a human, a machine has (relatively speaking) endless memory, does not forget, does not require sleep, and is backed by ever-increasing technological performance.

Impact on Core Responsibilities in Pharmaceutical Care

AI is set to revolutionize pharmaceutical care through connecting different pharmaceutical data sets, analyzing platforms of medical and pharmaceutical records, designing holistic treatment plans, or signaling adverse events or nonadherence. Also, AI may help automate repetitive pharmacy tasks, such as checking prescriptions or reviewing poly-pharmaceutical drug profiles (signaling, for example, overconsumption or interactions).

Therefore, it is to be expected that, of all the digital advances mentioned in this book and definitely with convergence of their data, AI is likely to be one that will disrupt the pharmaceutical care process most significantly.

Although AI in principle means artificial intelligence, some members of the AI community came to realize that it was really all about enhancing human capabilities and called it augmented intelligence. Taking this concept one step further, we introduce the term "*apothecary intelligence*": that is, augmenting human pharmaceutical expertise.

Here is the general impact that AI is expected to have on the five domains of pharmaceutical care provision (refer to Chapter 6 for a more detailed discussion):

 A. **Professional relationship between PCPs and patients:** This will be enhanced due to more integrated health data insights

 B. **Adequate collection and recording of health data:** This becomes a stronger prerequisite for feeding pharmaceutical AI in the most optimal way

 C. **Review health data and provide adequate PC proposal:** PC plan will need a roadmap denoting which data and which AI to use

 D. **Patient alignment and facilitate execution of PC plan:** Involves discussions on whether data and AI intelligence are accepted and how they augment the human care provider's role

 E. **Circular management of PC plan:** Care plan will be adjusted based on outcomes of personalized predictive and prescriptive monitoring models, driven by AI

Implementation in Daily Practice

One of the rate-limiting steps of AI in healthcare is the fact that, while it needs large training data sets, many of the health data sets that a patient generates are still stored in scattered technological applications, such as separate electronic medical records, pharmacy data, claims data, genetic profiles, and digital health trackers; and these health data sets are experiencing exponential growth.

Imagine what will happen if all these data sets are converged as described in Chapter 8. With the current pace of advancements in AI, it is, for example, assumed that by 2028 algorithms that analyze these big data sets will outperform humans by 80% in regard to classified diagnosis.

Examples of AI's Impact on Doctors' Activities

There are far too many excellent examples of the use of AI in healthcare to mention in this book. Therefore the following cases are meant for inspiration only and do not reflect their ranking in the level of disruption.

Machine learning can support analytic tasks like disease detection, usually by taking electronic health records and broader health-related data sets as its feed (Xiao et al., 2018). For example, in image recognition, as part of disease detection, AI has learnt to identify images that contain certain diseases by analyzing large training image databases that have been manually labeled as "cancer" or "no cancer."

In regard to predicting disease, in a 2017 win for AI medicine, researchers at the University of Nottingham in the United Kingdom created "a system that scanned patients' routine medical data and predicted which of them would have heart attacks or strokes within 10 years. When compared to the standard method of prediction (established algorithm of American College of Cardiology guidelines), the AI system correctly predicted the fates of 355 more patients out of 378,256 patients from UK family practices, free from cardiovascular disease at outset" (Weng et al., 2017).

In 2018 the first AI-based diagnostic system for the autonomous detection of diabetic retinopathy, a leading cause of blindness, was granted commercialization by the FDA. "The IDx-DR system can be used to provide a fast, immediate, reliable assessment for diabetic retinopathy, including macular edema, during a routine office visit in a primary care setting. It delivers a diagnostic interpretation and associated report, including care instructions that are aligned with the American Academy of Ophthalmology preferred practice pattern for diabetic retinopathy. This enables primary care providers to counsel patients regarding follow-up care while they are still in the office" (FDA, 2018d).

The company Babylon has developed an AI-powered diagnostic triage tool to 24/7 support patients to identify if they suffer from a disease (more extensively discussed in Chapter 12). It published in 2018 a paper stating that "their AI was able to identify the condition modeled by a clinical vignette with accuracy comparable to human doctors (in terms of precision and recall). In addition, they found that the triage advice recommended by the AI System was, on average, safer than that of human doctors, when compared to the ranges of acceptable triage provided by independent expert judges, with only a minimal reduction in appropriateness" (Babylon, 2018).

A study in 2016 at Beth Israel Deaconess Medical Center (BIDMC) and Harvard Medical School showed that AI isn't so much about humans versus machines, as it is often thought to be. Researchers trained an algorithm to identify metastatic breast cancer by interpreting pathology images. Their algorithm reached an accuracy of 92.5%, whereas the pathologists reached an accuracy of 97%. But used in combination, the detection rate approached 100% (approximately 99.5%). Thus the synergy between human knowledge and AI capacity is currently considered as the most optimal situation (BIDMC, 2016).

IBM Watson

 Watson is "a supervised cognitive system capable of learning from earlier interactions, garnering knowledge and value over time, thinking like a human. It works by combining AI and advanced analytical software for analysis of various forms of data, thereby providing optimal responses based on reasoning and interacting like a "question-answering" machine. Watson was in 2018 in clinical use in the U.S. and 5 other countries. It has been trained on a number of types of cancers with plans to add quite a number more in next years. Beyond oncology, the platform is in use in nearly 50% of Top 25 Life Science business, supporting genomics, clinical trial matching and drug discovery" (IBM, 2018).

Watson still requires substantial, laborious training, as experts are required to code vast quantities of well-organized data and feed them into the Watson platform in order to make useful conclusions.

Google

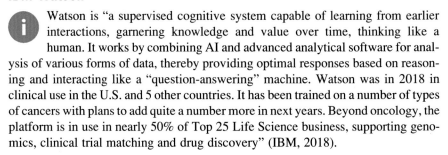 Google's DeepMind algorithms are based on unsupervised reinforcement learning and are applying AI to disease detection and to optimizing new healthcare data infrastructures.

For example, DeepMind Health entered into an agreement with the UK's National Health Service (NHS) to access patient records to train detection and prevention algorithms. DeepMind Health now works with NHS on mobile tools and AI research to help get patients optimally from test to treatment. Apps use mobile technology to send immediate alerts to clinicians when a patient's condition deteriorates, thus allowing physicians to take faster and more personalized action (Deepmind, 2018).

Scientists from Verily (former called Google Life Sciences) have also discovered "a new way to assess a person's risk of heart disease by analyzing scans of the back of a patient's eye. The AI is able to accurately deduce data, including an individual's age, blood pressure, and whether or not they smoke. Converged data can then be used to predict their risk of suffering a major cardiac event—such as a heart attack—with roughly the same accuracy as current leading methods" (Poplin et al., 2018).

The specific disease areas where Google is studying diagnostics and disease management include, among others, ocular diseases, diabetes, Parkinson's disease, and heart diseases. There are a number of initiatives to research aspects of medication, and more developments in the pharmaceutical environment may follow.

Google faced challenges in the United Kingdom for using de-identified health data, which do not ordinarily require an individual's consent, however, also this type of research is expected to go through rigorous medical research approval processes.

Microsoft

Microsoft's healthcare team NExT (New Experiences and Technologies) is designed to foster health industry partnerships and bring together Microsoft's research, AI, and cloud teams to focus on healthcare.

> "Researchers across Microsoft apply computer science expertise to enable data-driven healthcare, enhance wellness and accelerate progress in life sciences. Artificial intelligence, machine learning and exponential leaps in data availability and cloud computing fuel research initiatives to understand biology at molecular and cellular levels, guide the development of medical treatments and analyze data streams to detect health threats, predict disease outbreaks and counsel patients."

An example of a project the company is working on is Project InnerEye, an innovative machine learning tool that helps radiologists identify and analyze 3D images of cancerous tumors. "InnerEye is a research project that uses state of the art machine learning technology to build innovative tools for the automatic, quantitative analysis of three-dimensional radiological images. Project InnerEye turns radiological images into measuring devices" (Microsoft, 2018).

Microsoft also has a fitness band that is linked to its voice-user interface, Cortana, and makes use of AI, but it is still in its infancy and faces a number of user-related challenges that need to be solved.

AI to Fuel "Pharmacy-as-a-Service" Platforms

Introducing AI technology to analyze existing electronic pharmacy records (EPRs), combined with other data sets derived from technologies as described in Part 2 of this book, will create huge opportunities to build apothecary intelligence and deliver "pharmaceutical-care-as-a-service" platforms.

Conditional to success will be to identify at first whether unique and anonymized patient identifiers can be established to create a secure (patient) data platform on which AI can be built, while respecting the privacy of individuals. For instance, more standardized use of citizen identification numbers may create opportunities to combine all available data into one personal health application (preferably governed by the patient), as described in Chapter 8 as well.

With the use of a unique patient ID, different data sets may be connected that feed the AI, whereas working with open health databases and adoption of standardized interconnectivity standards like HL7-FHIR, as noted in Chapter 8, are vital prerequisites to make a convergence of data and technology happen.

Many pharmaceutical care teams are used to working in an EPR environment that connects with general practitioners' data, specialists' data, hospital data, wearables, and other digital health information.

These connected pharmaceutical data sets can be analyzed by AI technology, augmenting the pharmaceutical professional in various ways:

- **To support getting better patient outcomes:** For example, having access to the genomic profile of a patient and linking it to the data set of various other health data can provide professionals with a detailed prediction on how individuals are going to respond to medication and where to put extra attention to prevent, for example, nonadherence, adverse events, deterioration in illness, or suboptimal dosing.
- **To move from evidence-based to intelligence-based healthcare:** Although AI algorithms in the next decade most probably will not replace completely the need for clinical trials or postlaunch evidence data generation, significant insight on disease and behavioral patterns can be derived from real-world data analyses, gathered by consolidating large amounts of connected IoT healthcare devices.
- **To (re)organize patient routes or treatment plans more personalized:** This will be based on historical data, characteristics, and preferences of the individual.
- **To better informed advice physicians on optimal treatment:** This will involve AI results to augment existing clinical guidelines and balanced treatment decisions.
- **To create voice-controlled pharmaceutical coaching systems for patients:** This will emerge as natural language processing becomes increasingly more sophisticated and smart AI devices like chatbots can be managed via voice control (as described in Chapter 12). Various types of heterogeneous data sets may be added to these virtual coaches (e.g., scientific literature versus Facebook feeds versus facial recognition, each of which has very different contextual, semantic, and linguistic characteristics).

How to Start Tomorrow With AI?

In Chapter 20 the structured Digital-by-Design (DbD) approach is explained to identify whether technology can be a solution for a certain pharmaceutical care issue. In case of AI, not all business challenges require AI solutions, as statistics and database research often can do the job as well and may be much easier and less expensive to implement.

If AI is found to be a suitable option after running the DbD model, it does make sense to collaborate with data science experts at a project's early stage, for example, with consultancy companies, academia, big corporations, as well as with AI-in-healthcare startups, which are growing in number.

The majority of the AI-in-healthcare startups in recent years were found in the imaging and diagnostic area. Like the example box of Pacmed, the number of these promising startups aboard may supersede the development speed of the big corporate AI vendors, offering simpler and faster options to implement AI technology. Also, they are increasingly able to work with unprepared and incomplete data, as often is the case in healthcare.

AI Healthcare Startup Pacmed

Currently, evidence on the effectiveness of treatments is often based on average results on a very small number of patients, which is not always representative and does not cover the complexity and variety of the population a doctor sees in practice.

Patients and doctors are generating more data each day, which allows doctors to learn directly and objectively from every patient. Pacmed builds decision support software for doctors, based on the analysis of those observational health data. By combining medical expertise and machine learning techniques, the software computes and presents expected outcomes of relevant treatment options for the patient a doctor is seeing. Unlike other sources of medical knowledge, Pacmed algorithms learn every time they are applied in practice.

Pacmed identified the treatment of urinary tract infections at the GP-level in the Netherlands as the most feasible starting point for machine learning in the consultation room. The software that helps GPs choose the best treatment, based on data of over 250,000 urinary tract infections, is currently being used by over 100 GPs in a scientific implementation study. Pacmed is also developing software for optimal, personal, and outcome-based treatment choices in hospital intensive care units and in oncology, cardiology, and psychiatry.

The enormous wealth of smart healthcare AI startups is too broad to mention in this chapter, particularly as some are predominantly locally focused. However, before considering or even starting a new initiative in your pharmaceutical care pathway, it does make sense to run an analysis on available solutions in the market before starting from scratch to build the next own AI.

Kaggle to Answer Pharmaceutical AI Questions

An interesting platform to consider for a pharmaceutical care problem that may be solved by an AI solution is the Kaggle platform (QR Code 11.5).

Kaggle is a global crowdsourcing platform with public data sets for predictive modeling and analytics competitions in which companies and researchers post data and statisticians and data scientists compete to produce the best models for predicting and describing the data.

This crowdsourcing approach relies on the fact that there are countless strategies that can be applied to any predictive modeling task and that it is impossible to know at the outset which technique or analyst will be most effective. Contributors come from a wide variety of backgrounds, including fields such as computer science, computer vision, biology, medicine, and even glaciology.

Competitions have resulted in many successful projects, including furthering the state of the art in HIV research, chess ratings, and traffic forecasting.

QR Code 11.5

Kaggle.

Challenges to crowd-sourcing in 2018 in the healthcare environment are—amongst others—the complex and heterogeneous data sets as well as the sensitivity of dealing with patient data (Derrington, 2017).

Individual pharmacists of pharmaceutical care groups or chains may consider posting their pharmaceutical care questions (and strict anonymized data sets) on Kaggle or other competing platforms, initiating an environment where experts in big data programming can use their expertise to develop algorithms to solve the problem.

Considerations

Within the optimism about the opportunities of artificial intelligence, there is increasingly room for realism as well. AI has existed since the last decade of the 1950s, and although the current speed of computers and our advanced scientific approaches have increased the pace of applicability, there are still a number of hurdles to overcome before AI will have a secure, integrated, and trusted place in the field of healthcare.

Bias and Responsible Data Science

AI-based systems are as smart as the data that go into them and the programmers who build them. Thus, two forms are of specific relevance here: the bias caused by the programmer's vision and the bias caused by (poor) decisions in the past. The latter is particularly relevant for healthcare, as inadequate or skewed therapeutic guidelines, unequal gender admission in clinical trials, and many other selection biases may have led to inadequate outcomes in the past, which if fed into an AI program will reintroduce the bias. Being conscious of this phenomenon is essential when interpreting the results and further developing AI algorithms.

Additionally, AI systems may be skewed by variations and biases in diverging population data so that models trained in one pharmaceutical pathway may not be applicable in another, especially if they are in a different geographical region or disease population. And good data is hardest to collect in places that need it most, including low and middle-income countries (LMIC) lacking developed healthcare infrastructures. Critical data remain especially scarce in developing countries where electronic health records are not yet in wide use.

In this respect, to develop future-proof, responsible data science methods, more foundational research is globally needed, with a focus on FACT, which means questions related to Fairness, Accuracy, Confidentiality, and Transparency.

Lack of Differentiation in AI Providers

The huge increase in startups and established providers—all positioning themselves to offer AI products—is sometimes confusing to end users. In 2018 more than 1000 healthcare providers in the Western world with applications and platforms described themselves as AI vendors, or said they used AI in their products, whereas differentiation between focus areas is not always transparent.

In order to build trust with end-user organization like pharmaceutical care providers, AI providers are recommended to transparently publish research reports and case studies on the methods used and results achieved when implementing AI techniques. This will enable end-users to select an AI provider that best fits needs and provides a reliable solution for a pharmaceutical problem to solve.

Proven, Less Complex Machine-Learning Capabilities Can Address Many End-User Needs

Advancements in AI, such as deep learning, are getting a lot of buzz but may eclipse the value of more straightforward, already proven approaches. It is always recommended that programmers and researchers use the simplest approach to accomplishing a job rather than cutting-edge AI techniques.

This means that for pharmaceutical purposes many questions may already be answered by (relatively) simple, adequate statistical analysis of claims data, connected electronic health data bases, or prescription record databases built for pharmacoepidemiological outcomes.

For decades database analysis has created insight into disease epidemiology and provided the contextual background for the design of clinical trials. It can also provide evidence on safety outcomes, effectiveness, drug utilization patterns, burden of diseases, patient journeys, and adherence relatively easily. Additionally, different types of studies using longitudinal and real-life patient data have already helped in our understanding of management of health risks and have provided solutions for decision makers in the market access, health economics, and health outcomes sectors.

If processes are running well and solving the problems posed, sophisticated, complex AI and machine learning techniques are not necessary.

Ethical Challenges

In order to assure a sustainable balance between artificial and human intelligence, it is of utmost importance that AI applications remain under meaningful human governance and be used for socially beneficial purposes, as has been extensively emphasized by many stakeholders globally (Est van et al., 2017) (QR Code 11.6).

Technology is not value neutral, and in the slight overhyping that has been put on AI in last years, society ask technologists to take responsibility for the ethical and social impact of their work. Understanding what this means in practice requires rigorous scientific inquiry into the most sensitive challenges we humans face, and the inclusion of many voices throughout, in order to avoid misconception, misuse, and human rejection of AI implementation (Tegmark, 2017).

QR Code 11.6

Ethics and AI.

Also, transparency in how unsupervised learning mechanisms work, how algorithms are developed, and what human oversight is warranted are essential to create societal trust when working with AI. As noted in Chapter 16 regarding the use of robotics, in order to create trust, our future machines should be enabled to transparently communicate how their algorithms are programmed, how they are learning, and how suggestions, recommendations, and actions are being posed.

Additionally, as AI is going to help pharmaceutical stakeholders in making better predictions, it is important to realize that we humans make decisions in which we use both prediction and judgment (see Chapter 19). We've never really unbundled those aspects of decision making. Separating the process in the machine doing the prediction makes the distinct role of judgment in decision making clearer. As the value of human prediction decreases due to AI, the value of human judgment should go up, because that is something AI doesn't do.

The first big initiatives to warrant human governance in AI have already started. One interesting example is the installation of the Partnership on AI initiative (2017), which aims "to study and formulate best practices on AI technologies, to advance the public's understanding of AI, and to serve as an open platform for discussion and engagement about AI and its ethical influences on people and society" (Partnership on AI, 2018).

Also, the Future of Life Institute, founded in 2014, has a "strong mission to catalyze and support research and initiatives for safeguarding life and developing optimistic visions of the future, including positive ways for humanity to steer its own course considering new technologies and challenges. They have developed 23 principles to work responsibly with AI" (Future of Life Institute, 2017).

Much more information on how pharmaceutical care professionals deal with ethics in AI can be found in Chapter 18.

Competencies and Skills to Evaluate, Build, and Deploy AI Solutions

This is an important consideration within the time frame this book was written (2017–18). Currently, many organizations, including healthcare institutions, are built on traditional competency frameworks, since the organizations are expert in their own professional fields and may have had limited exposure to data science, machine learning, and platform management. Data sets, analysis, and adequate use are only as good as their creators; thus organizations need to adopt skills to make sure the workforce of the future is familiar with the data science and understands algorithms and the different ways of decision making.

In order to work adequately with AI data sets, pharmaceutical care providers may need to increasingly combine their pharmaceutical knowledge with technology perception and data science skills. Detailed information on the proposed competency profile of the future for pharmaceutical care stakeholders can be found in Chapter 19.

Privacy, Quality, and Security

While increased data collection and analysis in pharmaceutical practice may offer numerous benefits to patient care and healthcare business operations, these advantages also can come with a risk. As more sensitive patient data and algorithms are stored online, cyber threats present a growing challenge for the healthcare industry, as the example of the NHS reflects. As another example, a 2017 study by Accenture found that patient data theft is the most likely security risk to occur in pharmacy practice (Accenture, 2017).

In addition to causing financial loss due to legality issues, these breaches also decrease patient trust in pharmaceutical care stakeholders who aim to use digital health technology. Thus the detailed information on how to warrant security, privacy, and quality conditions by making a compliance blueprint prior to starting off—as discussed in Chapter 17—is noteworthy.

Privacy Breach in NHS
The Royal Free NHS Foundation Trust got a reprimand in 2017 for passing personal data on 1.6 million patients to Google's UK-based artificial intelligence unit, which taught the world that when working with AI platforms, informed consent and data privacy regulation is as valid as the previous manual on epidemiologic research (see also Chapter 17) (Deepmind, 2018). As has been done in other AI big data research, Google used de-identified data, which do not ordinarily require individual consent, but it still needs to go through a rigorous medical research approval process.

By now it should be clear why the sequoia analogy was used. Although AI is definitely not as mature and historical as those giants, both are overwhelming. Moreover, just as the sequoias have significantly influenced the Sierra Nevada landscape in North America, AI will have a large influence on how future human ecosystems are perceived.

The true beauty of AI in pharmaceutical care lies in the balance between the synergy of its decision support system and human healthcare leadership, making AI a true apothecary intelligence.

Probably AI's biggest influence in the upcoming years is the creation of smart virtual assistants, which is the topic of next Chapter 12.

This means for circular pharmaceutical care:

- Artificial Intelligence technology can feed pharmacy-as-a-service platforms, provided it has access to complete, adequate, and holistic health data sets.
- Apothecary intelligence is the use of AI to augment human pharmaceutical care.
- AI technology is not always required as a solution, as sometimes traditional statistical database research can do the job better and faster.
- Often it is not necessary to use AI technology at the starting point, as big platforms and a wealth of startups have a lot of AI experience to offer.
- When developing AI, algorithm transparency, detection of data bias, competency building, and ethical considerations are crucial conditions for success.
- Ensuring data privacy, quality, and security of both analysis and output are crucial to generate trust in AI algorithms.
- AI may help automate repetitive pharmaceutical care tasks and can augment personalized care plans with integrated decision support systems. This will increase providers' value for what they do best: make human judgment and provide empathic care.

An animation on the topic of AI in pharmaceutical care can be found on www.pharmacare.ai.

QR Code Animation

Artificial Intelligence.

Pharmbot canopies

12

Claudia Rijcken

Bots learn the same way as people learn, through progression.
Unknown

People in general don't like to go to the doctor. So, as mentioned in previous chapters, doctors are increasingly becoming home-oriented care providers. If needed, care is given in person, and if possible, a growing amount of support is offered via virtual personal assistants (VPAs) like chatbots or digital humans. Whether it is Molly, Ada, Melody, Tessa, or Mabu, they all aim to support your health in the virtual space, and they increasingly act as supports canopying healthcare service systems.

In this chapter you will read about how chatbots are conquering healthcare, how pharmaceutical chatbots called pharmbots can enhance patients' care experiences, and why it is essential for medication information to be drawn from a Single Point of Truth database.

And if the doctor is in the virtual space, why not have the pharmacist there, too?

Technology

In 2015 Gartner estimated that "30% of our interactions with technology will be through 'conversations' with smart machines by 2018." Although globally that figure has not yet been reached, in some regions of the United States the predictions are almost a reality, and comScore estimates that by 2020 a full 50% of all searches will be by voice. While it is not likely to replace all existing screen-based searches, voice search by chatbots and/or digital humans has become a factor that all businesses need to enter into the equation (Bentahar, 2017) (QR Code 12.1).

How Chatbots Work

 A chatbot is a digital application designed to simulate a digital conversation with human users through artificial intelligence and that may act via auditory or textual methods. Initially, chatbots were text-based, but because

Pharmaceutical Care in Digital Revolution. https://doi.org/10.1016/B978-0-12-817638-2.00012-2

QR Code 12.1

Healthcare chatbot example.

the techniques of voice-recognition and text-to-speech have improved significantly, the quality of spoken interactions with chatbots, called voice-user interfaces (VUIs), is quickly improving. The functionality as such can be called a virtual personal assistant (VPA) or digital human.

Typically, a chatbot will communicate with a real person, but applications are being developed in which two chatbots can communicate with each other. Some chatbots use sophisticated natural language processing (NLP) systems (see Chapter 11), but many simpler systems scan for keywords within the input and then pull out a reply with the most matching keywords, or the most similar wording pattern, from a predefined database.

Chatbots are currently used in many applications, such as e-commerce customer service, call centers, and internet gaming. So far they are typically limited to conversations regarding a specialized purpose and are not yet equipped to cover broad ranges of human communication. Nevertheless, in 2018 a Google Duplex algorithm was able to adequately plan and book a slot at a hair salon, based on the agenda of a businessman and the actual schedule of a local hairdresser, as communicated by phone by an employee. The VPA used a very natural speech pattern that included hesitations and affirmations such as "er" and "mmm-hmm" so that the virtual assistant calling was extremely difficult to distinguish from an actual human phone call.

Chatbots and AI

To execute conversations, chatbots require data inputs that through NLP and artificial intelligence (AI) may be translated into knowledge relevant for users. AI algorithms must understand the grammar in the language, and they also have to grasp the context in which they interpret the language, as in many languages semantics are well known for their ambiguity and may be easily misinterpreted, which in healthcare has the potential to lead to disastrous results.

Technologies that allow for programming VPAs are, for example, Amazon's Alexa, Google's Home Assistant, Microsoft's Cortana, and Apple's Siri. In addition, individual care robot systems and many other communication platforms and businesses are currently integrating voice-user-interfaces.

By smart NLP, VPAs can be programmed at the literacy level of the user, meaning that personalized advice on specific content can be provided.

There are two possible approaches to creating information from available data (see also Chapter 11). Let us explain the two approaches by the example of building chatbots for patient leaflets of drugs.

The first approach is referred to as the supervised route, in which the available data are manually encoded into domain-specific information categories, and an algorithm subsequently can analyze this information and create knowledge maps.

Often referred to as an "inventory of knowledge," these maps are organized using various interconnected nodes to make it easy to know where to look for information.

The coding can be labor-intensive and requires very solid, standardized classification of information and knowledge mapping. This approach is relevant in pharmaceutical care, for example, in the case of converting data from a patient information leaflet into a chatbot application. Currently, the regulatory-approved summary of product characteristics (SPC) text has yet to be coded and classified so that a chatbot can understand the context in a uniform way and make the ingoing data a Single Point of Truth (SPoT).

To simplify this procedure, a second way to convert pharmaceutical product information data to chatbot knowledge is a more statistical approach in which the computer is given a magnitude of SPC samples and then is allowed to identify patterns across this information. In this way intelligent chatbot context can be developed. However, this method requires an enormous amount of training data and computer power and also potentially even more checks for accuracy than the first approach does.

Complexity of Learning AI

The more data examples a chatbot gets, the more it has to learn. That means that if—for example, in healthcare—patients have a specific verbal accent, at the first interaction, a VUI chatbot will have to verify whether the patient asked a question known by the algorithm, however, with a different accent. Once the patient agrees that the question was correctly interpreted, the computer will store this information ("learn") and the next time will understand the question at once and will not repeat the verification process.

One can imagine the complexity in making healthcare bots work reliably for verbally impaired people (e.g., aphasia in dementia) using semantics that are not commonly known.

Therefore this type of chatbot learning may need programming and learning restrictions and thorough human oversight. In the coming years specific regulations will be required to ensure patient safety.

Because a chatbot in healthcare is considered to be a safety-critical application, tolerance for system mistakes ideally should be reduced to zero; thus the AI's conversion of data to knowledge process and output needs to be fully transparent and thoroughly checked by humans, as the example in the pink box reflects as well.

Chatbots in Healthcare and Pharmbots

By adding clinical triage and medical content into a bot framework, the virtual personal health assistants can interact with the user on topics regarding, for instance, well-being, experienced health, questions on diseases, and information about healthcare interventions.

Patient-oriented healthcare chatbots are now either patient-only applications (apps that help a patient track and make sense of health data) or patient-clinician applications (consultation apps that connect the two groups, for diagnosis support, treatment suggestions, etc.).

Assistive chatbots.

Additionally, chatbots can be great secretaries and customer-service representatives. They can provide communication solutions, with AI prioritizing and smart-routing requests to the right resource to meet the users' needs. An interesting example of an AI-enabled patient solution is the D.Assist in QR Code 12.2.

When chatbots are developed to support pharmaceutical care processes, they can be called Pharmbots.

 A pharmbot is a computer application that is designed to simulate pharmaceutical care with human users through artificial intelligence, and it may interact via auditory or textual methods. In other words, pharmbots are VPAs in pharmaceutical care. Pharmbots may help optimize adherence by answering drug-related questions, by telling a patient what to expect during the first weeks a medicine is taken, or by reducing the potential for medicine to taken other than as prescribed.

Avatars and Digital Humans

Chatbots on mobile technology are increasingly combined with avatars, that is, electronic images that represent and can be manipulated by a person using a device in a virtual space (as in a computer game or an online shopping site) and that interact with other objects in the space.

Digital humans.

Digital avatars, which more and more have human characteristics and are then called digital humans, are considered the future of customer support, and combined with bot technology, they would enable nearly humanlike interactions for pharmaceutical care. The advantage avatars have over written or device-driven interfaces is that communication is perceived as being more true to life (QR Code 12.3).

Considering that avatars are already able to run facial recognition models that can understand customers' moods and at the same time draw a number of conclusions based on people's facial expressions, the technology presents the possibility of always having an understanding virtual pharmacist accompanying you by way of your mobile phone.

Impact on Core Responsibilities in Pharmaceutical Care

Due to the growing quality of interaction and the 24/7 availability of chatbots, these systems may significantly augment the day-to-day interactions with patients. Many of the frequent questions a pharmaceutical care stakeholder gets have significant commonalities and thus may be standardized and offered to patients as needed in a reliable, programmed format as a chatbot.

Here is the general impact that chatbots are expected to have on the five domains of pharmaceutical care provision (refer to Chapter 6 for a more detailed discussion):

A. **Professional relationship between pharmacists and patients:** This will be enhanced with chatbot technology.

B. **Adequate collection and recording of health data:** Interactive chatbots may provide continuous personalized patient information.

C. **Review health data and provide adequate pharmaceutical care plan:** PC plans may be set up partially based on an analysis of chatbot interactions with patients.

D. **Patient alignment and facilitate execution of pharmaceutical care plan:** Patients will experience better pharmaceutical services as chatbots can be used if possible and human care can be added if required.

E. **Circular management of pharmaceutical care plan:** Chatbots may give PC adjustment advice to pharmacists.

Implementation in Daily Practice

As indicated previously in this chapter, there are many reasons why pharmaceutical care stakeholders will decide to deploy chatbot functionality. Whether it is to augment service experiences, to offer information on drugs, or to really be a virtual pharmacist that a patient can consult on 24/7 basis, chatbots can definitely help free up pharmacists' time for the most complex problems (as the simple questions can be answered by the chatbot) and also may assist in signaling which patients are in the most need of human intervention.

Logistic and Administrative Pharmacy Support

We are entering an era in which professionals can verbally consult a digital drug reference app on all aspects of medications (refer to Chapter 9 for more on this topic). One example is the Safedrugbot app, a chat messaging service that offers easily accessible drug information to health professionals who work with pregnant and breastfeeding women. It is a virtual assistant that can perform a variety of tasks, like providing information on drugs, active ingredients, or alternative drugs that are safer for women who are breastfeeding.

Also, a wealth of bot technology is under development that will support healthcare providers in their day-to-day logistical and administrative activities (refer to Chapter 9). Like the Google Duplex example mentioned earlier, these apps can answer voicemails, track patient dialogues, immediately update medical and pharmaceutical patient records, do claims management processing, support in inventory management, and plan agendas for healthcare professionals, all of which free up providers' time to do what matters most: care for patients.

Logistic and administrative tools mean that professionals will no longer have to search their desktops or books, in having to do administrative narrative tasks in patient health records or in activity planning.

Moreover, chatbot updates can be done with the click of a button. Thus a bot can scale up quickly and remain up to date, as long as all stakeholders upload relevant information in a timely way (sometimes in the past outdated books or reference documents were used).

Alexa, Can You Help Me With My Medication?

Alexa was catching up with Google Assistant in 2018, although a 2017 study showed that Google Assistant still led the field in accuracy, by faultlessly answering 5000 general knowledge questions (Dunn, 2017).

In 2018 Loup Ventures asked Siri, Google Assistant, Alexa, and Cortana 800 general questions. Again, Google Assistant was able to answer the most questions correctly: Google Assistant answered 86% of them correctly, while Siri answered 79% accurately, Alexa 61%, and Cortana 52%. To best of the authors' knowledge, this kind of research has not been done with medical questions.

Amazon's Alexa added medical advice to its repertoire for developers in 2017. WebMD announced that it launched its own skill for all Alexa-enabled devices, which can answer basic health-related queries. Topics include treatments for common ailments ("Alexa, ask WebMD how to treat a sore throat"), definitions of basic diseases ("Alexa, ask WebMD what diabetes is"), and the side effects of certain drugs ("Alexa, ask WebMD to tell me about amoxicillin").

The Advantage of a Virtual Personal Assistant

Take an elderly person, just having received a new knee, still on an anticoagulant, but happy to be released from hospital to go home. However, after 5 days in the homecare situation, the patient notices a number of blue spots on his arms and wonders what is causing them. Without having to call the doctor or navigate on a desktop while still rather immobile, just by asking the voice assistant what to expect 5 days after having surgery, the VPA can do a simple triage and reassure the patient that blue spots are known to occur with anticoagulant therapy and that there is no reason to worry.

Increasingly, more skills are programmed on the Alexa device, for example, a virtual nurse to ask questions, breast-feeding advice, triage protocol to assess symptoms, and hospitals interactions with patients in their homes; it is also expected that ordering medication will be possible via Alexa as well as other virtual personal assistants.

> Another example is from Boston Children's Hospital, which developed an Alexa-based app in early 2016 that provides parents with advice on how to care for a child with a fever. The KidsMD app, as it is dubbed, provides actionable health information while it collects data about symptoms and locations that could give public health professionals early warning signs of flu outbreaks.

Intelligent Chatbots to Support Triage, Diagnosis, and Screening

In a quest to improve patient safety, existing problems such as medication errors, healthcare-associated infections, and postsurgical complications have been better quantified in recent years. Diagnostic errors are also a well-known error, although true incidence rates are very difficult to calculate and rates seem to vary between 10% and 50% (Graber, 2013).

AI, in the form of structured image analysis, facial recognition, and triage chatbots, may provide strong supportive tools for doctors as well as pharmacists, both for reducing the incidence of diagnostic errors and for reducing avoidable harm.

The use of triage applications is growing exponentially; for example, in the United States primary care environment, it is expected that 5.4 million GP video consultations a year will be executed by 2020. This increase is driven by well-known triage tools such as iTriage by Aetna, Buoy, and YourMD, according to the US research firm IHS Markit.

QR Code 12.4

How Babylon Health works.

In Europe, for example, the ADA and Babylon chatbots are providing virtual doctor applications (more info on Babylon in QR Code 12.4). Both companies aim to put accessible and affordable health services into the hands of every person around the globe, thinking that up to 80% of physical consultations may be avoidable. By combining the ever-growing computing power of machines with the best human medical expertise, they have created comprehensive, immediate, and personalized health service.

By taking this route, the efficiency of offering doctors' knowledge is maximized by reducing the time doctors have to spend on administrative duties, as the apps store all patient information directly in the medical records. Doctors within Babylon Health are said to spend 93% of their time with patients compared with only 61% in Britain's public sector due to administrative duties.

Also, these chatbots allow easy triage in remote areas where access to healthcare facilities is difficult. Triage bots may prevent people from having to travel (unnecessarily) for days to reach facilities, and in the future chatbots may be augmented with drones that will provide the medication. As a result, a pharmbot may provide the pharmaceutical support required for adequate drug use.

Doctors Versus Chatbots

In 2018 Babylon released a paper in which they hypothesized that an AI-powered triage and diagnostic system would compare favorably with human doctors with respect to triage and diagnostic accuracy.

They demonstrated that the Babylon system was able to identify the condition modeled by a clinical vignette with accuracy comparable to human doctors (in terms of precision and recall). In addition, they showed that the triage advice recommended by the AI system was, on average, safer than that of human doctors, when compared to the ranges of acceptable triage provided by independent expert judges, with only a minimal reduction in appropriateness (Razakki et al., 2018).

Sensely
An interesting AI medical assistant is Sensely, which combines AI-based triage and support to specific groups of patients under the avatar name Molly. Molly supports patients with, for example, heart failure in their disease management, making use of both direct patient inputs (e.g., quality of life surveys) and inputs from digital health devices and medical records.

Closed Loop Medical Ecosystems Required

In order to have triage and online medical and pharmaceutical systems working as reliably as possible, a closed-loop ecosystem (as discussed in Chapter 8) comprising the health data of pharmacists, GPs, specialists, and other (paramedic) healthcare providers is essential. Also, adding other personal health determinants and goals, like those captured in the GAS score (refer to Chapter 6), or other lifestyle preference scores might further feed the algorithm with vital information, leading to more personalized care recommendations for patients.

Once both the medical and the pharmaceutical care process is viewed as an end-to-end data flow and approached this way, a holistic, integrated data set of patient data can be constructed that provides the backbone of a solid diagnosis and treatment analysis, partially facilitated by chatbots.

Moreover, integrating the triage app within a technology that patients are already familiar with (e.g., a smartphone that already tracks a number of health data in apps; see Chapter 9) may provide the highest likelihood for the adoption of chatbots. In 2018 it was announced that the Babylon Health app will be integrated in all UK Samsung phones and in WeChat.

By being in patients' home environments, we can begin to draw in all other relevant health determinants known about individual patients or a population in general. For example, screening large populations by triage bots may eventually allow for faster detection of rare diseases, outbreaks of epidemics, or occurrence of low-frequency adverse events.

Virtual Pharmacists

Once doctors and nurses' activities can be simulated in chatbots, it is very likely that the same will work for pharmacists' activities. Therefore pharmbots as VPAs can act as homecare coaches in a blended, synergistic approach to human care. Pharmbots are supposed to interact, like the triage apps, in a patient's natural language and offer continuous virtual pharmaceutical care as needed wherever the patient is located.

Pharmbot Vision

Although, to the author's knowledge, pharmaceutical bot applications for care purposes are still limited, we can imagine that future pharmbots will provide services to patients, such as mobile coaches via proactive and personalized communication of relevant changes in patient information leaflets.

Another example is personalized virtual care the first 10 days after a patient begins taking a medication, in which patients are thoroughly informed on what they can expect in terms of the medication's benefits and potential side effects, particularly because there is a high risk of nonadherence in this period of medication use.

The blended approach of digital support if possible and human care where needed does provide a patient's convenience, while also directing patients to the right level of care in a timely way (e.g., escalation to human care by chatbots is done in case of disturbing health signals). Additionally, providing these forms of virtual care may lower the number of calls to pharmacies, resulting in more time for pharmacists to focus on human care, where required.

As it would give patients access to 24/7 self-care, the pharmbot would also help healthcare commissioners and payers to cut down on any unnecessary patient visits to hospitals and pharmacies and reduce out-of-hour staff costs.

Considerations

When evaluating a pharmbot, a few factors are of particular importance:

- It should not use redundant text, as patients may not take a verbose bot seriously.
- Does it still work when a patient uses incorrect grammar or typos?
- Does it recognize synonyms, and does it have a sufficient understanding of the context?
- Can or has the bot dealt with accents, dialects, or diseases that impact the lingual centers in the brain?
- Does it encourage humans to learn or just tell them what they don't know?
- Is the advice given to patients understood by all, and is this sufficiently tested?
- Are the way the algorithms work transparent, and can they be made public?

- Are retention and engagement rates available to indicate why patients may or may not be satisfied with the service provided?
- Is it possible for patients to refuse a pharmbot if they prefer to speak with a human?
- Are optimum privacy and security ensured?

Security, Privacy, and Ethics

Data privacy and security challenges are increasing and will grow further and become sensitive conditional requirements for all digital health devices in the coming years. It is assumed that most patients will want to know how their privacy will be protected by bot-providing companies. In addition to being as cautious and strict with data as possible, providers must develop teams that observe regulations, create transparency, and follow data privacy requirements as explained in Chapter 17. As noted in Chapter 11 as well, future chatbots may explain clearly to users how they are structured towards giving recommendations, which data they have used, how the algorithm is programmed, and what data will be shared with whom. If chatbot technology aims to disrupt healthcare, it has to gain the trust of the end user, and that trust is largely built on providing transparency of algorithms and adequate use of data (both storing and analyzing).

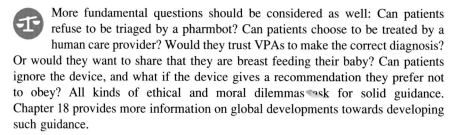 More fundamental questions should be considered as well: Can patients refuse to be triaged by a pharmbot? Can patients choose to be treated by a human care provider? Would they trust VPAs to make the correct diagnosis? Or would they want to share that they are breast feeding their baby? Can patients ignore the device, and what if the device gives a recommendation they prefer not to obey? All kinds of ethical and moral dilemmas ask for solid guidance. Chapter 18 provides more information on global developments towards developing such guidance.

SPoTs to Facilitate Pharmbots

When we look at pharmaceutical service skills currently built on VPAs, we see that the existing ones are used predominantly focused on services such as alarms to disseminate medication reminders or to provide very high-level drug- or disease-related information. Thus the possibility of using VPAs as true pharmaceutical treatment companions as envisioned in the earlier example is still limited.

An important reason for this is the earlier mentioned fact that the patient leaflet is currently not available as a Single Point of Truth (SPoT) medication information, in a format that allows consistent conversion to chatbot knowledge. In an ideal situation, all data on product information as approved by, for example, EMA or FDA would be centrally accessible and maintained as structured data. This SPoT can be uniform and always kept up to date on all digital derivatives used by all pharmaceutical care stakeholders, such as pharmacists, physicians, and adherence providers. In order to let the central data act as a SPoT as much as possible, up-front standardization of coding and classification is required. Now many mandated fields of medicinal product information are already standardized based on global standards like ICD-10, ATC codes, MedDRA codes, and so on.

Manufacturers would submit or update product information directly in the SPoT via authorized access levels and in a structured approach, which would be a large improvement over the current process, which is often driven by PDF files and Word documents.

Regulatory bodies can use the SPoT to run all required assessments and release SPCs and patient leaflets for use by third parties. Pharmaceutical care providers can use the SPoT as uniform data feed for artificial intelligent digital derivatives. Making the output of those derivatives (like pharmbots) HL7-FHIR-compatible would grant connectivity with EPRs or EMRS and thus patient leaflet updates may be connected via digital derivatives into patient health environments, allowing for personalized relevancy checks of medication updates.

This vision has another advantage as well, the SPoT would not only be the Single Point of Truth, but would also create a *single point of trust*, as it would be guaranteed that digital derivatives like chatbots are always up to date and based on the same, validated and approved product information.

Liability

As mentioned, triage tools and digital pharmaceutical care coaches may be seen as critical safety systems. Therefore when a pharmbot algorithm is not functioning adequately or a patient is not following advice, it is crucial to understand the legal environment. Unlike a face-to-face conversation, a pharmbot cannot yet implement emotional intelligence and may be less persuasive in convincing patients to follow advice. In the coming years it may become possible to apply facial recognition, but this feature may still lack some of the capacity needed to observe patients and interpret their answers, their comfort level, and their intuitive feelings that are based on decades of human experiences.

Legislation is required to determine the liability when the advice of a chatbot is not well understood and the patient's well-being becomes at risk due to misinterpretations or other reasons. Additionally, current regulatory systems are not yet positioned to adequately oversee and review the content of pharmbots and, for example, determine whether pharmaceutical-focused voice-controlled algorithmic content should be considered as advertisement, as direct-to-patient advertising is not allowed in many countries.

In conclusion, although there are still a number of hurdles to overcome, they are expected to be counteracted as soon as innovative pharmacists, regulatory, and big platforms all see the benefits of the canopy of chatbots, and this trend is expected to migrate into pharmaceutical care as well.

In the next Chapter 12, we will deep-dive into how virtual and augmented reality can enforce pharmaceutical care.

This means for circular pharmaceutical care:

- Chatbots are quickly finding their way into medical care to support systems and triage, diagnostic, and disease management applications.
- Pharmbots are virtual personal assistants in pharmaceutical care.
- Pharmbots can support blended pharmaceutical care as an augmentation of human care, for example, by providing drug information, adherence support, or adverse event signaling.
- Chatbots can also help reduce internal administrative burdens, offering pharmacists more time for situations that require human intervention.
- To ensure consistency in content of pharmbots, patient leaflet information should be coded and stored in a SPoT for all digital derivatives, like pharmbots.
- The conditions required for successful implementation of pharmbots (as a pharmaceutical intervention) are under development, and issues like security, privacy, standardization, liability, and reliability require an innovative, proactive, and entrepreneurial approach by regulating authorities.
- To enforce adoption, development of claim titles for pharmbots as insured support tools for blended pharmaceutical care is essential.

QR Code Animation

Pharmbots.

An animation on the topic of Pharmbots can be found on www.pharmacare.ai.

Savanna of virtual, augmented, and mixed reality

13

Claudia Rijcken

The power of imagination created the illusion that my vision went much farther than the naked eye could actually see.
Nelson Mandela

A savanna or savannah is a mixed woodland–grassland ecosystem, characterized by trees that are widely spaced so that the canopy never closes and allows a broad vision into the woods. The mixed community of trees, shrubs, and grasses offers beautiful insight into the realities of both forests and vegetation. It's like putting on your glasses and experiencing the synergy between the best of both worlds. Like an augmented reality.

In this chapter you will read about the fast-growing potential of virtual, augmented, and mixed reality to perform treatments, augment literacy in pharmaceutical care, improve patient experiences, and enhance educational techniques for pharmaceutical care providers.

Augmented reality as well as virtual and mixed reality are technologies that are quickly changing the perspectives we have on healthcare.

Technology

 Virtual reality (VR) is an interactive computer-generated experience that entails the user wearing smart glasses and that takes place within a simulated environment. Experiences are mainly auditory and visual, but other types of sensory feedback may be included, such as haptic sensors. The environments can be real-world experiences as well as fantasy worlds or a mix of the two. VR is used largely for gaming purposes and educational purposes. The sense of reality is enhanced when sound and smell are added (QR Code 13.1).

Augmented reality (AR) is best defined as a live, direct, or indirect view of a physical, real-world environment that is "augmented" by computer-generated or extracted real-world sensory input such as sound, video, graphics, or GPS

QR Code 13.1

VR to educate on the human body.

Pharmaceutical Care in Digital Revolution. https://doi.org/10.1016/B978-0-12-817638-2.00013-4

data. Augmented reality is related to what is called computer-mediated reality, in which a view of reality is modified (possibly even diminished rather than augmented) by a computer (QR Code 13.2).

Augmented reality enhances "one's current perception of reality, whereas in contrast virtual reality replaces the real world with a simulated one. Augmentation techniques are typically performed in real time and in semantic context with environmental elements, such as overlaying supplemental information like scores over a live video feed of a sporting event" (Wikipedia, 2017a).

Augmented reality can be depicted in smart glasses as holograms as well as in mobile applications, while the user hovers over real-world content. Most of the recent AR glasses make it possible to touch, grab, push, and pull 3D holograms.

Mixed reality (MR), sometimes referred to as hybrid reality, is the merged combination of real and virtual worlds to produce new environments and visualizations where physical and digital objects interact in real time and can coexist. Mixed reality is a mix of real and virtual reality, encompassing both augmented reality and augmented virtuality via immersive technology.

The differences between the three forms of reality are shown in Figure 13.1.

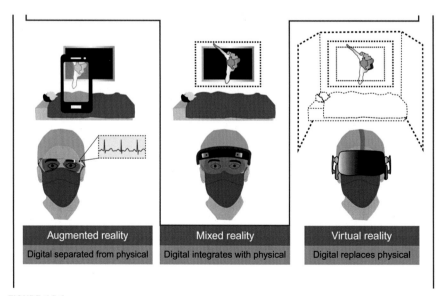

FIGURE 13.1

VR-AR-MR explained. Adapted from Silva et al. (2018).

In general, the concepts of serious gaming (refer to Chapter 7) are frequently integrated in VR-AR-MR applications.

Impact on Core Responsibilities in Pharmaceutical Care

Augmented and virtual reality experiences can help us determine how a drug works, visualize the expected prognosis of a disease or drug effect, translate the most probable experience of a pharmaceutical intervention, and depict a patient's status after adherent (or nonadherent) drug use.

Here is the general impact that virtual, augmented and mixed reality is expected to have on the five domains of pharmaceutical care provision (refer to Chapter 6 for a more detailed discussion):

 A. **Professional relationship between PCPs and patients:** This will be enhanced by better visualization of the impact of pharmaceutical care.

 B. **Adequate collection and recording of health data:** Health information may be collected via virtual or augmented experiences.

 C. **Review health data and provide adequate PC proposal:** Depending on individual patient preference, visualization by AR or VR may augment the PC plan.

 D. **Patient alignment and facilitate execution of PC plan:** Visual AR/VR experiences can facilitate an adequate mode of administering care, support adherence, and drive medication literacy.

 E. **Circular management of PC plan:** Visual AR/VR can enable visualization of adjustments in the PC plan to optimize literacy and the adoption of change.

Implementation in Daily Practice

Grasping the complex concepts of diseases and drugs in a 2D learning format is for many people a true challenge. Printed materials, pictographics, and animations or video can lack the immersive engagement needed for patients to truly understand the depths of their diseases and how best to treat and deal with them. Questions like how does the disease represent itself in different organs, what does the drug do in the body, or what will I experience after having taken the drug are most often explained verbally, with written documentation and sometimes with videos.

 According to a review of health literacy levels in England carried out by researchers from King's College Hospital and Keele University, the health information available to the public, including patient information leaflets (PILs)

in GP surgeries, are too complex for up to 61% of people (Totalhealth, 2014). Recent research suggests that PILs need to be shorter, better structured, and augmented with visual and textual explanations, which can lower the motivational threshold to use the leaflets, improve understanding, and empower patients (van Beusekom et al., 2016; Academy of Medical Sciences, 2017).

Because about half of our global population thinks and learns in a more visual way than in a written context, adding information via visual technologies may increase opportunities to augment the literacy of both patients and providers.

Moreover, focusing in interactive ways on the benefits of a medication—at least as much as on the risks—may ameliorate the trust of patients so that they start using the medication and make the effort to go through the PIL information.

VR-AR-MR as a Treatment Option

VR-based therapy exploits a psychological phenomenon known as "presence"—the illusion that you are really *in* an environment, not just looking at a picture or movie of it. If you turn your head, or stoop down, or walk forward, VR headsets detect that motion using built-in accelerometers or other position sensors and then shift synthetic images in a way that the computer calculates from the 3D geometry of the scene. Because this is exactly the way a brain expects the images on the retina to shift as one move through the real world, you will interpret the scene as real (Waldrop, 2017).

This phenomenon has shown particular benefits in treating psychological orders, like posttraumatic stress disorders, anxieties, or stress-related diseases. In 2010 a small study using fMRI brain scans found this kind of VR exposure therapy to be at least as effective as imaginal therapy at damping down the hyperactivity typically seen in a PTSD patient's amygdala and hippocampus—the first being the seat of the fight or flight response, and the second being a key site in memory formation and presumably the source of haunting flashbacks. Both therapies also seemed to restore normal activity in frontal lobe areas that are inhibited in PTSD and may account for the disorder's characteristic emotional numbing and social withdrawal. A much larger comparison with about 200 patients is now underway (Waldrop, 2017).

Anxieties like fear of flying and fear of vaccinations can be reduced by gradually exposing a patient to a "safe" frightening environment experienced with the use of VR smart glasses. This approach offers vivid forms of distraction and helps the patient to slowly get used to the concept of reducing anxiety to a lower level of dread. Step by step, this treatment reduces the paralyzing effects that anxieties can have and can diminish the need for high doses of anxiolytics, which are known for their serious adverse effects (QR Code 13.3).

The same sort of application is used in the care of severe wounds, where VR headsets offer gaming or relaxation environments that distract patients from the agony of their pain. VR is also used to reduce labor pain and perform drug-free deliveries.

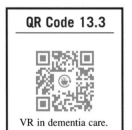

QR Code 13.3

VR in dementia care.

Interactive Learning and Pharmaceutical Care Support

People can be overwhelmed when trying to understand and select the correct over-the-counter medication in a supermarket or pharmacy. Without understanding dietary restrictions, drug interactions, or contraindication information at a glance, incorrect selections may occur, leading to further medical issues (QR Code 13.4).

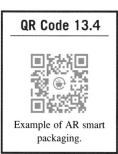

QR Code 13.4

Example of AR smart packaging.

In future days, people will be able to increasingly interact with products simply by looking at them through AR smart glasses or their smartphones. By hovering over a product, people will be able see information relevant to them, which may be data on allergies, on potential food–drug interactions, on possible side effects, and so on. Also, gaming aspects, such as ways to win awards or play against other users, may be integrated into the AR tool. By providing patients with such engaging and immersive experiences and offering new ways to optimally support adequate drug use, manufacturers and care providers can distinguish themselves.

App stores now have numerous medical and pharmaceutical AR/VR applications available to support a patient's educational program. These applications can be used in specific care consultancy, and VR experiences can be offered in general waiting rooms. Medical concepts may provide useful insights, such as why blood clotting is dangerous (e.g., with the Invivo Bloodstream Explorer VR app), how the anatomy of the ear works (e.g., with the Stanford Health Care Anatomy app), or how the human body works (e.g., with the Human Anatomy 4D MR Zone app). Or people can experience how it feels to have a certain disease (e.g., via the Virtual Dementia Tour) or how it feels to have a condition cured (e.g., getting over flight anxiety).

Also, as noted earlier, when patients start taking a medication, a lot of information is "pushed" through, which means that once they get home, they may find it difficult to recall how to use an asthma inhaler, how to apply ointments, what to expect when beginning a new medication, or when to alert a doctor in case of a serious adverse event. Through VR visualization patients can become more aware of what to expect from adequate drug use and thus be more engaged and integrated stakeholders in the disease management plan.

This approach could go as far as explaining, in a home kitchen environment, which foods may interact with individual drugs; for example, if a patient's medication should not be taken with grapefruit juice, and the patient starts to do so, the AR smart glasses could alert the patient and propose safer alternatives.

With AR technology medication reminders could pop up in the smart glasses in order to stimulate adherence. Or the technology could be used to inform polypharmacy patients which pill to take next. If they reach for the wrong bottle, they get a warning. When they have the correct medication in hand, they get a green light, along with directions for its use and other relevant information, such as interactions with alcohol, drowsiness risks, and so on.

Virtual Pharmacists

 The future blue sky scenario for AR most likely will introduce virtual pharmacy coaches in smart glasses that will guide patients through the situations that trouble them, ask them questions, and give them feedback and advice and that will personalize treatment experiences.

How to make this kind of support possible is basically a convergence of AR/VR with technology, which is described in other chapters of this book.

In principle this support involves programming each condition independently, knowing its various manifestations, tailoring the treatment conditions within a smart AI algorithm, and then connecting this algorithm with a patient's individual characteristics based on data in the Personal Health Application, but also potentially on additional, broader societal factors.

The coaching output may be projected in AR smart glasses, but may also fit in a digital therapeutic pharmbot, as explained in Chapter 12. The converged package of different technologies is a digital therapeutic on its own (see Chapter 15) and would require regulatory approval, given the sensitivity of risks if inaccurate advice is given.

Dynamic Education for Pharmaceutical Care Providers

Within the medical ecosystem, VR technology is already frequently used to, for example, assist in complex surgeries, in which surgeries can begin before a surgeon has lifted a scalpel or touched a patient. According to the Lancet Commission on Global Surgery, the surgical workforce will have to double by 2030 to meet the needs of basic surgical care for low and middle-income countries. Virtual reality companies anticipate that they will be asked to train thousands of surgeons simultaneously in virtual reality. Platforms enable doctors to remotely log into a shared virtual office to discuss patient cases and learn about specific surgical procedures.

QR Code 13.5

Example of VR/AR in pharmacy education.

Similarly, in cardiology teams are taking advantage of VR-AR-MR for education, preprocedural planning, intraprocedural visualization, and patient rehabilitation.

Extrapolating the VR-AR-MR advantages to the pharmaceutical environment, results, for example, in pharmaceutical students exploring the body via VR and visualizing in AR how receptors are acting and how the mechanisms of drug molecules work (as shown in QR Code 13.5).

An example of how to improve communication in the pharmaceutical profession is through the use of "pharmaceutical mannequins," which are virtual coaches in a training environment that can generate unlimited training scenarios and patient concepts, offering real-life practice on conflict-handling, counseling, and empathy to pharmaceutical stakeholders.

Another future use for VR is one in which pharmaceutical companies will train pharmacists in a global virtual VR community on how new, innovative drugs work, how to administer them appropriately, how to recognize specific side effects, and how to best inform patients.

Pharmaceutical industry representatives may use AR in brochures for tablet-equipped pharmaceutical care providers, which will provide easy access to up-to-date, in-depth drug and disease information.

Supporting the Work-Around in the Community and Hospital Pharmacy

Because in some cases pharmacy employees work with thousands of different prescriptions and bottles on a daily basis, there is a real risk for an error to be made on both a routine task and one done infrequently. With AR technology an employee can receive real-time input when a bottle is not filled according to prescription or the wrong medication is used. Currently, in most pharmacies this is done by barcode scanning (an extra step) or visual checking by peers (resources); however, AR could provide further accuracy and efficiency in the distribution process.

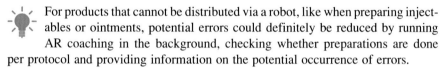 For products that cannot be distributed via a robot, like when preparing injectables or ointments, potential errors could definitely be reduced by running AR coaching in the background, checking whether preparations are done per protocol and providing information on the potential occurrence of errors.

Using readily available technology to improve safety when dispensing and compounding medication in everyday practice can create straightforward efficiency. In this light we can learn much from the construction industry, where technical documents are pictured as a layer of an instrument with an explanation of how to repair the instrument—or, for another example, in the case of a printer, how to replace ink cartridges.

Because the video stream of AR coaching can be stored, a rewind of the production process is possible and available for auditing purposes.

Using AR in pharmaceutical care consultancy will enable PCPs to view patient information through smart glasses while speaking with the patient and to have information at hand about any allergies, previous illnesses, or side effects experienced. Additionally, when the AR is connected to the PHA, the PCP immediately goes into an informed care dialogue, focusing on the human aspects of care.

Considerations

Although the promises of VR-AR-MR are huge, a number of factors still limit full adoption of the tools.

Adoption Challenges

These factors are largely related to the global feasibility, affordability, and accessibility of VR-AR-MR applications:

- For augmented reality in smart glasses, people will have to wear such glasses. Not everyone will consider doing so as convenient (or possible), and for patients who already wear correcting glasses, adding AR will mean needing a second set of glasses, at least for a period of time.
- VR-AR-MR applications are not yet available for all diseases and all use cases.
- Patients have limited knowledge about the advantages these tools can offer and may not be open to using ARs to their full potential.
- The cost of devices such as the Microsoft HoloLens, the Meta glasses, Oculus Rift, and other VR-AR-MR glasses are still relatively high. Also, compared with products entering the marketplace that are more easily used, such as Samsung Gear VR and Oculus Go, the slightly less convenient VR paper cardboards glasses are very low-priced and offer a nice VR experience as well (enabled by smartphones).

Potential Adverse Health Effects of VR-AR-MR

Notwithstanding the excellent opportunities VR-AR-MR can offer for healthcare, there are reasons for health-related caution as well.

One issue known with VR is a phenomenon called vergence-accommodation conflict, which can cause eyestrain. This is basically an eye-focusing problem that occurs because VR headsets create 3D images by showing left and right eyes images that are slightly offset. The eyestrain is usually temporary, though longer-lasting effects are worth monitoring, as only limited clinical research on extensive 3D use has been done.

Also, VR is known to potentially affect a person's psychological state, which can range from feeling temporarily dizzy, light-headed, and in a dreamlike state to more severe detachment that may last for longer periods. Again, this is probably relevant only when using 3D extensively, but it is important to keep in mind in personalized situations when starting to work with VR.

AR has also been correlated with misjudgment of real-life situations (think of the Pokemon Go issues with people ending up in very curious environments), underestimation of reaction times, and unintentional ignorance of the hazards of navigating in the real world. Shifting the view to the side of your vision (like when wearing glasses) for too long can distract focus in real-life situations. Even if the temptation to glance at a notification appearing at the edge of vision is avoided—waiting perhaps until finishing crossing a street—these intrusions still may present a danger, as they defocus the user.

AR wearables may as well affect the way a typical person perceives the world and thereby reduce focus. There are already various natural impairments to vision that affect focusing. For example, presbyopia, farsightedness, and nearsightedness all affect the ability to focus. Diseases like glaucoma, retinitis pigmentosa, and diabetes can create tunnel vision, which may mask objects in the peripheral visual field. Age-related macular degeneration causes the reverse, leaving only items in peripheral vision clearly defined.

A poorly designed AR interface could interfere with vision to the same degree as these types of ocular diseases do. Thus providing AR for this group of patients as well as considering the quality of the AR innovation are essential things to keep in mind when working with AR.

Therefore, as more applications become available and are used by a larger population, the boundaries for where to use or not to use particular types of medical and pharmaceutical ARs need to be further investigated. Safety measures are technicalities to consider, for example when developing AR tools like the stopping notifications in AR glasses for a user who is moving or limiting small children's access to AR.

Other Challenges to Solve

Just as malware can attack mobile software and the technologies covered in other chapters of this book, the same may happen with VR-AR-MR platforms. AR head-up displays can offer criminals a huge advantage on ways to develop scams that will potentially victimize innocent users, especially as healthcare-related data are extremely sensitive. This is why it will be essential for regulatory authorities to be involved and work with users and vendors to minimize any potential harms that could be unleashed and affect large populations at once or individuals in particular. Like the digital health compliance blueprint for other digital technologies (see Chapter 17), additional regulation may be needed to prevent the disadvantages of medical and pharmaceutical VR-AR-MR applications.

Last but not least, as other chapters address, reimbursement for medical and pharmaceutical VR-AR-MR applications is variable among countries. VR-AR-MR is still limited recognized as a valid therapy or care activity, and in order to support development of more patient-centric tools with a concrete healthcare intervention focus, reimbursement options must be further researched, based on the feasibility, reliability, and cost-effectiveness of VR-AR-MR tools.

In summary, these tantalizing insights in the savanna of VR-AR-MR show impressive opportunities for the future of healthcare; however, significant developmental work still needs to be done to fully integrate the principles these tools offer in pharmaceutical care pathways.

In the next Chapter 14, the opportunities regarding Blockchain in pharmaceutical care pathways will be explained.

This means for circular pharmaceutical care:

- Virtual, augmented, and mixed reality (VR-AR-MR) are proven tools that can be used as autonomous patient treatments and are crucial in future training of physicians as well as other healthcare stakeholders.
- VR-AR-MR can support pharmaceutical care providers by visualizing medical and pharmaceutical care concepts, which can lead to better understanding and improved literacy among medication users, thus reducing mistakes and optimizing outcomes.
- VR-AR-MR technologies may not only support customer services but also augment educational pharmacy programs or the efficacy of daily operations.
- Feasibility, affordability, and accessibility of VR-AR-MR applications are aspects that influence broad global adoption.
- Health risks associated with VR-AR-MR applications should be well considered before integrating the technology into a patient care solution.

Blockchain taiga

14

Claudia Rijcken

I will engage in no transaction which does not benefit all whom it affects.
Napoleon Hill

The taiga is the world's largest biome apart from the oceans, interlinking all high northern latitudes and primarily consisting of similar coniferous forests, making it a relatively structured and noncomplex biome.

In this chapter you will read about how a blockchain is an immutable, decentralized, and transparent record of all transactions throughout a peer network. The technology offers a promising solution for solving the siloed structure of healthcare, thus facilitating secure data flows required for pharmaceutical care, and may also speed up the financial management of care and reduce the number of errors made in medication interventions.

The fast-expanding biome of the blockchain, interlinking transactional activities in a structured and noncomplex way, make blockchains potentially the next taiga in the digital ecosystem.

Technology

A blockchain (originally block chain) is a continuously growing list of records, called blocks, that are linked and secured through the use of cryptography. Records or blocks can contain any form of data, such as digital money, real estate (ownership) data, and healthcare data. Each block typically contains a hash pointer (digital fingerprint) as a link to a previous block, a timestamp, and transaction data. By design, blockchains are immutable; that is, they are resistant to any modification of the transactions.

Functionally, a blockchain can serve as "an open, distributed ledger or "shared record book" that can record transactions between multiple parties efficiently and in a verifiable and permanent way. As a distributed ledger, a blockchain is typically shared by all the computers in a decentralized peer-to-peer network collectively adhering to a protocol for adding and validating new blocks. Once recorded, the data in any given block cannot be altered retrospectively without the alteration of all subsequent blocks, which would require collusion or compromise of the majority of computers in the network (QR Code 14.1).

QR Code 14.1

Blockchain explained.

Pharmaceutical Care in Digital Revolution. **https://doi.org/10.1016/B978-0-12-817638-2.00014-6**

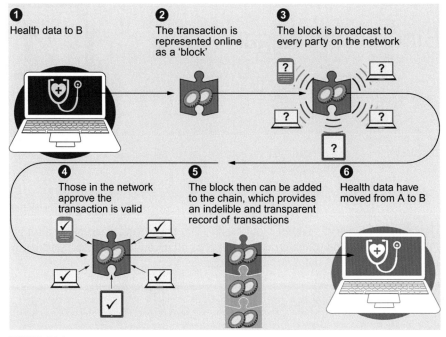

1 Health data to B

2 The transaction is represented online as a 'block'

3 The block is broadcast to every party on the network

4 Those in the network approve the transaction is valid

5 The block then can be added to the chain, which provides an indelible and transparent record of transactions

6 Health data have moved from A to B

FIGURE 14.1

How the blockchain works.

Blockchains are secure by design, and decentralized consensus is a main characteristic. This makes blockchains suitable for recording transactions of events, medical data, and other record management activities (Wikipedia, 2017b).

Figure 14.1 shows what a financial transaction on a blockchain network looks like.

It is important to mention that in a regular blockchain every transaction (a smart contract) is open, although in Europe transactions are not allowed to be made public. In a permissioned or private blockchain, users (in healthcare this may be the patient) are in the lead and determine who sees which type of information in their blockchain.

Decentralization Can Facilitate Security

Blockchains' decentralized, open, and cryptographic nature can prompt people to trust the system and transact peer-to-peer, eliminating the need for trusted intermediaries. Blockchains also generally provide security benefits. Hacking attacks that commonly impact databases of large, centralized intermediaries like banks are less likely to be successful on blockchains, at least not at the same scale. It is not impossible to hack into a large blockchain (smaller private, permissioned blockchains will be more vulnerable), and the amount of personal data held by any one user is very small compared to the large data stored in a centralized mode.

This is especially true for unauthorized alterations of data. For example, if someone wants to hack into a particular transaction in a blockchain and change information, not only would that person need to create a fake version of the specific block with that transaction but also of all subsequent blocks in the blockchain. And the person would need to do so on a majority of ledgers in the network almost simultaneously. Based on the current state of cryptography, the chances of that happening are very unlikely and would be incredibly expensive, which means that so far such systems are rather safe (Thompson, 2016).

To keep a blockchain consistent, complete, and unalterable by repeatedly verifying and collecting newly broadcasted transactions into a new group of transactions (blocks), the computers in the network perform validations, also known as "mining." Mining uses the processing power of the computers in the blockchain network to collectively secure the network against fraudulent transactions. A successful mining computer, that is the first to compute a new block, is rewarded with cryptocurrencies, for example Bitcoin (when mining for the Bitcoin network). Bitcoin was created as a digital payment network, which is increasingly used globally for ordinary payments of services and goods, as well as for storing value as a speculative investment. Meanwhile, many more cryptocurrencies have been developed, each linked to separate blockchain environments.

Smart Contracts

One of the biggest advancements in blockchain technology is the smart contract, which enables self-execution of conditional transactions in a machine-to-machine network. A smart contract is a set of promises specified in digital form, including protocols within which the parties perform on these promises. The contract allows communication of terms and conditions that multiple parties have previously agreed upon. Smart contracts are far more functional than their inanimate, paper-based ancestors in which no use of artificial intelligence is implied.

Smart Contracts in Pharmacies

Suppose a patient enters a pharmacy with a prescription and orders medication. The distribution can be done through a blockchain and payment can be considered by format of cryptocurrency.

The patient gets a receipt that is held in the virtual contract between the pharmacist and the patient; the pharmacist gives the patient the drug, which is sent to the patient at a specific time.

If the drug doesn't arrive on time, the blockchain releases a refund once the patient denies receipt of drug.

The system works on the if-then premise and is used by hundreds of computers (in an anonymized way), so people can expect faultless delivery.

For the pharmacist this system ensures payment; for the patient (after payment by insurer, who is automatically in the loop) the system ensures adequate drug delivery, after automatic checking of conditions like adverse events or contraindications.

The transaction's code cannot be changed by the parties after the smart contract is put on the blockchain, so neither can renege on their obligations.

Moreover, smart contracts don't define the rules and penalties around an agreement in the same way that a traditional contract does; instead they automatically execute those obligations.

A smart contract is not necessarily related to the classical concept of a legal contract, but can be any kind of computer program for all sort of situations, like financial derivatives to insurance premiums, breach contracts, property law, credit enforcement, financial services, legal processes, or pharmaceutical transactions (e.g., a prescription can be a smart contract, as reflected in the example).

Impact on Core Responsibilities in Pharmaceutical Care

Once a blockchain enters the pharmaceutical environment, a number of pharmacists' activities may be further automated, such as patient record management, patient information distribution, and reimbursement management.

Here is the general impact that blockchain is expected to have on the five domains of pharmaceutical care provision (refer to Chapter 6 for a more detailed discussion):

A. **Professional relationship between PCPs and patients:** Blockchain can provide better data interoperability and higher trust in adequate patient data processing

B. **Adequate collection and recording of health data:** Decentralized, secure data flows integrated into PHAs will provide a more holistic overview on the patient's health

C. **Review health data and provide adequate PC proposal:** PC plans will include all safe, connected data that patients want to share

D. **Patient alignment and facilitate execution of PC plan:** Continuously updated data will provide more holistic insights and will drive better personalized care

E. **Circular management of PC plan:** More secure interoperability of data will lead to quicker adjustments in care when needed

Implementation in Daily Practice

In the healthcare environment, we often talk about a blockchain in terms of its ability to securely, privately, and comprehensively track patient health records.

Traditionally, the interoperability of medical data among institutions has followed three models: push, pull, and view, each of which has its strengths and weaknesses.

Blockchain seems to offer a fourth model with the potential to share secure, lifetime medical records across providers.

Blockchain in Healthcare

A patient's medical history is often like a puzzle with its pieces dispersed across multiple providers and organizations. For example, one piece is held by GPs, several pieces are held by different specialists, and another data set is held by wearables or other digital health technology.

By providing private and immutable ledgers of transactions, cryptographic tools for data security and integrity and "smart contracts" to manage health data access, blockchain appears to be a good solution to connect the pieces of the patient's data puzzle.

Thus blockchain can change how medical records are stored and shared, ensuring fraudulent activity is reduced in all medical activities.

Blockchain also offers a means to interoperate in a seamless way. Because all users of a network can access the same shared blockchain, all pieces of information are verified, and the blockchain stores a reliable history of transactions (although European Union regulations do not allow open distribution of such data).

Benefits of Blockchain in Healthcare

Whereas cloud solutions offer centralized possibilities to create a personal health application, blockchain enables creation of a decentralized permanent log of online health transactions or information exchanges, meaning that, once a patient approves to share specific data, every stakeholder in the healthcare pathway gets up-to-date, reliable information at any point in the patient's journey. This situation has the potential to significantly reduce errors and fatalities in healthcare, particularly when patients use geographically distributed care providers.

> **Medication Records on Ethereum Offer Research Opportunities**
>
> MIT Media Lab is developing a prototype system called MedRec, using a private blockchain based on the Ethereum platform. It automatically keeps track of who has permission to view and change a record of the medications a person is taking. MedRec also solved an issue facing many who want to take blockchain outside the realm of digital currency: miners.
>
> With cryptocurrencies, miners use computers to perform calculations that verify data on the blockchain—a crucial service that keeps the system functioning. In turn, they're rewarded with some of that currency.
>
> MedRec incentivizes those who are doing the mining—generally medical researchers and healthcare professionals—to perform the same work, but by rewarding them with access to aggregated, anonymized data from patients' records that can be used for epidemiological studies (as long as patients consent) (MIT Media Lab, 2018).

Blockchain also has the potential to improve the way healthcare payments and insurance contracts are executed. When an insurance provider and a patient are dealing with an insurance contract, the blockchain can automatically verify and authorize information and the contractual agreements. There is no more back-and-forth haggling about what was paid, why it was paid, or whether it should have been paid. With transparency and automation, greater efficiency can lead to lower administration costs, faster payment of claims, and less wasted money.

Another potential healthcare application of blockchain is managing population health. Instead of relying on large health information data exchanges, database providers, or other forms of aggregated data, organizations can eliminate the middleman or institutional role and access anonymized patient databases on a large population scale. For research (as in the MedRec example) as well as for trend identification, this kind of management can be a big step forward. Optimally, patients in a blockchain will decide whether they want to make their data accessible for research or keep it private for themselves.

Blockchain technology may also be able to improve Internet of Health (IoH) security. According to the Protenus Breach Barometer Report, there were a total of 450 health data breaches in 2016 globally, affecting over 27 million patients. About 43% of these breaches were insider-caused, and 27% were due to hacking and ransomware (Das, 2017). As noted in Chapter 8 by 2020 more than 20 billion IoT connected devices are expected to be used globally of which a significant part involves health data. Blockchain-enabled solutions have the potential to bridge the gaps in device data interoperability, while ensuring security, privacy, and reliability in IoH use cases (Das, 2017).

Blockchain in Different Pharma Domains

Blockchain can be integrated in different domains of the pharmaceutical patient journey. Although the principle scope of this book is the pharmaceutical care patient pathway, here we want to further elaborate on the different pharmaceutical domains to show the diverse opportunities that blockchain can provide.

- **Drug supply chain integrity**

Based on global industry estimates, pharmaceutical companies incur an estimated annual loss of $200 billion due to counterfeit drugs. About 30% of drugs sold in LIMC countries are considered to be counterfeits. A blockchain-based system could ensure a chain-of-custody log, tracking each step of the supply chain at the individual drug or product level. Furthermore, add-on functionalities could help build in proof of ownership of the drug at any point in the supply chain and manage the certifications of different parties (Das, 2017).

- **Pharma clinical trials and population health research**

It is estimated that nearly half of all clinical trials go unreported, and investigators often fail to share their study results (e.g., nearly 90% of trials on ClinicalTrials. gov lack reported results). This may create safety issues and knowledge gaps for patients, healthcare stakeholders, and health policymakers. Blockchain-enabled, timestamped, immutable records of clinical trials, protocols, and results could potentially address the issues of outcome switching, data snooping, and selective reporting, thereby also reducing the incidence of fraud and error in clinical trial records. Further, blockchain-based data witnessing systems could help drive collaboration between participants and researchers around innovation in medical research in fields like precision medicine and population health management (Das, 2017).

- **Blockchain in health claims and insurance management**

Blockchain-enabled solutions that streamline the exchange of data among and between contractual parties in pharmaceutical care contracts would increase efficiency. Rather than independently collecting and reconciling data related to contractual terms and obligations, insurance companies and pharmaceutical care providers could share contractual updates via a private, shared transactional ledger that is jointly operated by the network of players in the value chain.

This will promote real-time transparency in health claims transactions, reduce need for clearing houses, and improve flow of currency after the transaction has taken place, meaning that PCPs or patients are paid in nearly real time after the prescription transaction takes place.

- **Patient data exchange and reliability of prescriptions**

The process of delivering medication to a patient is a complex process for almost all prescriptions, and certainly for specialty medications. Multiple parties, including the payer, the dispensing pharmacy, and the manufacturer, engage in repetitive exchanges of information to determine the suitability and sustainability of a given drug therapy. These steps include but are not limited to clinical guidelines benchmarking, step therapy requirements, patient support assessment, patient education, medication therapy management, and prescription adherence tracking.

> **Moving Lab Data Securely Between Hospitals**
>
> Exchange of blood values is a day-to-day problem for many hospitals. In many countries, most lab-to-lab communication is still done via postal mail, which is expensive, slow, and error-prone.
>
> Labchain, a permissioned (privacy) blockchain that is used to identity and manage transactions, is fully decentralized and consists of two parts, a decentralized file exchange and a permissioned blockchain.
>
> Health data is stored off-chain and is sent directly to other hospitals via peer-to-peer networking.
>
> Labchain is legally approved by the Dutch state law firm Pels Rijcken.

Currently, the majority of the steps take place in isolation for every stakeholder, often requiring repetitive collection of the same data and at great expense in time and patience on the part of the patient. A series of blockchain-enabled solutions would instead treat a prescription as a joint file, to be accessed and added to by the variety of players in the ecosystem with the goal of improving access and ease for the patient.

Bringing the patient directly into this joint process as an active participant adding transactions into the blockchain, the healthcare ecosystem would benefit from a stream of patient reported outcomes and adherence data, which would benefit providers as well as PCPs in outcome-based improvement programs.

It would also remove the need to set up separate real-world evidence registries as anonymized data could be deducted from the blockchain.

Blockchain applications may also help improve detection and prevention of fraud and illegitimate drug transactions. Some patients, in an effort to obtain additional amounts of legitimately prescribed drugs, alter the physician's prescription. Also, computers are sometimes used to create fake prescriptions for nonexistent doctors or to copy legitimate doctors' prescriptions. A blockchain application will not allow for these illegitimate actions anymore, as the transactions will have to be verified in strict coded blocks by all computers in the healthcare network before the drug is provided to the patient.

Considerations

Although blockchains offer many opportunities for improved, secure transactional management, there are a number of things to consider before starting to explore their use.

If 90% of Functionality is Database-Like: No Blockchain

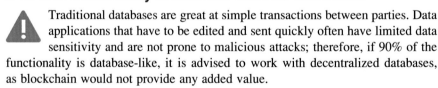 Traditional databases are great at simple transactions between parties. Data applications that have to be edited and sent quickly often have limited data sensitivity and are not prone to malicious attacks; therefore, if 90% of the functionality is database-like, it is advised to work with decentralized databases, as blockchain would not provide any added value.

Only the need to manage the longer-term behavior of assets in a transparent and secure way justifies altering the database application and potentially converting it to a blockchain model (like interconnecting decentralized data sets in healthcare).

Speed and Capacity of Blockchain Networks

Because of the nature of blockchains, they are slower than centralized databases. To digest the large amount of data flowing into the healthcare ecosystem, the capacity of blockchain's current protocol needs to be further improved.

The major blockchain platforms (Bitcoin, Ethereum) are already working on solutions to make their networks scalable, based on side chains and shading—that is, not putting every small transaction in the main blockchain immediately, but bundling them together in smaller chains and then timestamping them as one transaction to the main chain only as needed.

The Challenge of Identity and Privacy

To use blockchain in future pharmaceutical care chains, the big challenge is probably to secure the identity and privacy of the user (patient), as public ledgers currently do not afford this privacy by default. Therefore in healthcare environments only private blockchains seem to be feasible.

In this context identity on the blockchain is the means by which one can make "claims" to rights, membership, and ownership of healthcare and pharmaceutical data. Identity is increasingly secured by using biometric authentication, which can uniquely identify you within a given set of users.

A number of companies are actively working on identity solutions independent of a central authority, such as a governmental body or enterprise or a physical representation. All of these solutions involve identity claims residing on a blockchain to achieve decentralization, executable contracts, secure encryption, and consensus.

Biometric Identification Via Blockchain

Businesses often store user credentials in centralized databases that can be targeted by hackers. Centralized passwords create a single point of failure and have remained the #1 cause of mass breaches and credential reuse—until now.

The company HYPR develops solutions for this problem. Rather than storing fingerprints, facial features, iris images, or voice patterns, the company is working on an end-user's biometric signature that is encrypted and stored on-device in a decentralized manner.

This solution is expected to eliminate credential reuse and minimize the risk of a breach.

Biometric tracking is also an emerging trend in healthcare, and its reach extends to patient identification, giving organizations more flexibility, accuracy, and confidence when locating, aggregating, and sharing patient records.

The low cost, yet sophisticated technology can be deployed in various environments, from self-service (pharmaceutical) kiosks to the emergency room, enabling rapid identification of patients and access to their clinical information accurately across the ecosystem.

Biometrics could become a primary method for linking natural persons with their associated identity claims on these blockchains, as it offers the most convenience in the most secure way.

From a pharmaceutical care point of view, this would mean that the patient is in the driver's seat for deciding which healthcare provider is able to see which part of her medical information, but only if such modularity and selective encryption and decryption of information are built in at the design stage.

The questions lie in how we are going to deploy the solutions, how we protect the biometric data independently of the blockchain, and whether patients are always literate enough to understand the importance of allowing access in the public, open structure of a blockchain.

Uncertainty in Regulation

The amount of regulatory uncertainty on blockchain legislation is hindering the uptake of blockchain to a certain extent. National and European regulations that support the use of blockchain for business purposes such as contracts and financial audits will likely tip the scales in favor of mass adoption. Legislation will need to provide answers on a number of questions, for example: Does private blockchain activity represent an inherently reliable confirmation? Can a smart contract represent the execution of a legal contract in a court of law? Who are the responsible persons when the blockchain is used for illegal practices? (Schatsky and Piscini, 2016). Providing clarity in those questions will require changes in regulations, laws, practices, and protocols; however, with these answers scaling of blockchain will be quicker and easier to facilitate.

Development Stage Technical Standards

Outside the financial sector blockchain technology is still a rather new technology, and both standard taxonomy and (global) technical standards are in their beginning stages. As noted in Chapter 8, standards will be required to guide governance models for managing new digital technologies like blockchain networks and applications. Also, once standards do become available, systems can establish procedures to manage and resolve disputes, which will help the regulatory process as well.

It is expected that standards will become available in the near future; for example, ISO is working on standardization of the definitions of blockchain and ledger technology under the ISO/TC 307 technical committee (Frank, 2016).

Making Changes in Blockchain Transactions

It remains yet unclear how required changes in a blockchain transaction can be handled retrospectively. Suppose, for example, patients want certain data removed from the blockchain. In that case, the transaction cannot be withdrawn from a blockchain-based platform, since immutability of the transaction is a key design principle of the technology. It is preferred that a workaround is found for this problem in healthcare; for example, people have the right to have certain information removed from their PHA.

In conclusion, the taiga of blockchain is a fertile environment that is expected to grow towards the largest global transactional biome. Nevertheless, in healthcare specifically, a number of hurdles need to be overcome before fast upscaling is possible.

In next Chapter 15, the inspiring and fast emerging field of Digital Therapeutics will be explained.

This means for circular pharmaceutical care:

- Blockchain is an immutable, decentralized, and transparent record of all transactions throughout a peer network.
- Blockchain technology can enable trusted and secure transactions within healthcare systems, facilitating up-to-date and transparent data flows and thus decreasing siloed data parts.
- Registration on a private blockchain could offer reliable cradle-to-grave healthcare data transaction solutions, putting patients in the lead to facilitate a more efficient and up-to-date information flow between different healthcare providers.
- When and how blockchains will be best suitable for healthcare in general and pharmaceutical pathways in particular must be further established, although early pilot projects in distribution and logistics are being successfully implemented around the globe.
- Blockchain applications in pharmaceutical care may lead, among other benefits, to more secure PHAs, improved health claim management, and faster reimbursement of services.
- Blockchain technology by itself will not automatically solve all data-related problems that have plagued healthcare information systems for decades. A number of hurdles have to be overcome before blockchain technology can help pave the way to a secure and interconnected healthcare system.

An animation on the topic of Blockchain in pharmaceutical care can be found at www.pharmacare.ai.

QR Code Animation

Blockchain.

Digital therapeutic mangroves

15

Claudia Rijcken

Synergy and serendipity often play a big part in medical and scientific advances.
Julie Bishop

The fast-growing ecology of numerous digital therapeutic applications often propagates the drive to create symbiosis with traditional well-immersed pharmaceutical interventions. This symbiosis is similar to how trees in mangroves long time ago adapted to become salt tolerant and develop complex root systems to create synergy with salt water immersion and wave action. The symbiosis led to a highly fertile forestry environment in which many species bloomed. Digital therapeutics (DTx) may develop a symbiotic relationship with medication treatments as well.

In this chapter you will read about digital therapeutics (DTx) developed to support behavioral changes in favor of health optimization. They can be used as autonomous treatments or may augment the effects of drugs. Pharmaceutical care providers may consult future digital health management teams on the synergy between drug and DTx use.

DTx use app technology to optimize patients' well-being and health status, often from a behavioral and lifestyle perspective, and sometimes in conjunction with wearables and virtual reality. In addition to stabilizing disease, many DTx companies aim to decrease the dosage of drugs or even eventually eliminate the need to take medications.

Some refer to DTx as the new specialty pharma. Andreessen Horowitz, a venture firm, predicted in 2017 that "digital drugs" will become "the third phase" of medicine, meaning the successor to the chemical and protein drugs we have now, but without the significant cost and time of bringing them to market.

Pharmaceutical Care in Digital Revolution. https://doi.org/10.1016/B978-0-12-817638-2.00015-8

Technology

 DTx, a subset of digital health and often a combination of the digital techniques described in previous chapters, is a health discipline and treatment option that utilizes a digital and often online health technology to treat a medical or psychological condition. This approach engages patients and can lead to clinically relevant outcomes. DTx relies on behavioral and lifestyle changes that are usually spurred by a collection of digital impetuses. Because of the digital nature of this methodology, data can be collected and analyzed both as a progress report and as a preventative measure (Wikipedia, 2018b) (QR Code 15.1).

Digital therapeutic solutions consist of patient-facing wellness or disease management as well as direct treatment applications. Many of the products include clinical assessment and outcome tracking and improvement tools, with data feeding into clinician monitoring dashboards. When these capabilities are integrated into clinical practice, physicians and other healthcare providers may prescribe these products just as they do with any other medication or intervention.

 DTx may have applications on mobile platforms, and some wearable health devices connect their wearable to online behavioral support tools, making them a digital therapeutic platform as well (see examples later in this chapter).

First FDA Approved Digital Therapeutics

In early 2017 the company WellDoc released a prescription-only version of its BlueStar phone app for managing diabetes, which was referred to as the "first FDA-cleared mobile prescription therapy." Nevertheless, the application did not claim therapeutic benefit.

In this respect, Pear Therapeutics clearly stands out in their FDA submission with claims around therapeutic benefit in substance use disorder all supported by the clinical trial results. They received FDA clearance in 2017 and may be considered as one of the first approved DTxs.

Certified DTx products, which promise a true clinical intervention, are supposed to undergo rigorous clinical testing through randomized clinical trials and real-world pilots to demonstrate their safety, efficacy, and economic benefit. These DTx solutions are positioned as medical devices, and to distinguish them from "wellness" gadgets, they undergo a thorough review and regulatory clearance process by federal agencies such as the US Food and Drug Administration (FDA) and European Medicines Agency (EMA) (DTX Alliance, 2017). The regulatory compliance conditions for DTx can be found in Chapter 17.

Digital therapeutic treatments are being developed for the prevention and management of a wide variety of diseases and conditions, including Type II diabetes, congestive heart failure, obesity, Alzheimer's disease, dementia, asthma, COPD, substance abuse, ADHD, anxiety, depression, and several others. DTx often employ strategies rooted in cognitive behavioral therapy.

QR Code 15.1

What are digital therapeutics?

Impact on Core Responsibilities in Pharmaceutical Care

DTx, as do individual apps or other technologies, may have a significant effect on the activities that take place in a pharmaceutical care pathway.

Thus pharmaceutical care providers should be aware of the fact that a patient is supported by a digital therapeutic and that as a consequence drug dosages and patterns may need to be changed over time.

Here is the general impact that Digital Therapeutics are expected to have on the five domains of pharmaceutical care provision (refer to Chapter 6 for a more detailed discussion):

 A. **Professional relationship between PCP and patients:** This relationship goes beyond medication and considers DTx as an optional treatment

 B. **Adequate collection and recording of health data:** DTx devices and data are considered in PC plans

 C. **Review health data and provide adequate PC proposal:** If required, care that blends DTx and medication is considered

 D. **Patient alignment and facilitate execution of PC plan:** Offer the possibility of using DTx if feasible, and align it with informed consent for data sharing

 E. **Circular management of PC plan:** Use DTx data to measure outcomes and adjust plan, if required

Implementation in Daily Practice

A number of digital therapeutic interventions have been introduced that patients, pharmaceutical care providers, and doctors did start working with.

Digital Therapeutics to Enhance or Replace Medication

Digital therapies tend to fall into two categories, which are often called "medication augmentation" and "medication replacement." The therapies either optimize the effect of the drug intervention chosen or are so effective that medication can be tapered or stopped completely at a certain point in time.

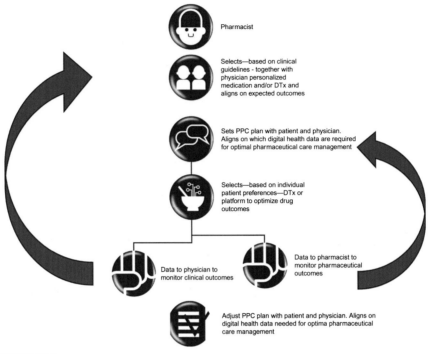

FIGURE 15.1

Choosing a digital therapeutic in a pharmaceutical pathway.

Figure 15.1 shows a potential process flow for choosing a DTx in a pharmaceutical care chain.

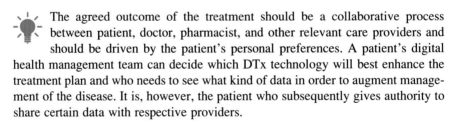 The agreed outcome of the treatment should be a collaborative process between patient, doctor, pharmacist, and other relevant care providers and should be driven by the patient's personal preferences. A patient's digital health management team can decide which DTx technology will best enhance the treatment plan and who needs to see what kind of data in order to augment management of the disease. It is, however, the patient who subsequently gives authority to share certain data with respective providers.

The Role of the Pharmacist in a Digital Health Management Team

In Chapter 6 we note that a pharmacist's role can be regarded as an optimizer of medication treatments. Thus it is that pharmacists acquire the knowledge needed to determine which DTx can augment medication outcomes.

In addition to knowing what kind of tools are available and understanding certain technical details, in the future pharmacists will work in a domain that requires them to understand which patients will benefit most from a synergy between DTx and medication. To make such a determination will also require setting up structured pilot studies in pharmaceutical environments, in which pharmacy software data is linked to digital therapeutic outcome data, as explained in Chapter 8.

With these networks in place and a scientifically sound pilot study format, statistics including integrated trend analyses can be used to predict which DTx provide value for which category of patients.

Next we review a number of digital therapeutic interventions that may fit well in pharmaceutical care pathways. The interventions discussed are not all-inclusive, but are representative of those relevant to pharmaceutical care.

An examination of the increasing number of DTxs and the difficulty in understanding their differences indicates the future need of a "comparison and overview database system," as we discuss in detail in Chapter 10.

Diabetes

A number of interesting digital therapeutic examples can be found in the diabetes area. Evidence shows that certain lifestyle changes give people with diabetes better control of their disease (and prevents most people with prediabetes from developing the disease), so this created an opening for digital lifestyle support services focused on prevention of disease and reduction or enhancement of medication use.

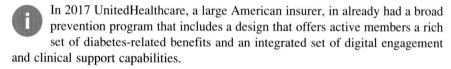 In 2017 UnitedHealthcare, a large American insurer, in already had a broad prevention program that includes a design that offers active members a rich set of diabetes-related benefits and an integrated set of digital engagement and clinical support capabilities.

Members receive a welcome kit and a mobile diabetes application that provides a set of robust features to track and share blood glucose levels, with access to a care team (wellness coach and nurse) within the app, as well as fitness, nutrition, and medication tracking and reminders. A secure microsite gives members a Personal Health Summary and trending analyses and reports that can be printed in PDF format and emailed to a doctor or caregiver (UHC, 2017).

A Diabetes DTx Platform

Onduo, a joint venture of Google's healthcare venture, Verily Life Sciences, and Sanofi, a French pharmaceutical firm, was set up in 2016. Onduo started by developing a virtual diabetes platform to help people with diabetes make better decisions about their use of drugs and their lifestyle habits. The services include digital insulin dose recommendations and coaching systems, cloud-based software that evaluates blood glucose and patient attributes to adjust insulin dosages, cellular-enabled glucometers, and cloud-based data systems.

In its next phase Onduo wants to help those who are at risk avoid developing diabetes. The startup gained the interest of the pharmaceutical company Sanofi, whose blockbuster insulin medication, Lantus, was steadily losing its market share and recently lost its patent protection. Onduo and Sanofi now jointly provide integrated diabetes solutions focused on synergistic prevention and care delivery.

Meanwhile, Onduo is partnering with Blue Shield to be integrated in standard health plans.

Another digital support program for diabetes is called Livongo, which aims to be a catalyst for behavioral change to treat diabetes and hypertension. It uses bite-sized personal contextual and clinical data to drive lifestyle optimization, empowering people to better manage their diabetes. By combining the latest connected technology with real-time, personalized support and live coaching, people with diabetes are able to improve their outcomes, optimize their drug dosage, and make their life experiences better.

Also, with an AI-powered software platform, the FDA-approved DreaMed Advisor Pro assists healthcare providers and patients in management of Type 1 diabetes. The software includes insuline delivery recommendations based on analyzing the information garnered from pumps and glucose monitoring. Medtronic is as well a highly innovative company in the diabetes digital therapeutic ecosystem.

Also, there are many other established diabetes companies as well as startups which invest in developing new diabetes DTx in order to improve the life of diabetes patients.

Substance Abuse

Pear, as indicated in an example earlier in the chapter, is a company that integrates clinically validated software applications with previously approved pharmaceuticals and treatment paradigms to provide better outcomes for patients, smarter engagement and tracking tools for clinicians, and cost-effective solutions for payers. Pear's lead product, reSET, is an FDA-approved, 12-week interval prescription therapy for substance use disorders to be used as an adjunct to standard outpatient treatment. reSET has been shown to increase abstinence from abused substances during treatment and also when used as part of an outpatient treatment program. The product uses a patient-facing smartphone application (providing behavioral support tools for the patient) linked with a clinician-facing web interface.

Further research on the product is ongoing for integration in opioid use disorder and additional prescription DTx in schizophrenia, combat posttraumatic stress disorder, general anxiety disorder, pain, major depressive disorder, and insomnia. In 2018 Novartis and Pear announced what the latter claims to be the first development deal between a pharma and a digital therapeutic company. The agreement affects two therapeutics: Pear's Thrive for schizophrenia, and another targeting mental health conditions affecting multiple sclerosis that will be developed jointly between the two companies. Such a collaboration is a nice example of the mangrovic symbiosis analogy presented at the beginning of this chapter.

The Pear example introduces a new paradigm, in which in the future healthcare providers, including pharmacists, may receive synergistic intervention packages for patients, consisting of both a conventional drug and a digital therapeutic intervention.

Pain, Stress, and Mental Disease Management

Halo is an example of a digital health and therapeutic system shown to help treat conditions in which patients experience a great deal of (often pharmaceutically untreatable) pain through a proven cognitive behavioral therapy called biofeedback. Biofeedback-assisted relaxation training has been clinically proven to be equally or more effective than drugs for treating tension headaches, migraine headaches, and pain, but without any of the negative side effects caused by medication. The sensor, in combination with an app, senses muscle tension, displays actionable feedback in real time, coaches relaxation techniques, and supports the patient in a convenient and comfortable way.

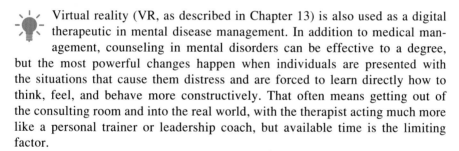

Headache-Reducing Headband

Muse is a brain sensing headband that claims to elevate a meditation experience. It gently guides the user through meditation through changing sounds of weather based on the real-time state of a brain. This allows for obtaining a deeper sense of focus and motivates to build a highly rewarding practice. Meditation has been scientifically shown to reduce symptoms associated with stress, depression, and anxiety as well as improve focus, performance, and quality of life. Thus synergy between this DTx and conventional therapies is something to study in the years to come.

Virtual reality (VR, as described in Chapter 13) is also used as a digital therapeutic in mental disease management. In addition to medical management, counseling in mental disorders can be effective to a degree, but the most powerful changes happen when individuals are presented with the situations that cause them distress and are forced to learn directly how to think, feel, and behave more constructively. That often means getting out of the consulting room and into the real world, with the therapist acting much more like a personal trainer or leadership coach, but available time is the limiting factor.

Here, virtual reality may offer digital therapeutic help as it can immediately create powerful simulations of the scenarios in which psychological difficulties occur. Suddenly, there's no need for a therapist to accompany a client on a trip to a crowded shopping center, for example, or up a tall building.

Situations that are more or less impossible to build into a course of therapy—flying, for example, or the shocking events that often lie behind posttraumatic stress disorder, or the potential frightening side effects of a drug—can be conjured at the click of a mouse. The in situ coaching that's so effective for so many disorders is now delivered in the consulting room or even in the pharmacy environment, with the simulations graded in difficulty and repeated as often as necessary.

Having this opportunity available means that psychologists and psychiatrists may decide less often to initiate medical treatment directly or that they have tools available that may help reduce drug dosages, leading to a better tolerance profile for the patient. Moreover, when a medical treatment is chosen, explanations for what to expect when a drug is first used can be better guided through VR training, potentially resulting in better compliance and acceptance profiles.

Digital Contraceptives

After extensive clinical research, in 2017 Natural Cycles became the world's first digital birth control app to receive FDA approval. The app allows users to gain knowledge about their body and supports them in truly understanding how individual menstrual cycles work. The app is positioned as providing protection with more sexual freedom, minus the side effects of contraceptives.

The app stores information on every cycle, as every cycle can be different, and determines when a woman ovulates and is most likely to get pregnant, with pregnancy generally possible six days (five days before ovulation and about 24 hours after ovulation). The woman takes her temperature in the morning and enters the information into the app; the app then emits a red light (fertile days) or a green light (nonfertile days), indicating when the woman needs to use protection or abstain from sexual intercourse.

In 2017 Neura Inc. developed a similar type of application under the name of MyDays. Through artificial intelligence, Neura equips MyDays with user awareness. Machine learning algorithms transform data from users' phones and devices into information about activities in the physical world (e.g., when they wake from sleep). MyDays uses this information to adapt its behavior to the users' to achieve better health outcomes.

Considerations

Defining exactly what a digital therapeutic actually is remains a fluid space that many companies are trying to categorize. The general consensus among researchers in the field of DTx is that the discipline of DTx requires more clinical data and investigation to be fully evaluated. Subsets of analyses are done on individual tools used as DTx, for instance, research on the effectiveness of wearables or virtual reality. Information on those results can be found in the respective chapters.

The number of product as well as regulatory developments in the digital therapeutic sector are expected to expand in the near future. Digital therapeutic systems will be tested for their efficacy and for their added value from both the perspective of their benefits to patients and their cost-effectiveness in the healthcare system.

Gamification

Gamification or serious gaming is the transfer of game concepts in a nongaming context, as explained in Chapter 7. For example, level crossings, avatar upgrading, and competition to get to a reward are becoming methods to make people do specific activities in the most diverse sectors, including health where gamification has found its way in recent years.

Apps or wearable devices incentivized by insurers and governments, such as those that persuade people to walk a certain distance every day, are far less expensive than years of taking medications and visiting doctors and hospitals. Even though wearables frequently end up in the back of a drawer, they can and do motivate some people to get off the sofa.

The best example of this motivation may be the success of the players of Pokémon GO, who collectively walked nearly 9 billion kilometers between 2016 and mid-2017. In the diabetes area it is a big challenge to develop a digital therapeutic gamification method such as that used by Pokémon GO to get people moving to improve their lipid and sugar levels and thus their overall health outlook and need for medication.

Gaming is also used in neurohabilitation; for example, MindMotion GO was approved in 2018 by the FDA as a means of providing 3D virtual environment–based therapy for neurorehabilitation to patients in the United States. Patients get a much more personalized, stimulating environment than they would with traditional rehabilitation treatments, which motivates them to get the most from their therapeutic exercise training regimen. With real-time multisensory feedback, patients can monitor their own performance and also, for example, manage painkiller needs better than with the DTx platform.

Another interesting example is Akili's video game, which fosters compliance and has a therapeutic effect in ADHD; the game is delivered through a creative and immersive action gaming experience. Treatments leverage art, music, storytelling, and reward cycles that keep patients engaged and immersed for the delivery of therapeutic activity. The company is known as a prescription digital medicine company, combining scientific and clinical rigor with the ingenuity of the technological industry to reinvent medicine for a number of indications in the neuroscience field.

Once studies provide clinical evidence of the game's effect, it is likely that the results will have an effect on clinical guidelines, potentially resulting in some patients being treated via digital tools rather than or in addition to ADHD medications (which are well known for their side effects). At the time of this writing, Akili is planning to seek FDA approval of the video game specifically designed to treat pediatric ADHD. This is one of the first serious medical games considered as a legitimate treatment option for disease (Graafland, 2014; Akili, 2018).

Regulatory and Reimbursement Framework

Software development is not a linear, one-and-done process. It is an iterative process that goes much faster as compared to the timelines known to development of innovation medication (>12 years).

Not all DTx need to satisfy the rigors of regulatory review and approval. As noted in Chapter 10 noninvasive devices that are intended for general wellness use, hardly ever undergo strict certification, whereas medical wearables with a clear clinical purpose do, because if they are not used properly, a user's health can decline. The PreCert program, which the FDA will further built on in 2019, exemplifies a framework that may set the regulatory scene for the future of DTx systems (for more information, see Chapter 17).

Currently, the business of DTx is still in the early stages, including matters of reimbursement. Many authorities and healthcare payers still mainly reimburse only the cost of drugs and traditional interventions and are still in the process of getting used to compensating for DTx.

Gradually, in a number of countries healthcare providers are being compensated for DTx implementation. In 2016 in the United States, Omada Health broke new ground when MCO Medicare agreed to reimburse the cost of the company's digital diabetes prevention program. In 2017 MCO Big Health charged people $400 a year to use certain FDA-approved digital insomnia programs, whereas its best sleeping pill cost $73 for six tablets.

This approach plays into the hands of payers, who may encourage their customers to use digital interventions (that are shown to be effective in clinical studies) in the early stage of treatment and move to pharmaceutical products only at the second stage (or in parallel with adjusted dosing). The approach may completely disrupt therapeutic guidelines in days to come.

It is essential that governments develop structured health technology assessments on what is considered appropriate cost-effectiveness for DTx in order to achieve reliable reimbursement for both pharmaceutical and digital interventions.

One organization that is pushing the ecosystem's progress in this respect is the Digital Therapeutics Alliance, a global nonprofit trade association with the mission of broadening the understanding, adoption, and integration of clinically validated DTx into healthcare through education, advocacy, and research.

Owner of the Prescription of Digital Therapeutics

How pharmaceutical care providers will perform their future role in digitally managed healthcare is still unclear. A structured approach will be necessary to define who in the patient journey is the key responsible healthcare provider to prescribe and integrate digital therapeutic interventions in individual treatment programs, including medication.

Many commercial providers develop their own DTx platforms currently and in that roll-out differences in approaches are evolving between hospitals, regions, and countries.

 It may be very confusing for patients to be prescribed a digital lifestyle support program one day by a physician and the next day by a pharmacist, not to think on lack of communication and siloed structures between different providers and patients ending up with different digital therapeutic solutions, potentially with contraindicative effects. Thus working in one data-and-prescription ecosystem with close alignment between all care providers is essential.

In this respect, the responsibility of the patient also comes into play, as DTx ask for a secure and updated virtual environment, as well as retention and user accuracy to bring them to their full potential.

Another interesting aspect here is that many adverse events are known only to the patient, as they are often not formally communicated. With the quantified-self era having DTx at hand, these events become known to the entire virtual disease management team the minute they happen. This requires a completely different business setup in order to adequately and timely follow up on events and comply with prevailing pharmacovigilance regulation.

Thus in the next couple of years it is to be expected that the symbiotic mangroves of DTx with medications will be further entangled and that strong contributions from pharmaceutical care providers are required in order to valorize DTx systems to support adequate and appropriate use of drugs.

In the next Chapter 16, we will look at digital health technologies that promise great patient outcome improvements, but concrete and validated use will most probably only be globally seen in some 5 years from now.

 This means for circular pharmaceutical care:

- DTx is a fast-growing health discipline and treatment option that utilizes a digital and often online health technology to treat a medical or psychological condition, thus engaging a patient and leading to clinically relevant outcomes.
- DTx can exist as stand-alone technologies or as integrated platforms and are sometimes provided in a synergistic combinatory package with drugs.
- Certified DTx products have undergone rigorous clinical testing through randomized clinical trials and real-world pilot projects to demonstrate their safety and efficacy.
- Reimbursement structures for DTx are in their early stages, and further regulation should ensure that a comparison of health technology with traditional medication is done appropriately and that the value of DTx is quantified.
- Pharmaceutical care stakeholders are recommended to become knowledgeable about which DTx can augment the impact of drugs and how they do so in order to contribute optimally to a digital health management team.

An animation—kindly adopted by the Dutch Association Innovative Medicines—on the topic of digital therapeutics can be found on www.pharmacare.ai.

QR Code Animation

Digital Therapeutics.

Digital vegetation beyond 2024

16

Claudia Rijcken

What is coming is better than what is gone.
Arabic proverb

Thus far this book has dealt with digital innovations that are expected to disrupt the pharmaceutical ecosystem significantly between 2019 and 2024.

Although looking into a crystal ball is always tricky, it is already possible to envision that other innovations will further change the way we organize pharmaceutical care.

In this chapter you will read about digital health technology that is already showing great promise along with some early 2019 examples. However, technologies such as precision medicine, 3D printing of drugs, and social robots in every home are not expected to reach their full potential until 2024 and beyond.

The content of this chapter is not meant to be all-conclusive but is meant as an inspiring view of what lies ahead. We focus on three technologies under significant development, that are expected to further grow in next decade and will create paradigm shifts in future healthcare.

- Precision medicine
- Regular use of 3D-printed drugs
- Social robots in every home

Precision Medicine

Precision medicine, as also discussed in Chapter 5 and visualized in QR Code 16.1, is an emerging model that aims to customize therapy to subpopulations of patients, categorized by shared molecular and cellular biomarkers, to improve patient outcomes. Precision medicine differs from *personalized medicine* in that the latter refers more to the tailoring of procedures and therapeutic interventions at an individual patient level.

Computational pharmacotherapy is supportive of precision medicine and incorporates multiple sources of raw data (e.g., clinical electronic medical records,

QR Code 16.1

What is precision medicine?

Pharmaceutical Care in Digital Revolution. https://doi.org/10.1016/B978-0-12-817638-2.00016-X

laboratory data, pharmacogenomics, metabolomics, imaging, microbiome, nutrigenomics, personal health application data, digital health data, and so on), extracts biologically and clinically relevant information from those data, and subsequently uses mathematical models at the levels of molecules, individuals, and populations to generate diagnostic inferences and predictions.

The methods used in precision medicine and computational pharmacotherapy technology are driven largely by AI (refer to Chapter 11).

Computational pharmacotherapy technology can present clinically actionable and relevant knowledge to users through dynamic and integrated reports and interfaces, enabling pharmacists, physicians, patients, and other healthcare system stakeholders to make the best possible medical and pharmaceutical decisions.

The output of such technology will help providers select the most appropriate and efficient laboratory tests, run a multidimensional diagnosis, drive faster and more accurate preventive management, and target therapeutic intervention and follow-up for individual patients.

Pharmaceutical care providers are experts in applied therapeutics and are uniquely positioned to understand, integrate, and utilize diverse experimental approaches to realizing precision medicine.

The historical one-size-fits-all approach is no longer valid, and patients and healthcare systems greatly need and will benefit from research and implementation of precision medicine.

Considerations

In many countries having the DNA profile of a patient scanned and integrated into medical information systems is still prone to regulatory, ethical, and procedural challenges. Data privacy requirements and complex informed consent procedures can limit access to a precision medicine approach.

Cost is also considered as a major hurdle. Precision medicine initiatives, such as those President Obama introduced in the United States in 2015, have over the years cost many millions of dollars. Using technologies such as sequencing large amounts of DNA is also expensive (although the cost of sequencing is decreasing quickly), and that doesn't include the costs related to effectively linking these data into electronic health records (EHRs), electronic pharmacy record (EPRs), or Personal Health Applications (PHAs).

Nevertheless, implementing precision medicine may well be a worthwhile investment because the prevalence of and therefore costs for adverse events, nonresponding users, and deterioration of disease are expected to decrease significantly when precision medicine is adopted.

It is expected that, with the integration of current population-based data sets with the broader genotypic and phenotypic data sets, precision medicine will be gradually further implemented towards 2024 and beyond.

3D-Printed Drugs

Once computational pharmacotherapy becomes a reality, personalized 3D printing is the logical next step towards precision medicine.

To envision the potential of 3D-printed drugs, think about the fact that most people get a "general" drug dosage that is, however, not aligned with their personal profile, which can lead to a number of the previously mentioned issues. Or think, on another level, about the aggravation of having to stand in line at a pharmacy. Wouldn't it be more convenient for people to make their particular medicines safely at home, have a dose that is calculated exactly for them and never have to queue up again? That future will be here once 3D printers become mainstream in pharmacy and maybe even home environments and enable local synthetization of pharmaceuticals and other chemicals from widely available compounds and feed these products directly into smart reactors.

Multiple techniques for 3D printing are now being developed and tested, for example, layer-to-layer printing by combining powdered medications and liquid droplets; or by applying heat and pressure to melt a polymer and print drugs into different geometric shapes, which due to the reduced surface area may help to fasten the release of the active ingredient; or via organic vapor jet printing, which deposits nanostructured films of small molecular pharmaceutical ingredients with accuracy on the scale of micrograms per square centimeter onto different drug carriers, such as tabs, needles, and adhesives.

QR Code 16.2 exemplifies how 3D printing can work for manufacturing of theophylline. Another drug, Spritam, the first 3D-printed drug to treat epilepsy, received FDA approval in 2015. The manufacturing technique allows rapid dispersion of the tablet, high drug-loading, and modified release.

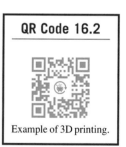

As an another example, the University of Glasgow plans to follow the tactics Spotify did with music (and Uber did with transportation) for the discovery and distribution of prescription drugs in which a prototype 3D printer capable of assembling chemical compounds at the molecular level is used. The device is designed and constructed by using a chemical-to-computer–automated design that enables the translation of traditional synthesis into platform-independent digital code. They demonstrate the potential of the system by the production of the drug Baclofen, establishing a concept that could pave the way for the local manufacture of drugs outside specialist institutions (Kitson et al., 2018).

3D Printing Towards Individualized Dosing

Spritam is now printed commercially in a number of fixed doses. The ultimate blue sky result would be to print tablets that are customized according to the genetic profile of a given patient and other factors influencing optimal individual doses (e.g., concomitant medication, food preferences that influence the metabolism of a drug, environmental circumstances like allergen load, etc.). Such opportunities are particularly promising for drugs with a narrow therapeutic dose, as personalized 3D printing may prevent overdosing and occurrence of adverse events. Also, a 3D-printed drug can be tailored to patients in terms of its size, appearance, and delivery, all of which can make the drug safer and more effective.

 After receiving a digital prescription from a doctor, patients will go to an online drugstore, buy the blueprint and the chemical ink materials needed, and then print the drug at home in the prescribed dose; or go to their local pharmacy, where a pharmacist will take their physical measurements, perform a finger-prick blood test, and input the data online on the pharmacy's 3D printing medicines portal. Instead of storing and distributing packets of tablets, pharmacists will have reels of filaments of the base product (the prescribed drug) and will customize the dose and shape of tablet to individual needs.

New techniques in printing may also make it possible to print multiple drugs in one pill (Brown, 2017). Although there are still many hurdles to overcome, like the potential impact of drug–drug interactions within a pill and the shelf life of combined compounds, the technique could reduce the number of pills that poly-pharmacy patients have to use every day and thus improve their quality of life and the likelihood they will adhere to taking the drugs.

Added Value of 3D Printing

Compared with the way drugs are manufactured and distributed now, 3D printing may solve a number of issues:

- The cost of drug development may be reduced by allowing faster customization of trial material in R&D phases.
- Faster disintegration of a drug may make it easier for patients to swallow it.
- No longer will stocking large quantities of nonpatient-specific pills be needed.
- Personalizing the dose, size, appearance, smell, and so on will make it possible to tailor a drug to the (pharmacogenomics) profile of a particular patient.
- The potential for printing customized pills 24/7 in a home setting will be possible.
- Counterfeit drugs will be reduced, as drugs will be printed from digital databases (however, the raw chemical materials are prone to fraud).
- Waste of medications will be reduced, as necessary adjustments of dosing can be done in a more agile way and thus, less amounts of fixed-dosed drugs have to be destroyed in case patient dose changes (provided that chemical ink cartridges can be redistributed or delivered in small-quantity drug packages).
- Pharmacy waiting times will be reduced, potentially saving lives in time-sensitive situations.

Considerations

Before 3D printing can take off in consumer markets, a real challenge is fully digitizing the chemistry so that a digital blueprint exists for all molecules and so that computers can build drugs from scratch. Those blueprints should be encrypted to ensure that drugs are always produced according to a validated blueprint and to eliminate the use of counterfeit chemicals as much as possible. Here is where the security of blockchain-type data transferal (refer to Chapter 14) may offer possibilities.

 With respect to the encryption of blueprint and further security, both pharmacy-delivered and home-printed 3-D drugs need to be strictly governed and controlled. Only login codes with a complexity similar those for bank accounts or biometric access techniques should allow access to domestic 3-D printing machines used for medication. In addition, integrating transactions done with a device (e.g., a doctor's prescriptions being directly referred to a domestic 3D printer) into, for instance, a blockchain environment may provide better safety for patients.

Also, 3D printers may be hacked, and securing them from unauthorized access will be important. In a world where even cruise ships' navigation systems can be hacked, it is clear that 3D printers can be threatened to disrupt individual lives, to steal personalized data, or to disrupt larger operational systems where networked 3D printers are used.

Drug regulation authorities will need to establish strict and guaranteed guidelines to ensure that future mass marketing of 3D-printed drugs is safe, reliable, secure, and safeguarded against human error. Risks need to be adequately mapped, requirements for safety and security settled, and guidelines made to prevent all cybersecurity-related risks.

As with more digital health technologies described in previous chapters, in the case of technical errors or malfunctions that result in physical harm to patients, legal authorities will need to determine whether the 3D printer's manufacturer, a drug company, or another party is liable. It may still take years of trial and error, or case-by-case studies, before satisfying solutions are found.

An additional complexity of the technology is its global, decentralized distribution. It will be difficult for drug companies and pharmacists to ensure that the right packaging and user instructions are made accessible to patients in a timely way. Virtual assistants, like those noted in Chapter 12 and augmented reality as noted in Chapter 13, may offer connected digital pharmaceutical solutions that provide holistic care that includes both the product and the service.

Big Opportunities Ahead

Assuming that the conditions for safe and reliable use of 3D printing are in place, providing patients with the exact amount of the drug they need, supporting them with continuous digital and human care services, and subsequently enabling them to measure outcomes with customized digital health technologies are the panacea for pharmaceutical care.

Printing drugs via 3D printing is likely to increase from 2020 on, but true integration in healthcare systems and printing mass-marketed drugs may still be years away.

Social Robots in Every Home

As discussed in previous chapters, we are on the verge of building machines that don't need sleep or food (though they do need electricity), don't have biases, and that can give us interrupted help with the things that matter to us.

The principle definition of a robot is a machine—especially one programmable by a computer—capable of carrying out a complex series of actions automatically. Robots can be guided by an external control device, or the control may be embedded within, mainly driven by AI algorithms (Wikipedia, 2018d). Robots increasingly substitute human tasks in predominantly repetitive situations. Gradually, as more algorithms like machine learning and deep learning (see Chapter 11) are added, their value will spread to broader services and care tasks as well.

A large percentage of current robots are still industrial step-and-repeat machines designed to perform a task in industry or at home with no or limited regard to how they look or interact with humans.

For some decades integrated pharmacy automation systems that automate partial or entire processes for delivering packages or for dispensing unit-dose medications have existed in the pharmaceutical industry. Those pharmacies using dispensing robots are augmented in such a way that the robots' increased speed and efficiency allow the human labor force to spend more time with patients or other healthcare professionals and to focus on better patient outcomes. Also, robots help to decrease medication errors, as the variability of robots' preciseness is usually less than that of humans.

Some special forms of robots are microscopic and nanorobots (10^{-9}) robots. Microscopic robots were inspired by insects such as spiders and could one day be capable of migrating through and performing delicate medical tasks inside the body. Nanorobots can be swallowed and assist in, for example, targeted drug delivery. An example are origami robots built into medication capsules. When swallowed, the capsule containing the robot dissolves in a patient's stomach and unfolds itself. These robots are most often controlled by an external technician and with the help of magnetic fields; they, for example, patch up wounds in the stomach lining or safely remove foreign items such as swallowed toys.

Attitudes Towards Robots

Different cultures have various attitudes towards robots and artificial intelligence. In the European Union, the attitude is rather positive with 61% of people seeing value in robots (EU, 2017). More than eight in ten respondents agreed that robots are needed as they can do jobs that are too hard or too dangerous for people (84%), while 68%

agree robots and artificial intelligence are a good thing for society because they help people do their jobs or carry out daily tasks at home.

The United States has the highest level of robot utilization at home and in retail stores. Nevertheless, in the United States adults are roughly twice as likely to express worry (72%) as enthusiasm (33%) about a future in which robots and computers are capable of doing many jobs that are currently done by humans (Pew Research Center, 2017).

Japan is the world leader in robotics, and demand is high for robots, which could help fill the huge shortfall in nursing care due to the country's aging population. The country is, for example, home to Erica, one of the first realistic female humanoids in existence; and (as shown in QR Code 16.3), Azuma, a holographic girl in a jar that combines virtual personal assistant functionality with a cute look and a simulated, deferential personality. Japan's labor shortage will hit service industry jobs like eldercare with ferocity; therefore future caretakers currently may be under development in a Japanese factory (Ross, 2016).

QR Code 16.3

Example of a social robot.

Robots in Hospital Care

During a hospital stay many patients prefer to frequently interact with human nurses. Nurses draw blood, check your vital signs, check on your condition, and take care of your hygiene if needed. They are often exhausted by physically and mentally daunting tasks, and the result of people being overworked is often an unpleasant experience for everyone involved, including the patient.

Robotic nurses can help carry this burden in the future, as certain robots can, for example, take blood samples or support with dressing or grooming. Also, social companion robots may entertain and reassure people, where possible. Supported by these robots, the staff may conserve the energy needed to deal with issues that require human decision-making skills and empathy.

A few countries have already established themselves as "robotic" societies, with Japan, China, the United States, South Korea, and Germany in the lead.

Social Companion Robots in Healthcare

Alongside industrial robots, the number of aesthetically appealing and even adorable social robots is growing.

A social robot is a specific kind of AI system that is designed to interact with humans and possibly also with other robots (QR Code 16.4).

Social (companion) robots come in different forms:

- Monolithic voice-user interfaces like the ones noted in Chapter 12
- Anthropomorphic devices, with tangible body frameworks, holograms, or avatars that exhibit adorability and that excite human empathy
- Humanoids or androids with faces resembling humans (see QR Code 16.4)

QR Code 16.4

Example of a humanoid robot.

In light of an aging population combined with a smaller workforce available to meet the increasing need for care, the use of robots may solve a number of issues in home-situated or hospital healthcare.

Social companion robots may act as a sort of jack of all trades and thus freeing up time for care providers to focus on the human touch in the (health) care system. Social robots may entertain, may perform small household tasks, may remind people of drug-related activities, and motivate physical action.

In hospital or community care situations where the amount of attention given to patients is driven by restricted resources, the results may be unnecessary deterioration of a disease or unnoticed adverse events. In such cases social robots can play a caring and alerting role, making sure patients feel comfortable and cared for as much as possible.

Additionally, in homecare settings social isolation and loneliness can be soothed by certain forms of companion robots. Many home healthcare environments are already equipped with an increasing number of smart robotics, and these machines may simultaneously and in real time analyze large sets of data, using a combination of deep learning, machine reading, and data augmentation to identify trends that create a holistic vision of a patient's status. Based on these data, the robots are able to anticipate a patient's needs, signal alerts in case of medical abnormalities, and provide companionship when asked for. Thus they help to ensure safe environments where patients can feel comforted.

Social robots are often made to look adorable in order to increase the level of trust and the likelihood people will follow advice offered by the robots. Humanlike robots tend to increase a person's comfortable level, and they may be perceived as being easier to communicate with it than another person. A potential disadvantage is the expectation that a robot can to do a broad set of human activities, which is still not the case. Moreover, if robots are too humanlike people may "forget" the difference between a human and a machine, which may be experienced as scary by some.

Social Robots in Pharmaceutical Care

QR Code 16.5

Example of an adherence robot.

Within a pharmacy, tasks like those a receptionist performs (with smart AI integration) may be conducted by social robots. In fact, Chinese hospitals already have hospitality robots at the entrance to the hospitals. Robots also may be a combination of an anthropomorphic device and personal assistant technology that in the future can perform triage activities, for example, helping patients with straightforward, over-the-counter medication questions.

Robot technology is also increasingly used to help in homecare settings with medication adherence programs (like Mabu in QR Code 16.5), with using drugs according to prescription, and with providing educational support. When part of a domestic environment, some robots are able to learn the interactions specific to a household and adapt to offer more personalized support.

Considerations

In-home virtual care assistants will never replace human interaction or the human touch, but they are programmed to reduce many of the inefficiencies associated with healthcare today, which may contribute to an increase in value-driven healthcare.

As with 3D printers, with robots safety and security are essential, and it must be nearly impossible for unauthorized people to access a robot's infrastructure. Also, biometric patient recognition and fully secure encryption of data sharing with external care providers are still big challenges; however, solutions for them are expected in the future.

Ethics in the Time of Robotics

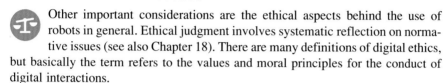 Other important considerations are the ethical aspects behind the use of robots in general. Ethical judgment involves systematic reflection on normative issues (see also Chapter 18). There are many definitions of digital ethics, but basically the term refers to the values and moral principles for the conduct of digital interactions.

In his 1942 short story *Runaround* science fiction writer Isaac Asimov introduced the Three Laws of Robotics, engineering safeguards, and built-in ethical principles that he would go on to use in dozens of stories and novels.

 The laws of Asimov are

- a robot may not injure a human being or, through inaction, allow a human being to come to harm;
- a robot must obey the orders given it by human beings, except where such orders would conflict with the First Law; and
- a robot must protect its own existence as long as such protection does not conflict with the First or Second Laws.

Using robots in healthcare may raise fundamental questions regarding the responsible use of digital technology, such as the unintentional discovery of confidential information in medical scans or database searches, or algorithms supporting clinical decision making without transparency of validity and evidence.

As such digital technology including robots is not neutral. Rather, they enshrine a vision and reflect a worldview, as they are programmed by humans, living in certain ecosystem. For instance, social robot technology from Japan may not land in other contingents, as cultural backgrounds and beliefs may imprint the actions that social robots execute.

Thus, when using social robot technology in pharmaceutical care, it is recommended that providers understand the way the algorithms are programmed and to ask for transparency in machine learning mechanisms and how they are connected to what is considered "good care" by individual patients (as discussed in Chapter 5).

The principles of the profession (see Chapter 19) and the moral values linked to the pharmacist's role may serve as guides at the current time, as digital ethics standards are not yet sufficiently developed.

The Value of Humans

Additionally, the more basic question should be posed: Will human beings be allowed to choose to be treated by a human professional rather than a robot?

Although it promises tremendous societal and economic benefits, as this technology is implemented it may become more and more difficult for people to act in a self-determined way, and thus their freedom of choice and action may be put at considerable risk.

Human compassion is central to the welfare of people, and in fact the human touch is considered to be vital in the practice of medicine. It is an integral part of the patient–pharmacist relationship, in which patients feel that they are taken care of by a fellow human being and are not alone in their time of need.

Even if ethical frameworks are built such that future robotic applications are empathic, they will never be able to relate as a human does. As in the movie *Ex Machina,* the question is asked: Would you believe it if a robot could show authentic emotion?

Artificial intelligence and robots may outpace human intelligence from a hardware perspective, but humans, definitely the ones who are ill, may want to choose on the side of human judgment; a caring, warm arm; an empathic ear; or a calming, soft hug. Moreover, there is also the phenomenon of trust, in which humans are not sure robots really can make the right choices for human healthcare, in spite of the fact that human choice is itself not always infallible.

A good way forward will be to develop people's trust in robots, which can be done by creating transparent understanding of how the algorithms are fed with data, how the robots are programmed, how they analyze, and how they provide reasons for actions.

However, even if an adorable-looking social robot displays full transparency by way of adequate data and structures and consistent decision-making trees, some real-life situations ask for intuitive human consideration and judgment that will never be programmable. Thus it becomes our challenge to develop models fitting for a synergistic society in which robots and humans live in creative cooperation.

Full integration of social robots within the pharmaceutical care journey is not expected to take place prior to 2024.

In the next Part 3 of this book, we will describe the conditions to drive combinatoric pharma-digital innovation and to make adequate and ethically sound digital pharmaceutical care implementation happen.

This means for circular pharmaceutical care:

- Computational pharmacotherapy will help healthcare providers drive precision medicine, leading to optimal individualized treatment patterns.
- Multiple techniques for 3D printing can offer tailored drugs to patients in terms of dosage, size, appearance, and delivery system.
- Social companion robots come in different forms, that is, monolithic voice-user interfaces, anthropomorphic devices, and humanoids.
- Social companion robots may act as a sort of jack of all trades and, for example, may entertain, may perform small household tasks, and may remind people of activities and motivate physical action.
- Robots free up time for healthcare providers so that they can focus more on the human touch, an empathic touch that cannot be simulated by robots.
- To warrant ethical use of social robotic technology in pharmaceutical care, it is recommended that we understand how the algorithms are programmed, how machine learning mechanisms work, and how the connection is made to what individual patients consider to be "good care."
- Both 3D printing and robotics are prone to privacy and security challenges, and the future challenge is to provide safe systems that can be trusted by both providers and patients.

How: Conditions to drive combinatoric pharma-digital innovation

Heathlands of digital health compliance

17

Rob Peters, Barry Meesters

If you think being compliant is expensive, try noncompliance.
Paul McNulty

Medical devices monitor medical adherence, measure medical conditions, determine medical diagnoses, analyze anomalies during treatments, and produce big (health) data for scientific research purposes. A few examples of how technological innovation can improve future care pathways are discussed in depth in previous chapters. Innovations are necessary to face the increasing demand for (health) care and exploding costs in the (near) future.

In this chapter you will read about the principles of data privacy, quality compliance, and information security. By following a strong compliance blueprint in the design of your product, you find that adhering to regulation becomes a true business enabler.

Many believe in the potential of these game-changing technologies, but nevertheless, patients and medical specialists sometimes seem to be reluctant in using and adopting the innovations (Deloitte, 2017b).

Questions are posed like:

• Is this medical device reliable?
• What will they do with my data?
• Who is liable if the device does not work?
• Why do they give or sell my data to a (pharmaceutical) company?

In the heathlands of innovation adoption, many rules and regulations prevail and may seem overwhelming at first. This chapter aims to provide a concrete view of the regulatory principles relevant to developing digital health applications and explain how to create a compliance blueprint that is feasible for everyone.

 A compliance blueprint is a risk-based overview of the aspects that must be considered in digital health applications weighted against the prevailing rules and regulations.

Pharmaceutical Care in Digital Revolution. https://doi.org/10.1016/B978-0-12-817638-2.00017-1

195

From the standpoint of the principles of risk management, a compliance blueprint consists of one or more of the following most common elements:

- laws and legislation on data privacy;
- regulations and quality standards for medical devices;
- guidelines and best practices for security; and
- organizational rules.

At the end of this chapter you will find a structured procedure for developing a compliance blueprint. But first let us deep-dive into the details of the four items above, whereas it is important to mention that even more details on the regulations can be found in the Appendix.

Managing Risks

Apart from their potential to create value, successful innovations in pharmaceutical care journeys are built upon the pillars of privacy, quality compliance, and information security. They establish what is most important in health ecosystems: trust. Trust in the functions of medical devices (e.g., "how an algorithm is working"), in security (e.g., "is my data safe"), and in privacy (e.g., "is data treated confidentially").

Proving compliance is therefore crucial in order to stimulate use and acceptance of innovations and also to reduce the risk of using them for unacceptable purposes.

A current challenge in compliancy is the difficulty that regulatory agencies have keeping up with the upsurge of digital health innovations. In general, practice and innovation set the scene and regulation follows. In healthcare systems this process has frequently led to the perception that current regulations for health devices or services are somewhat obsolete.

However, this regulatory backlog is not at all an obstacle for innovation. The principles behind all regulations are transparent: protecting patients from risks related to privacy, security, and quality (patient safety). Adhering to these principles will guide the way to develop proper innovations.

It all starts with a thorough risk analysis

 Risk is the potential of gaining or losing something of value. The two aspects of risk are

- the probability of occurrence of harm; and
- the consequences of the harm and the severity.

Evaluating risk is often difficult and subjective by nature. Stakeholders may place different values on the probability of risk and the potential impact (damage) of the identified risks. At some point in time, risks will have to be weighed and balanced. Therefore involving all stakeholders (including patients and other end users) up-front in the risk analysis of an innovation is highly recommended.

This approach means that different interpretations of identified risks are considered in the developmental phase. (See the section Quality: Trust in Patient Safety later in the chapter for more details related to implementing a proper risk management process in accordance to the ISO 14971 standard.) As further background for identifying risks and prioritize actions, specific for General Data Protection Regulation (GDPR), the European Commission has developed a guidance website to help organizations understand, prioritize actions, and comply with the requirements of GDPR (EU, 2018a).

When balancing risks in digital health innovation, the principles behind privacy, quality, security, and organizational rules determine the appropriate compliance blueprint. These principles are explained in the following paragraphs.

1. Privacy: Patient Always in Control of Own Data

Patient data are considered by many as the new gold in healthcare. As these data accumulate and data analysis techniques become increasingly better (as discussed, e.g., in Chapters 8 and 11), the ability to create a holistic view of individuals is becoming easier. This trend offers many advantages; however, safeguarding the privacy of individuals is under increasing pressure.

 When patient data fall into the wrong hands, the consequences can be serious. It may impact jobs, relationships, sponsorships, insurance, and so on. To protect the individual (patient) against such risks, governments all over the world have introduced privacy laws and legislation.

Privacy Case 1: Nike+ Running app

The Dutch Data Protection Authority concluded in 2015 that the Nike+ Running app violated the Data Protection Act.

The app, which was downloaded globally 10–50 million times on Android devices, helped people keep track of their running activities.

Nike was accused of not providing sufficient information to the app's users about the processing of their health data (for Nike's own analysis and research purposes).

Also, Nike had not obtained lawful consent of required explicit consent and had not determined retention periods for the data.

Nike took measures to update the app in order to become compliant with applicable regulations (DPA, 2015).

The most relevant laws and legislations for pharmaceutical companies and developers related to privacy aspects are, in general:

- the GDPR, restrictive from May 2018 onwards in Europe;
- the Health Insurance Portability and Accountability Act (HIPAA) in the United States; and
- the Privacy Act (Australian Privacy Principles) in Australia.

There are also laws and legislation for specific groups, such as children, for example, the Children's Online Privacy Protection Act (COPPA) in the United States.

The objectives of laws and legislations such as GDPR, HIPAA, and COPPA are comparable. These objectives:

- give (back) transparency and control to patients on their (healthcare) data;
- create transparency in how analytics are built up and where they are used;
- gain the trust and confidence of patients and healthcare providers; and
- create and simplify a stable legal environment for technology adoption.

Although the GDPR violations in the aforementioned Nike+ case may seem innocent, it does exemplify what can happen when organizations processing health data, such as personal health records, DNA results, or psychological reports, are not compliant.

The Nike+ case indicates some of the most important aspects of the general privacy laws and legislation:

- informed consent;
- transparency;
- data minimization; and
- awareness.

We will now consider these aspects in more detail.

Informed Consent

The most general concept of informed consent means that the organization responsible for the data processing, gives appropriate information to the person consenting in order to inform and empower them to make a voluntary choice to accept or refuse a specific processing of data.

Within the privacy laws, informed consent relates as well to the fact that the user (either patient or healthcare provider) understands which data are collected during the intervention and how these data are being used. In the aforementioned Nike+ example, Nike had to modify its privacy statement in such a way that users are appropriately informed about the (personal) data that are processed, for what purposes, and the retention period of the data.

Under GDPR informed consent can be collected by different media. Under HIPAA, the requirements are stricter and must be received in written form before any analysis can start.

Transparency

In order to gain trust and avoid misinterpretation, companies have to take appropriate measures to disclose all information related to which data are collected and how they are processed.

Companies must be able to inform the person whose data is being processed in a concise, transparent, intelligible, and easily accessible way, using clear and plain language understood at different levels of society (Intersoft Consulting, 2019).

Data Minimization

Nowadays many organizations collect all possible data from the perspective that the data might become useful in the future. However, aforementioned privacy laws and legislation set limits to this practice. Both the principle of data minimization and purpose limitation raise specific challenges for such limitless data collection. Data minimization means that organizations responsible for the data processing, identify the minimum amount of personal data that is needed to fulfill the purpose of the data processing (e.g., data that is needed for the correct functioning of the application). The organization is only allowed to process that (minimal) amount of data.

By default, only essential personal health data is allowed to be processed and retained. In healthcare this minimization aspect has a clear advantage as it reduces the administrative burden on appropriate data cleaning and storage, one of the biggest challenges in healthcare. Additionally, data which is not obtained cannot be misused, stolen, or lost.

Pharmaceutical stakeholders have to *keep their promise* and process only the data they included in their agreed-upon disclosure and consent statements. When product owners or healthcare providers decide to broaden the objective of their intervention and thus need more data from a patient, they need to re-consent every individual to obtain approval.

Awareness

It is recommended that all healthcare providers and product owners review their mindset on matters of privacy and put the protection of their patients and customers first. Therefore during the development phase, it is best (in the EU it is even to obligated) to embed the aspects of privacy in structured designs such as *privacy-by-design* and *privacy-by-default*. (See Chapter 20 for more on the broader principle of development-by-design.)

In principle, no digital solutions should be launched without a formal "privacy" approval. By implementing the privacy-by-design principle, penalties due to breaches and violations can be avoided at an early stage.

Continuous training and education are essential cornerstones to keeping the workforce aware of privacy priorities. For example, the Norwegian Data Protection Authority has developed guidelines to help organizations understand and comply with the requirements of data protection by design and by default in article 25 of the GDPR (Datatyilsynet, 2018).

 Conducting a privacy assessment (based on one or all mentioned frameworks) and following up on the observations could directly affect topics that are regulated by other legislation as well, such as retention terms of retention periods of medical data or medical secrecy.

2. Quality: Trust in Patient Safety

The general objectives of quality regulations and standards are to

- ensure a consistent high level of health and safety protection; and
- ensure trust of patients and healthcare professionals in the safety and reliability of medical devices.

As mentioned earlier the impact of poor-quality digital health tools on patient health and safety may be significant. It could result in physical injury or even death. Also, an incident may have significant impact on the reputation of the digital solution, the pharmaceutical provider, and the industry in general.

A Blood Collection Device

Theranos, a once successful startup in Silicon Valley with a value of $10 billion, set out to revolutionize blood testing industry. With a capillary tube nanotainer, the company claimed that it could run over 200 tests with just one finger prick and a few drops of blood. After an investigation by the FDA, it appeared that, in addition to analysis accuracy questions, the blood collection device was sold as a class I device but in fact was a higher classified medical device. The FDA concluded that Theranos did not adequately document risk or hazard analysis for its products, which resulted in immediate risk for health and safety of patients. Allegations against Theranos are still pending, and the company is on the verge of bankruptcy, laying off from 800 to 25 employees (Wasserman, 2015).

With the significant growth of digital devices and solutions, both medical professionals and patients have more and more questions about which digital devices are reliable and safe and which ones are not.

Therefore it is not surprising that more quality regulations have been released recently. The most relevant quality standards for pharmaceutical care stakeholders are, or written by, nowadays:

- Software as a Medical Device (SaMD) in the United States;
- Therapeutic Goods Administration (TGA) in Australia;
- Medical Device Single Audit Program (MDSAP);
- ISO 13485—Quality Management System—Requirements for regulatory purposes;
- ISO 14971—Application of risk management to medical devices; and
- Medical Software Regulation in Europe: Medical Device Regulation.

In the European Union the MDR will be effective as of 2020. As one of the consequences, in a risk-based approach medical software such as mobile applications will be more quickly assigned as medical devices and therefore will face additional quality requirements. Under MDR a categorization of devices is made, ranging from class I (low risk for patients), to class IIa (low/medium risk), to class IIb (medium/high risk), to class III (high risk). Medical devices with a higher risk category require stricter regulatory controls to provide reasonable assurance of the device's safety and effectiveness.

The FDA introduced, in 2018, a precertification program (PreCert), which will support the development of a regulatory model to assess the safety and effectiveness of software technologies without inhibiting patient access to these technologies. All the questions in this model relate to patient safety, quality, and so on, and can be used as the first baseline to identify gaps and key priorities related to quality in an organization. More information on the program can be found in QR Code 17.1.

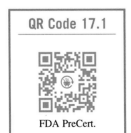

QR Code 17.1

FDA PreCert.

More detailed information on the regulatory frameworks can be found in the Appendix.

A topic that is presenting a more frequent dilemma is the difference between wellness and medical devices. The general approach of most regulators is that they will not regulate general wellness products as they do with medical devices. As long as products are intended only for general use and present a low risk to users' safety, they only have to undergo product or company certification processes like ISO (ISO, 2018) or CE (CE, 2018).

Nevertheless, devices like the wearables discussed in Chapter 10 are being increasingly introduced in care environments and may require further regulation in the future.

Quality Management

Quality is not only a result of regulations, it preferably is an integrated business process, like privacy awareness embedded in the DNA of developers. Quality management systems support a structured approach. Once policies and procedures are in place, it is easier to continuously deliver the required levels of quality and patient safety.

Quality management systems, among other things, include risk analysis, complaint management procedures, and quality audits based on an audit schedule. In the Theranos example, most of these parts were lacking, reflecting the risks that both the company and the users were exposed to.

ISO 13485 specifies the requirements for a quality management system for medical devices, to which many digital health tools will belong. The standard is applicable to organizations regardless of their size and type and is designed to be used in the design, production, installation, and delivery of medical devices and related services.

An Insulin Pump

In 2016 Johnson & Johnson informed doctors and about 114,000 patients in the United States and Canada about a security vulnerability in one of its insulin pumps. It was possible to hack this device, which could allow a hacker to exploit it to overdose diabetic patients with insulin. Although the probability of unauthorized access was extremely low, the risks associated with a cyberattack are huge. J&J appropriately informed patients how to diminish the risks to the bare minimum (Finkle, 2016).

Quality management also means informing patients about poor quality or vulnerabilities. In the insulin pump example, J&J decided to inform all 114,000 patients and explained the probability of misusing the vulnerability. Risk management and incident response are the correct approach to dealing with quality issues. By doing so, lives as well as reputations could be saved.

The Appendix covers the quality regulations and standards in more detail.

3. Security: Data Protection as the Foundation for Building Trust

In recent years theft of personal (including medical) records increased as the digital revolution gave more access to more data. A report by IT Governance Ltd estimated that by mid-December 31, 2016, a total of 3,154,135,541 data records had been leaked worldwide. This estimate included the largest breach ever reported, that is, the one billion user records stolen from Yahoo (Cyjax, 2017).

Due to the increasing amount of data breaches, patients and medical specialists have growing concerns about the protection of their data. Cybersecurity is the practice of protecting systems, networks, and programs from digital attacks. These attacks are usually aimed at accessing, changing, or destroying sensitive information.

In addition to individual harm, cybersecurity incidents can also impact the availability, continuity, and correct functioning of digital solutions. If someone gains unauthorized access to digital solutions, data can be modified, critical algorithms can be changed, or devices can be shut down, with all having the potential to result in wide-scale injury.

Figure 17.1 exemplifies the broad scope of daily security threats which (healthcare) personnel are facing.

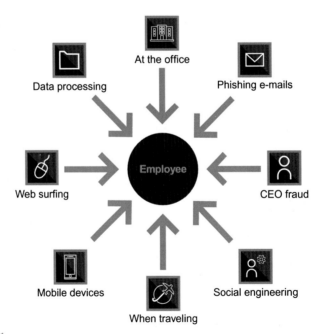

FIGURE 17.1

Security threats.

To decrease such cybersecurity incidents, the quest for laws and legislation and enforcement of these rules is increasing. Security is a fundamental part of laws and legislation related to privacy and quality. In many cases it is said that we need to take suitable security measures. However, what is suitable is not always clearly defined, although specific cybersecurity laws are more and more developed (such as the, nowadays, proposed NIS directive and Cybersecurity Act on a European level).

Despite that cyber security laws will come in to affect more and more the upcoming years' authorities support organizations in defining and implementing appropriate security measures based on globally accepted standards, guidelines, and best practices such as:

- ISO/IEC 27001 Information security management system (ISMS);
- Open Web Application Security Project (OWASP);
- Guide to securing personal information in Australia; and
- National Institute of Standards and Technology (NIST) guidelines.

The main goals of these security standards, guidelines, and best practices are always linked to globally recognized standard models. One of the most widely accepted models, which is also used in ISO standards such as ISO 27001, is the confidentiality, integrity and availability (CIA) triad (Network World, 2008):

- **Confidentiality:** Prevents unauthorized disclosure of sensitive information. It refers to the capability to ensure that the necessary level of security is enforced and that information is concealed from unauthorized users. When it comes to security, confidentiality is perhaps the most obvious aspect of the CIA triad. Encryption is a method to ensure the confidentiality of data transferred from one computer to another.
- **Integrity:** Prevents unauthorized modification of data, systems, and information, thereby referring to providing assurance of the accuracy of information and systems.
- **Availability:** Prevents loss of access to resources and information and refers to responsibility to ensure that information is available for use when it is needed.

Connected Pacemakers

The FDA in 2017 recalled about 500,000 internet-connected pacemakers manufactured by Abbott Health, formerly St. Jude Medical, due to hacking fears. The security vulnerability of the pacemakers could allow an unauthorized user to remotely access a patient's implanted, connected pacemaker and could result in patient harm and, in the worst case, death from rapid battery depletion or administration of inappropriate pacing or shocks.

Rather than having patients remove or replace the device, the manufacturer released a firmware update. During the update the device ran in backup mode and loss of diagnostic data or settings was possible. Patients were requested to talk to their doctors about the risks and benefits of updating their pacemakers (FDA, 2018b).

QR Code 17.2

Cybersecurity.

QR Code 17.2 and the Abbott example underline the necessity for adequate design of medical devices' security, including digital solutions.

 Security-by-design is a structured approach to make digital solutions as free as possible from vulnerabilities and impervious to attack through measures such as continuous testing, authentication safeguards, and adherence to best programming practices.

OWASP contains many guidelines to implementing security-by-design principles (OWASP, 2017). They contain, for example, the use of nondefault passwords and best-encrypted USB devices and involve intensive vulnerability testing on servers.

Humans are still considered a weak, if not the weakest, link in any system that contains risks, and this also applies to the security chain. QR Code 17.2 shows various examples of why awareness of cybersecurity risks is essential. Security awareness is considered to be the knowledge and attitude that members of an organization possess regarding the protection of the physical and, especially, the informational, assets of the organization.

 In a world where all devices are connected to the internet (as reflected in Chapter 8), the possibility of a cyberattack is always present. One hundred percent security may never be possible, so *assume you are being hacked.*

Preventing cybersecurity incidents starts with awareness, both upfront while designing as well when breaches are identified. Implementation of an adequate incident response process and communication (including training) of the protocol during a cybersecurity incident is also part of an adequate awareness program.

Last but not least, during the development of digital tools, best practices and guidance advice need to be used, as described in the Appendix (including for encryption methods). These best practices are published by well-known security parties and communities. Using the time and effort that they have put into the development of such practices is probably more valuable than developing individual encryption methods.

4. Organizational Rules

In addition to external rules and regulations, compliance with one's own business and organizational rules, for example, standard operating procedures and guidelines, is essential as well. Although noncompliance with these rules may not result in a penalty by an authority, they are fundamental to the culture, efficiency, and consistency of every organization.

Internal company rules are often described in documents or procedures such as standards of integrity, standard operating procedures (SOP), conflicts of interest, codes of conduct, mission and core value statements, and other corporate governance documents.

Compliance Blueprint: What to Do Tomorrow

At this point, we want to provide an overview of what will be required in the near future in order to remain compliant on all aspects of privacy, quality, and security. Taking a structured approach may be best called making a "compliance blueprint," as shown in Figure 17.2.

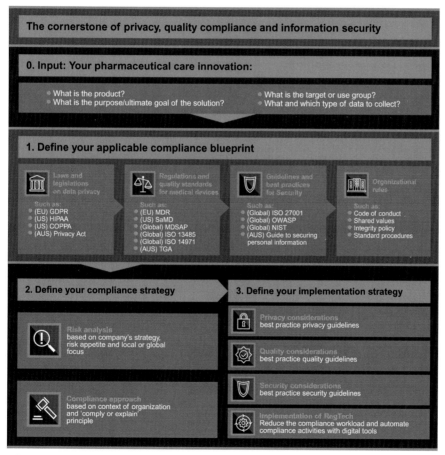

FIGURE 17.2

The steps in a compliance blueprint.

Before starting always remember that laws and legislation exist on global, regional, and local levels. Before executing a digital pharmaceutical care initiative, identify the applicable laws and regulations (your compliance blueprint starting point) that must be complied with.

In Table 17.1 shows some of the key considerations for making an adequate compliance blueprint.

Table 17.1 Some of the Key Considerations for Making a Compliance Blueprint

Make a Proper Risk Assessment (Based on ISO14971 Methodology)			
Privacy	Quality Aspects	Information Security	Organizational Rules
Take a compliance-by-design approach for all four elements into account			
Document privacy impact analysis with template of HIPAA/GDPR	Identify whether the quality standards are applicable; for example, is my solution a medical device and if so which class of medical device?	Encrypt all data connections	Determine which organizational rules you need to comply with
Consider privacy-by-design approach	Determine intended use (wellness or health) and classification	Run periodic security tests	
Document how transparency is provided	Follow quality management system rules (ISO 13485)	Secure and encrypt data storage	
Obtain consent on what will be tracked and analyzed (processed)	Prepare documentation on operational, technical, and legal controls (technical file)	Use best practices as mentioned earlier in the chapter	
Minimize data to the essentials	Implement processes and specific requirements	Create a high level of security awareness in the organization	
Create a high level of privacy awareness in the organization			
Automate where possible and efficient Remain compliant-aware on all four levels and adjust where required			

Compliance Within the Context of Your Organization

Laws and regulations are generally not black and white. Most of them contain room for interpretation, such as "the organization should have suitable measures." Thus, being compliant is also about including the *context* of the organization or innovation.

For example, a company or institution's economic situation (what investments can be justified to guarantee the continuity of the organization) and the state of its technology (what technology is proven and affordable) are considerations that need to be taken into account once products are audited or inspected (EU, 2018b). A small pharmacy's requirements to compliance frameworks are different from those of a multinational pharmaceutical company. Nevertheless, patient privacy, safety, and security requirements are the same for all.

Figure 17.3 can be used to assess whether an organization's compliance lies in the immediate stage or in a future stage. This information makes it possible to set goals and understand expectations when a digital health solution becomes a commercial success.

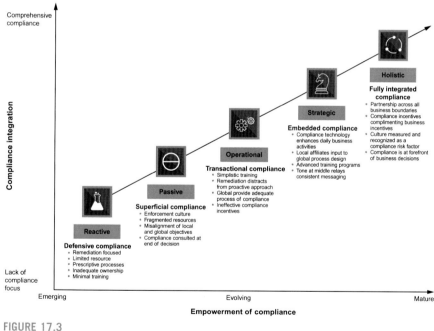

FIGURE 17.3

Compliance Maturity Model (Deloitte, 2015).

The model also shows that potential compliance risks are defined in the context of the organization (a small company does have fewer risks and lower budgets to mitigate risks than a larger company does).

Defining Your Compliance Approach

Based on the context of an organization, the respective proposed digital innovation, and a thorough risk analysis, a compliance approach and, in the extension thereof, control measures can be identified. From this perspective, the principle of *comply or explain* applies.

 This principle means to let the market decide whether a set of standards is appropriate for individual companies. Since a company may deviate from the standard, this approach rejects the view that "one size fits all."

If a company finds that a certain rule is inappropriate due to particular circumstances, it can choose another solution than that found in the law or regulation. This principle is in line with the changing, more open, approach of overseeing authorities and may be accepted based on a balanced risk score as shown in Figure 17.4.

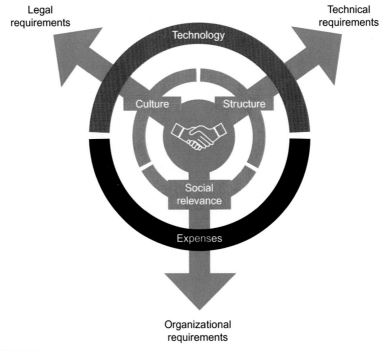

FIGURE 17.4

Balanced compliance strategy.

Reduce Compliance Costs and Work

A recent industry study showed that 97% of pharmaceutical industries indicated that they already use or plan to use digital health technologies (Deloitte DCoHS, 2017). Although this number may be lower in hospitals and community pharmaceutical care environments, this book provides examples that strongly suggest the disruptive adoption of technology in the next decade. As indicated previously, this fast uptake will drive the need to have newer types of rules and regulations.

The fast and ongoing innovations require large investments from stakeholders who want to develop and use digital health tools in a compliant way. Depending on the size of your organization, this means investment in (dedicated) compliance factors such as privacy officers, security officers, and data protection officers. It also means investment in processes and controls to mitigate the (security, privacy, and quality) risks of noncompliance. Also, technology to protect the confidentiality, availability, and integrity of health data is required.

All these investments ask for resources that might otherwise be spent on other business processes.

> However, if you think compliance is expensive, think about the higher cost of noncompliance. The risk of immediate loss of revenue, delayed product launches, costly remediation programs, fines, and long-term damage to your reputation are not just theoretical threats, as examples in this chapter have indicated.

There are also positive triggers for compliance. Compliance "inside" refers to a situation in which compliance is experienced as a strategic asset rather than a liability. It means that by smart working and with the right mindset, compliance is experienced as a natural competence that enables a business. Because of this embedded insight (hence inside), the organization can focus on client-facing processes and R&D, and it might even develop into a competitive advantage based on the ability to respond more quickly to regulation and build trust with clients and other stakeholders.

RegTech

As a potential solution to the increasing regulatory burdens, professionals in the banking and finance industries have begun to use artificial intelligence to manage regulatory compliance. Machine learning and natural language processing (NLP), as explained in Chapters 11 and 12, are particularly powerful tools for this purpose; blockchain systems may fit in as well.

QR Code 17.3

RegTech.

These solutions are called RegTech, which stands for Regulatory Technology and contains digital solutions by which compliance activities can be executed in a more automated and cost-effective way. More information on the principles of RegTech can be found in QR Code 17.3.

RegTech companies in healthcare ecosystems focus on analyzing and embedding regulations that are specific to this industry (as reflected in this chapter) and are growing in number. Some pharmaceutical stakeholders have already started collaborating with RegTech firms to, for example, digitize compliance activities and analyses.

Although RegTech solutions initially will require investments, in the long term RegTech is expected to create transparency in the heathlands of ever-changing laws and regulations and is expected to help make compliance reliable, affordable, and scalable for many stakeholders.

In the next Chapter 18, the ethical considerations for implementing digital pharmaceutical care will be given.

This means for circular pharmaceutical care:

- In a world full of disruptive healthcare innovations, following regulations is crucial in generating trust among all pharmaceutical care stakeholders.
- Digital health compliance always starts with a thorough risk analysis, integrated in a structured privacy, quality, security, and organizational assessment.
- A compliance blueprint means placing the digital solution within the context of an organization and helps to define a competitive compliance strategy that fits the developer's profile.
- RegTech solutions, based on AI and blockchain, are supportive technologies that can optimize a digital health compliance environment by keeping it reliable, affordable, and scalable.
- With a compliance blueprint and RegTech, regulatory requirements no longer have to be considered dissatisfiers for innovation, but can become true business enablers.

QR Code Animation

Digital Health Compliance.

An animation—kindly adopted by Deloitte—on the topic of Digital Health Compliance can be found on www.pharmacare.ai.

Ethical practice: Fostering trees of life

18

Wilma Göttgens, Claudia Rijcken

Educating the mind without educating the heart is no education at all.
Aristotle

Trees must share resources to survive. For example, they use a fungal network to exchange nutrients and communicate with other trees when defense mechanisms are needed. However, some plants use the underground root system to support their offspring, while others hijack it to sabotage their rivals (see QR Code 18.1).

QR Code 18.1

The Wood Wide Web.

> *In this chapter you will read about how the core values of pharmaceutical care professionals are the fundament to provide care that patients consider as good and meaningful. We also delve into why appropriate use of data and integer scientific research supports ethical framing, what is considered a meaningful life, and why human rights may become more pivotal in the digital age.*

This ecosystem is somehow similar to how the world wide web functions in our technology-driven world, and it also applies to our digital revolution. That is, we can use the Fourth Industrial Revolution for future prosperity, or we can abuse it. If we go the latter route, this revolution may result in the next extinction, as described in this book's Introduction.

Ethical Practices in a Technological Culture

The traditional philosophy of ethics does address the highly dynamic character of today's technological culture and its values. Insight into the moral significance of technological tools and systems is hampered by the intimate intertwinement of technology, individuals, and society, resulting in what is sometimes called "technological blindness."

Science and technology studies tend to show a "normative deficit" and resistant attitude towards ethics (Keulartz et al., 2004). The first question is: how can our pluralistic society address value conflicts in current and future technological landscapes?

Contemporary philosophy is built on the rational and empirical tradition that understands humans as autonomous and conscious subjects who use science and technology to achieve social and material progress. Depending on the underlying ethical theory, research is focused first and foremost on the underlying principles (deontological) or on the consequences of our actions (consequentialism). These theories are further discussed later in this chapter.

The next questions are whether underling principles can be universalized and to what extent actions contribute to aggregating individual welfare. Conceptual restrictions of contemporary philosophy may obstruct our view of the bigger picture of the social and moral order of societies.

The same holds for Beauchamp and Childress in their book, *Principles of Biomedical Ethics*, in which they propose four principles: autonomy, beneficence and nonmaleficence, and justice. These principles look at technology as being instrumental to human welfare. In both clinical medicine and scientific research, it is generally held that these principles can be applied, even in unique circumstances, to provide guidance in discovering moral duties in certain difficult situations.

However, nowadays it is increasingly thought that these principles alone may not be sufficient for ethics of healthcare. For example, in the provision of healthcare, theories related to ethics of care and virtue ethics have shown us that choices and deliberations cannot be made exclusively from the perspective of the four bioethics principles. Finding the right ethical framework, what is sensible, and what is the right thing to do also requires pragmatic wisdom based on ongoing education, professional expertise, and meaningful life experiences.

Thus alternative ethical approaches were developed based on pragmatic conceptions, feminist perspectives, and caring professions such as nursing. Interpretations of virtue ethics and social practices were also developed (MacIntyre, 1985).

In this chapter we build on the ethical perspective of digital pharmaceutical patient care as a professional practice. As reflected in Chapter 1, Cipolle et al. (2012) provide the explanation of the underlying philosophy of practices and concepts in pharmaceutical care.

 Ethics can be defined as a branch of philosophy that involves systematizing, defending, and recommending concepts of morality: that is, establishing what is a good and flourishing life.

As every individual is unique (see QR Code 18.2) and worldviews are open to change, as they do under the influence of digitization, views on ethical frameworks change as well. Thus there is no static description of "a good life."

To align views on what is a good life with changing paradigms, practitioners must embrace the concepts of professional, social, and scientific integrity. The philosophy of practice sets the values that guides a practitioners' behaviour by defining the rules, roles, relationships and responsibilities of the practitioner (Cipolle et al., 2012).

QR Code 18.2

The human game.

The Core Values and Virtue-Based Practice of Pharmaceutical Care Providers

Science, like other well-established cultural practices, has an inherent normative structure: a set of values, both epistemic and ethical, that guide and govern its practice (Douglas, 2009). Many medical science professions have a specific value set, often based on a code of conduct that is similar or strongly related to the Hippocratic Oath.

The Hippocratic Oath is an oath historically taken by physicians. It is one of the most widely known of Greek medical texts. In its original form, it requires a new physician to swear and to uphold specific ethical standards. The Oath was the earliest expression of medical ethics in the Western world, establishing several principles of medical ethics which remain of paramount significance today. These include the principles of medical confidentiality and nonmaleficence (Wikipedia, 2018e). The nowadays often used "first-do-no-harm" principle was not part of the initial text of the Hippocratic Oath, but the current use of that phrase is a continuous reminder that we need high-quality research to help better understand the balance of risks and benefits for the tests and treatments healthcare professionals recommend.

A Hippocratic Oath for scientists is an oath which is somehow similar to the Hippocratic Oath for medical professionals, however, adapted for scientists and addressing potential concerns with the ethical implications of scientific advances.

The topics of ethical practice and autonomy are nowadays especially important to the practice of pharmacy, because the profession is in transition, moving in many countries from a supply-oriented practice to a more patient care-oriented practice. In this context, the International Pharmaceutical Association has acknowledged that pharmacy cannot achieve its full potential, and patients will not benefit from that potential, unless pharmacists are committed to the highest standards of professional conduct and have sufficient autonomy to serve patients' best interests (FIP, 2013).

In some countries documentation for pharmaceutical care professionals regarding the expectations of a professional virtue-based practice is available. Such a document generally describes professional standards on how every care practitioner is expected to set priorities for the expectations and needs of an individual patient and the care for all citizens.

Pharmaceutical care practitioners are expected to contribute towards the efficiency of care and pharmacotherapy (treatment with medicines) and are facilitated in this role with information and knowledge about medicines, conditions, and patients. With the aid of knowledge systems, the pharmacist translates this complex data set into appropriate care for individual patients (KNMP, 2012).

The knowledge within these systems as well as the data they generate have grown exponentially over time due to health technology innovations, as described in previous chapters.

Uncertainty and sometimes limited theoretical and empirical proof of the true value of these innovations, incompleteness of data, and lack of clarity on how these digital health tools influence outcomes with regard to good care require pharmaceutical care practitioners to daily assess whether an innovation is sufficiently aligned with ethical practice.

Additionally, in many current worldviews, economic and regulatory frameworks tend to dominate professional care matters, which can make healthcare situations even more complex for practitioners and emphasize the need for an awareness of ethical considerations and the competency to autonomously make professional responsible decisions.

Although pharmaceutical care practitioners have autonomy, they work within a broader setting that includes other care practitioners, healthcare insurers, and patients who have a right to self-determination. Pharmaceutical care professionals are responsible for their decisions and for adhering to the frameworks established by society. They ensure good pharmaceutical judgment, while maintaining a balance between their commitment to patients and a socially responsible course of action (De Gier et al., 2013).

In finding responsible course of action in ethical dilemmas, pharmaceutical care providers need to be aware of and act according to the core values of their profession. The adjacent example box shows an example of how these values were formulated for Dutch pharmacists.

> The Royal Dutch Pharmacists Association drafted a charter that described the core values of the pharmacist:
>
> * Commitment to the patient's well-being
> * Pharmaceutical expertise
> * Social responsibility
> * Reliability and care
> * Professional autonomy
>
> These values are considered as the foundation of the professional practice of care (KNMP, 2012).

The expressed values of professional practice may differ semantically among countries, but in general their contents are quite similar. Core pharmaceutical values are usually developed at a country level and cover individual pharmaceutical care practitioners as well as professional associations. The professional code of ethics and professional standards are based on the philosophy of practice and the core values of the profession.

Such values act as beacons in the open-ended journey of ethical decision making (as opposed to norms and regulations, which generally have a more restrictive character). The values will support a professional, virtue-based practice that delivers care that patients perceive as good care.

Digital Ethics

 Literature contains numerous definitions of digital ethics. The essence of those definitions define the field of digital ethics as a framework in which to work ethically with digital technology by understanding the background, methods, principles, procedures, regulations, and institutions that determine the responsible use of digital technology.

Digital ethical concepts include, for instance, confidentiality, risk, privacy, and responsibility. Also, issues related to, for example, causality versus correlation as output of (scientific) data analysis are part of the digital ethical equation and are discussed later in this chapter.

There is a clear-cut reason why digital ethics is getting so much attention. First of all, the increase in the global amount of data creates concerns, as is reflected in the example box.

Meta-analysis of the literature on big data has identified five ethical concerns related to big data analysis.

- Informed consent (obtained in a timely way).
- Privacy (including anonymity and data protection).
- Ownership (who owns the data).
- Epistemology and objectivity (of the data used).
- "Big data divides" which are divides between those who have and those who lack the necessary resources to analyze increasingly large data sets (Mittelstad and Floridi, 2018).

Also, as technology like AI grows, so does the magnitude of its effect on society. As noted in Chapters 11 and 12 all industries, including healthcare, are using algorithms increasingly to assist, augment, or even replace human decision making.

These decision making support tools raise more questions about the appropriateness of data processing; the adequacy of artificial intelligence (AI) systems that interact, such as chatbots; and the integer support of automated decision making systems.

For example, imagine that an algorithm identifies a correlation that later is proved to be unfounded, for example, between two data groups, such as gender and the fatality rate among individuals who have a certain symptom. Without adequate scientific background checks and analysis, such digital findings might lead to inaccurate, potentially fatal recommendations. For example, the advice to proceed with a surgical intervention when it actually is not needed.

As such, AI algorithms may be regarded mainly as complementary mechanisms that augment human cognitive intelligence and that require meticulous human judgment before being used.

As discussed in Chapters 8 and 11, for algorithmic support to gain trust, full transparency of the quality of the data analyzed and of how an algorithm's decision-making tree is built are required. Additionally, to warrant ethically sound treatment decisions, algorithmic output must be synergized with human competency in order to understand both the context of the treatment situation and the scientific methods used (to distinguish causality from correlation) and thus supported by the defined core values, provide personalized treatment advice that adheres to the principles of the Hippocratic Oath.

Technology Versus Humanity

The need for such a multivariate ethical framework shows that digital health technology has an intrinsic moral significance, as it actively influences the ecosystem and perception of all its stakeholders. However, although it has a moral impact, technology in and of itself is amoral and is not associated with the human experience of empathy and compassion. For example, when a computer first became the best AlphaGO player in the world, it did not cry or scream or get goosebumps.

This inertia may have advantages in situations where human emotions may lead to subjective, suboptimal choices and a "neutral" decision making support system is valued. But there we move into the next dilemma (Roeser et al., 2012). Technology is never value-neutral, as it depends on (most often historical) data that may be biased, skewed, or outdated. Also, algorithms created by humans with particular worldviews. Extrapolating the output of such algorithms will always require an educated human to critically understand the context and to support a patient's perception of what constitutes good care.

Technology such as chatbots and digital humans, as described in Chapter 12, may also challenge the distinction we have long made between the human and the nonhuman and bring us to the boundaries of what we understand as humanity, of what is mankind and what is machine-kind. Patients may increasingly feel uncertain about what or whom to trust and how to carefully consider their treatment options.

Although digital tools can support pharmaceutical care practice, it is the ethical responsibility of the autonomous healthcare practitioner to enable a patient to guard the boundaries of digital treatment and a timely alert for human care when needed. This is also where the humanity part of the STEM+ education of pharmaceutical care practitioners comes into critical play, as described in Chapter 19.

Both pharmaceutical and digital technology are based on a STEM education; however, the + element in STEM+ refers to the social competency needed to effectively contextualize technical knowledge so as to provide a safeguard for patients' pharmaceutical care pathways. The latter asks for human skills like translating knowledge at different literacy levels, reading social cues, showing empathy and compassion, and balancing broader societal challenges towards the best-accepted solution.

This human touch is the key part of practicing medicine or pharmacy. It is an integral part of patient–doctor and patient-pharmacist relationships.

A Principle-Based Approach Is Not Sufficient to Safeguard Holistic Ethical Decision Making

Making a balanced care decision means much more than complying with regulatory conditions and communicating them. Digital compliance mechanisms (see Chapter 17) are being developed worldwide. At first blush this seems to make sense: perhaps the most obvious, straightforward method of preventing unethical or damaging behavior is to increase the number of rules designed to curtail it. However, one of the more unsettling and unintended consequences of a singular focus on ethics-as-compliance is a checkbox mentality that gives the illusion of reducing risk without really doing so (Rea et al., 2016).

Making a balanced care decision means internalizing pharmaceutical care values, acting with integrity, and taking a virtue-based approach. Human integrity is characterized by consistency in attitude, actions, expectations, principles, and values. Consistent alignment of professional integrity with individual *and* societal needs is central to the development and sustainability of a professional practice and can be experienced at different levels—in relation with oneself, with patients and peers, and with society at large. For pharmacy as a values- *and* science-based practice, it comes as no surprise that the principles and values of research are well aligned with the core values of pharmacists. Moreover, a "good" pharmacist knows how to find his way in difficult decisions, balancing values of patients, peers, and society and at the same time maintaining the core values of the profession. It may as well emphasize pharmacists' historical reputation as trusted and well-recognized members of the healthcare team.

Acting with integrity in complex ethical situations requires continuous interaction and alignment with the needs of the patients and with the perspectives of peers, experts, and policymakers. The ability to do so is predominantly acquired in daily practice. The foundation for a virtue based practice was set by Aristotle, and also Plato emphasized a virtue-based approach 2400 years ago in his Academy. Virtues are generated best through deliberative practice rather than through statements and proclamations.

 Therefore global communities of deliberative practice are to be stimulated, thus pharmaceutical care practitioners can share and discuss their concerns about ethical dilemmas due to the adoption of digital innovation.

In this way practitioners develop new roles and relationships with corresponding responsibilities to adjust the standards of professional practice.

Responsible Research and Use of Technology

While studying the use of technology around the world, we often found that two questions were being asked: how to guarantee the appropriate use of patients' health data and how to ensure that digital health tools are adequately researched before being adopted for use.

Responsible Use of Data

As noted in Chapter 8 the International Data Corporation forecasts that by 2025 with the rise in connected devices, the global data sphere will grow to 163 zettabytes (IDC, 2018), all of which we must digest in order to make sense of information sources within a specific context. We treat data as the new gold, and in doing so, tend to overlook how personal these data are and that they relate to identified or identifiable living individuals. With the current use of social media sensitivity to the ownership and privacy of data is an increasing topic of debate.

In the spectrum of global data, health data are considered as sensitive data and are expected to be handled with the greatest possible care. In Chapter 17 we explain some of the most prominent data privacy regulations, how they protect persons, and how they relate to informed consent.

Many people are happy to share their healthcare data for research on better care options, provided appropriate safeguards are in place to protect their data and privacy. Both patients and ethical committees prefer that steps are taken to ensure that patients provide informed consent when their health records or other data are used for clinical management or research. Because this may not always be possible (e.g., when dealing with historical data sets), methods based on analyzing only aggregated, anonymized data sets with no unique identifiers have been introduced.

However, individual health data are also increasingly shared in a type of unaware or "implied" consent. Big platforms like Google and Amazon, which have billions of users, tend to form partnerships with health technology vendors, and by combining user databases, create big data sets of pivotal health data. Big platforms generally do acknowledge that data may be used for research purposes; however, users often do not read this "fine prints."

The combination of big data mining and big platforms' vast influence and increasing pharmaceutical interests is a global concern for both individual patients and policymakers.

Even if the reasons behind selling data is truly to enhance care for patients, inappropriate commercializing of data can result in profiling patients without their knowledge or a proper informed consent. The next step might be that some doctors wind up using inadequately acquired data sets and may even recommend drugs based on such data. Merged data may result in the development of algorithms (called "profiling") that predict which healthcare professionals are most likely amenable to using such data to treat patients and to share patient data to improve care.

Patients may not be opposed to this practice as long as their care is improved. However, according to data privacy regulations as well as ethical considerations, everyone is entitled to know how their data is used and should be able to make an informed decision about whether and with whom their data can be shared.

The number of dilemmas in this area is increasing, and it is in this context that the professional autonomy and values of pharmaceutical care providers can help both patients and big platforms make responsible use of sensitive health data.

Tools and systems have been established worldwide that help healthcare professionals determine that data are used in an ethical way in projects and in the development of digital products. In addition to addressing the quality of data (as explained in Chapter 8), these systems and tools address questions such as whether the data are adequately anonymized, whether results are appropriately visualized, whether the data are easy to access, whether the data will be reused, and whether an expiry date is designated.

Open sharing of health data for medical and pharmaceutical research, policymaking, and humanitarian purposes is increasingly recognized as a crucial means to improve private and public life in mature, data-driven societies. At the same time, competing tensions concerning data control and ownership, respect of individual rights and consent, and lack of appropriate frameworks for coordination and ethical governance pose serious challenges to what is called "the safe donation of data," which remains virtually impossible today.

In Europe the Digital Ethics Lab at the University of Oxford is researching whether an ethical code for data donations will offer the necessary guidance to meet these challenges and shape data donation practices to ensure respect of users' individual rights and consent, foster transparency and trust, as well as harness the value of data to spur scientific research, public debate, and private and public well-being (DEL, 2017).

Another possible consideration is to draw examples from the Global Alliance for Genomics and Health, which has developed a framework for responsible sharing of genomics and health-related data based on the "human right to science and culture," one of the economic, social, and cultural rights claimed in the Universal Declaration of Human Rights and related documents of international human rights law. The framework promotes responsible data sharing, indicating that data-intensive science may gradually come to be founded on a more communal ethos (Ga4gh, 2018).

Responsible Scientific Research

The European Code of Conduct for Research Integrity (BBACH, 2017), describes research as "the quest for knowledge obtained through systematic study and thinking, observation and experimentation."

Principles serve as basic values of integrity in research. They should guide individual researchers as well as other parties involved in research, such as the institutions where it is conducted, publishers, scientific editors, funding bodies, and scientific and scholarly societies—all of which, given their role and interest in responsible research practices, may be expected to foster integrity (see adjacent box for example of principles).

> Different principles of integrity in the world's research community are, for example, those in the European Code of Conduct for Research Integrity:
>
> - **Reliability** in ensuring the quality of the research, including, for example, the design, methodology, analysis, and use of resources.
> - **Honesty** in developing, undertaking, reviewing, reporting, and communicating research in a transparent, fair, full, and unbiased way.
> - **Respect** for colleagues, research participants, society, ecosystems, cultural heritage, and the environment.
> - **Accountability** for the research from conception to publication; for its management and organization; for training, supervision, and mentoring; and for the scope of its impact (BBACH, 2017).

In data-driven societies research is moving from empirical evidence-based to statistic data-driven concepts. Establishing causality, as opposed to correlation, is probably the most difficult task in both models, as the probability of inadequate output is high. In big data analysis, due to the magnitude of data sets, correlations may be found more quickly; however, proving causality is something completely different and much more complex as the boundaries of statistics are being sought.

 Correlation suggests an association between two variables. Causality shows that one variable directly affects a change in the other. Although correlation may imply causality, it is different from a cause-and-effect relationship. For example, if a study reveals a positive correlation between happiness and liking digital health technology, this doesn't mean that an affinity for digital health technology causes happiness. In fact, correlation may be entirely coincidental, such as a correlation between Napoleon being small in stature and his rise to power. Conversely, if an experiment shows that a predicted outcome unfailingly results from manipulating a particular variable, a causality is more likely, and also denotes a correlation.

Scientific research in contemporary medicine is characterized by an evidence-based approach, meaning conscientious, explicit, and judicious use of the available evidence in making decisions about optimal care patterns. The evidence is based on observations that come from clinical studies of populations to establish cause-effect pairs. The gold standard is the double-blind, randomized clinical trial (RCT; see also

Chapter 6), where an adequate sample of patients is selected, some are given a particular treatment, and others are given either a different treatment or a placebo (and no one, neither the patients nor the researchers, knows who gets what). Subsequently, a predefined, measurable endpoint is analyzed.

Randomized controlled trials have high internal validity but can have limitations, such as those related to expense, speed, reproducibility, generalization to routine practice, selection bias, characterization of confounding factors, and ethical constraints. Also, trials that are "checklist" in nature may limit the ability to choose the most appropriate trial design.

If running a randomized experiment is not possible (e.g., either due to logistical reasons or to ethical considerations), existing data sources may be used in what is called an observational study design. The events compared in such studies happen without any control and the selection process is most often not randomized.

Big data analysis with observational event data present resources and methodologies that can be incorporated into the design of RCTs in order to augment and extend them and to address the RCT issues previously described.

Use of supervised learning techniques may help to improve accuracy in the analysis of big data, as classification and standardizations in, for example, designation of key data elements or nomenclatures may reduce the complexity introduced by variability and increase the reliability of consistency checks on inputs and outputs (see Chapter 11). Use of standardization in routine clinical care and in trials facilitates the development of sharable automated curation algorithms to flag outliers or longitudinal variation in data entries that may signal errors (Mayo et al., 2017).

An increasing number of digital health technologies, such as digital therapeutic solutions (see Chapter 15), are expected to undergo thorough scientific study in order to gain regulation-approved certification as medical devices. Understanding how these digital health technologies prove their value in clinical trials or big data analysis is an essential part of the professional expertise of pharmaceutical care practitioners and is a pivotal aspect for analyzing ethical dilemmas related to data and science matters.

In future thought eight (see the "Final Discussion" chapter), we further elaborate on how pharmaceutical care practitioners take up a caring value-based approach and balance deontological with consequentialistic perspectives to establish whether research (either RCT or Big Data analysis) are justified means to humanistic endpoints.

A Meaningful Life and Human Rights in the Digital Age

As Friedrich Nietzsche addressed, mankind has a commitment to instituting some set of higher values. The cost of not doing so is vitiating our deepest aims and precluding a central form of happiness.

But what is happiness in the context of a meaningful life? And in the digital age, which human rights are essential to ensure a life in which individual meaning is possible?

A Meaningful Life

In philosophy a meaningful life is a way of human being having to do with the purpose, significance, fulfillment, and satisfaction of life. Definitions of meaning have focused on several components, two of which appear central and unique to meaning in life, suggesting a conceptual framework of meaning in life comprising two pillars: comprehension and purpose. Comprehension encompasses people's ability to find patterns, consistency, and significance in the many events and experiences in their lives, and their synthesis and distillation of the most salient, important, and motivating factors. Purpose refers to highly motivating, long-term goals about which people are passionate and highly committed (Steger, 2009).

Meaning in general is mostly related to concepts like sense-making. When something that has meaning is gone, a feeling of loss will occur. This is especially applicable to health experiences, where disease and disability are generally considered as a loss of life value. A main goal of all healthcare practitioners is to minimize this feeling of loss by taking care that interventions first will do no harm.

In Chapter 6 we note that successful health interventions ideally target individual goals to which patients feel committed. This is where the core value of "commitment to patients' well-being" addresses the professional approach pharmaceutical care practitioners take when providing a personalized treatment that aligns with a patient's key beliefs. This approach means identifying what matters most to the patient (as described in Chapter 3 under value-based healthcare) as well as, for example, determining which part of treatments can be done digitally and which part should be performed by humans.

Also, many of the 10 factors that patients consider as essential for good healthcare (as described in Chapter 5) reflect aspects that support either the comprehension or the purpose of a meaningful treatment pathway. For example, the selection of effective treatment refers to a treatment that matters to the individual patient, ideally enabling the patient to continue her preferred lifestyle and to achieve personal goals (e.g., career and sports-related goals and as providers of care).

Digital health tools can support good care and individualized treatment pathways, as has extensively described in Part 2 of this book. The merge between humans and technologies may affect how we perceive ourselves as humans, as it creates what is referred to as a techno-human condition.

Electronic coaches like the chatbots described in Chapter 12 and the social companion robots described in Chapter 16 facilitate self-monitoring and treatment, but these systems' data may also be used to profile human beings in all kinds of ways with the explicit commercial goals of intervening in human processes. Also, virtual care approaches may blur the quality and intrinsic value of human relationships, which are essential to foster experiences of meaningful life. These factors raise the question of how to protect the rights of individuals in the digital age.

Human Flourishing in a Digital Age

Much of the bioethical debate on health technology and related human rights has so far focused on technologies that work inside the body. The Oviedo Convention was shaped around this premise. The convention created common guiding principles— such as the protection of private life, respect for autonomy, and the right to information and informed consent—to preserve human dignity in the way humans apply innovations in biomedicine. As already noted, a broad range of technologies that work outside the body exist, and those also impact the bodily, mental, and social performance of human beings (Council-of-Europe, 1997).

With the fast convergence of nano and biological data and cognitive technologies in the Internet of Things (see Chapter 8), each type of interaction between humans and those "intelligent artifacts" can raise various human rights issues.

The Rathenau Institute in 2017 submitted a report to the Council of Europe with the recommendation to adopt two new tracks toward ensuring human rights in the digital age. The first recommendation relates to the right not being measured, including the need to protect the privacy of data by respecting private and family life and people's ability to refuse to be subjected to profiling, to refuse to have their location tracked, or to refuse to be manipulated or influenced by a "coach." The second proposed new right was to have the opportunity, within the context of care and assistance provided to elderly people and people with disabilities, to choose to have human contact rather than a robot (Est van et al., 2017).

Although these rights are not yet formalized, they may give healthcare providers clearer guidance on where patients' rights need to be safeguarded. Most of the information in this book aligns with these two fundamental perspectives, reflecting that digital pharmaceutical care is an option but should be considered only after patients provide their informed consent to do so.

Pharmaceutical care practitioners' professional standing and value-based work is what enables them to support patients on moral choices (see the example in QR Code 18.3), to alert patients where rights are potentially infringed, to help them stay self-determined in the digital revolution, and to serve those patients who demand human care rather than digital help, even in an economically restricted environment.

QR Code 18.3

Moral choices of driverless cars.

Final Thoughts for Ethically Sound Digital Pharmaceutical Care

Unfortunately, space in this book does not allow a more comprehensive discussion of the ethical issues being presented in the digital age. However, you can find more comprehensive and detailed information online and most probably in your direct environment, where ethical communities debate the constantly emerging ethics in response to the exponential growth in technology (particularly, AI and robotic technologies), as well as new insights, frameworks, and thought patterns.

In many countries biomedical research is controlled by national consultative ethics committees. Similar bodies may be put into place either nationally or regionally to govern the ethics of digital health technology. Although these bodies may not monitor the regulatory compliance blueprint as described in Chapter 17, they may address ethical boundaries such as those described in this chapter.

Initiatives like the Partnership on AI (Partnership on AI, 2018) and the Future of Life Institute (Future of Life Institute, 2018) are examples of frameworks that aim to serve this purpose. They are a result of societal concerns about how to keep our digital revolution benevolent, how to warrant unified digital literacy, and how to protect individuals in a fully connected ecosystem.

Organizations and humans who want to proceed ethically must further scrutinize their actions and go beyond compliance and aim for the highest ethical standards. More institutions are drafting extensive codes of conduct, but it is questionable if these efforts will be a panacea for ethical difficulties. However, cultural factors such as feeling confident enough to speak up, balancing care with commercial pressures, identifying conflicting goals, or improving role modeling may accelerate the creation of ethical codes of conduct and create intrinsic understanding of ethical standards.

During their academic studies most healthcare professionals internalize ethical standards such as those based on the principles in the Hippocratic Oath. Healthcare practitioners should be granted time to focus on this important aspect of care, and they should be rewarded for investing time to facilitate making the right decisions together with patients.

Time to Care

In many of today's healthcare systems, patients are viewed as numbers and symptoms in overcrowded waiting rooms. Doctors sometimes allow only a few minutes for a patient, and at times patients do not see a pharmacist. Many healthcare practitioners are overwhelmed by administrative burdens, the lack of collegial consultations, and the number of repetitive tasks they perform, all of which can lead patients to think that these practitioners don't really care about individual patients.

However, when asked, many healthcare practitioners say that they chose their profession primarily to care for and give time to people in need of healthcare. These practitioners honestly would like to have more time to make the ethical considerations needed in healthcare systems and to support personalized treatment of patients based on professional knowledge and values.

Let us foster and further root a system of ethical, well-grounded human care providers so that they are fully embedded in society and ultimately have the tools they need to determine the boundaries of what good healthcare is, to take care for their fellow creatures, and to prevent sabotage of these human-inspired roles by digital interventions, even while using them to patients' advantage.

The authors realize that one chapter in a broad-spectrum book does not allow us to elaborate in more detail some of the major topics of digital ethics. Therefore we have set for ourselves the goal to continue working in and studying this field and in the future contribute to the specific, research-based literature on the evolving digital ethics in pharmaceutical care.

In the next Chapter 19 we will further elaborate on education, required to be prepared for the digital revolution.

    This means for circular pharmaceutical care:

- Every pharmaceutical care practitioners is expected to responsibly balance the expectations and needs of individual patients with those of society.
- Pharmaceutical care practitioners' core values are meant to act as beacons in the open-ended journey of ethical decision making.
- Digital ethics provide the concepts to work ethically with digital technology through an understanding of the background, methods, principles, procedures, regulations, and institutions that govern the appropriate use of the technology.
- The human touch, potentially augmented by digital technology, is the key part of practicing medicine and pharmacy. It is an integral part of the patient-pharmacist relationship.
- Helping patients protect their data is a core task of all professional caregivers.
- The combination of consecutive data mining and the big platforms' vast influence and increasing pharmaceutical interests are, to say the least, a global ethical concern for professionals, policymakers, and patients.
- Successful health interventions ideally target individual goals that patients feel committed to and that support a meaningful life.
- Healthcare practitioners should be facilitated, rewarded, and granted time to solve ethical dilemmas that come with the digital revolution.

An animation—kindly adopted by Service Apotheken Nederland—on the topic of Digital Ethics for Pharmaceutical Care can be found on www.pharmacare.ai.

QR Code Animation

Digital Ethics.

Educational biome

Claudia Rijcken

Learning never exhausts the mind.
Leonardo da Vinci

The Fourth Industrial Revolution has brought us advanced robotics and autonomous transport, artificial intelligence and machine learning, advanced materials, biotechnology, genomics, and much more. Those technologies have significantly changed the pharmaceutical biome. A biome is characterized by a variety of different habitats, and in healthcare many, if not all, professional habitats are experiencing serious changes. In light of these large-scale changes, the educational requirements needed to function adequately within this healthcare biome must change as well.

In this chapter you will read about competencies and skills of pharmaceutical care providers, how they are expected to change in the digital epoch, and which ones are required to lead circular pharmaceutical care.

The digital revolution transforms the way we live, the way we work, and the way we learn. We know that some jobs will disappear due to AI, that others will grow, and that many jobs that don't exist today will become commonplace. We also know that the future workforce will need to align its skillset with these changes to keep pace. Moreover, we know that the winners won't be those who can run the fastest, but those who are the most agile and can adjust their journey successfully.

Let's take a look at what this new environment means for pharmaceutical practice. We will look at knowledge domains, competencies (defined as the proficiency to act within a certain domain successfully or efficiently), as well as skills (defined as the ability to do a certain task or activity well and which are developed through training or expertise).

Characteristics of a Professional Practice

As shown in Chapter 6, a professional practice is the application of knowledge that is guided by a philosophy and purpose towards the resolution of specific problems. This precise knowledge held by a practitioner is applied according to a standard that is accepted by professional review. Moreover, practice in the case of pharmacy means the experience a practitioner encounters during the process of caring for a patient (Cipolle et al., 2012).

Pharmaceutical care providers are professionals, as they become competent in their role through substantial academic training; they maintain their skills through continuing professional development and commit to behaving ethically to protect the interests of both the individual and the public.

Knowledge Domains in Pharmaceutical Care

Three knowledge domains are the basis for pharmaceutical care providers: knowledge of medicine, of the human body, and of human behavior (KNMP, 2016). Through their extensive understanding of the interactions among these domains, pharmacists add value to the care continuum.

The study of pharmacy comprises knowledge of medicines in the broadest sense, both inside and outside the human body. The knowledge of medicines outside the human body includes the characteristics of products in terms of storage and use, development, production, quality control, and control of biopharmaceutical properties such as bioavailability and absorption.

Pharmaceutical knowledge also includes comprehension of the effects of medicines inside the human body and the implications of their use and administration. This means that a clear understanding of the human body and human behavior in illness and in health are also included within the knowledge domain of pharmacy, which requires proficiency in anatomy, physiology, pathophysiology, and psychology. The tenets of this discipline enable the pharmacist to develop a clear understanding of the actions and effects of medicines in the body.

In many countries, community and hospital pharmacies have evolved from a product-oriented profession to a more patient-centered profession. Thus understanding human behavior is considered of growing importance in the provision of pharmacotherapy and the goal to achieve optimal patient outcomes (KNMP, 2016).

Competencies

The International Pharmaceutical Federation (FIP) places competencies of pharmacists in four categories: pharmaceutical public health, pharmaceutical care, organization and management, and professional/personal (FIP, 2012).

Moreover, in several countries up-to-date standards and assessment tools are published to describe the competencies, skills, attitudes, and attributes essential to a practicing pharmacist (KNMP, 2016; Australia PSA, 2016; Singapore MoH, 2017; South African Government, 2017; Canada CCocEip, 2017; Pharmacy Council NZ, 2015; Irish Institute of Pharmacy, 2017).

In the majority of these standards, there is a consistency in the essential competency domains, which can be categorized as follows:

- Expert professional patient care
- Public health and integrated working relations
- Leadership and management
- Product and distribution excellence
- Education, training, and quality
- Research, innovation, and evaluation

Digital health literacy as an individual competency is not yet separately described; however, in some countries an integrated subset of competencies fall in the six preceding categories.

Skills

In 1999 the WHO developed the concept of the "seven-star pharmacist," detailing the skills and attitudes required of pharmacists to be effective members of the healthcare team. In 2000 the FIP adopted this concept in its policy on pharmacy education.

The required skillsets of a pharmacist are described as

- caregiver;
- decision maker;
- communicator;
- manager;
- lifelong learner;
- teacher; and
- leader

The WHO and FIP later added the function of researcher in their 2006 handbook entitled *Developing Pharmacy Practice: A Focus on Patient Care* (FIP, 2009).

After graduation, pharmacists can develop a generalist profile (as many community pharmacists are) or can specialize in a specific topic or range of skills (as seen more often in clinical pharmacies). The level of patient focus can vary significantly within these profiles.

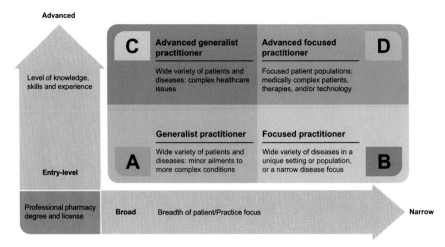

FIGURE 19.1

Skills in terms of patient and practice focus (Council on Credentialing in Pharmacy, 2010).

Figure 19.1 shows how skillsets can develop depending on the role and expertise, as can be seen in a community pharmacy.

Shift From Product-Orientation to Patient-Centricity

Pharmacists who intend to play a more active role in direct patient care shift their focus from products to helping people use the products in the most optimal way.

As Cipolle and colleagues noted in 2012, pharmaceutical care is a service that starts with understanding patients' concerns, beliefs, and behaviors associated with their medication and beyond (Cipolle et al., 2012).

It is a service beyond the distribution of medicines; however, in many countries the care-responsibility is not yet mainstream, mainly driven by the fact that the responsibility for this service is not everywhere institutionalized as a formal role of pharmacists (as there is overlap in knowledge and skills with other patient care providers) and therefore, often not or not fully reimbursed.

Nevertheless, many studies on pharmacy practices have shown that in an integrated approach with physicians, pharmacists are instrumental in improving patients' adherence and health outcomes through interventions such as counseling, pushing reminders for adherence, driving medication surveillance, or running medication reviews to optimize treatment profiles.

In countries which have a legal responsibility in patient treatment and treatment outcomes such as the Nordic countries, the Netherlands, and Canada, pharmacists are allowed to and rewarded for intervening and discussing treatment with a patient and the patient's other healthcare providers. Skillsets related to understanding human behavior like mastering effective human dialogue, understanding the psychology of interviewing, demonstrating empathy, active listening, and effectively anticipating patient and customer needs are expected to become ever-more important skills, as we explain later in this chapter.

Lifelong Learning Paradigm and Adopting Digital Change

While the fundamental competencies linked to the three knowledge domains will remain of vital importance, many, if not all, pharmacists around the world acknowledge that after they entered the labor market, a number of additional competencies and skills did become also very relevant to grow fast in their professional leadership.

As in all professions, a lifelong learning attitude is essential, but it's particularly the case in the health field, where we must adapt to nearly constant innovations, such as new, advanced methods of administering medication, progress in cell and gene therapy, the demand for precision medicine, and changes in the dynamic relationship between patients and healthcare providers.

Pharmacists may benefit from an initial broader set of skills related to understanding the (local) healthcare system, ethical scoping, and balanced communication, which are increasingly domains that become more important in the digital pharmaceutical care process.

Additionally, as explained in Chapter 6, initial and ongoing education on digital abilities and digital health literacy may bridge potential gaps with the fast developing digital global ecosystem.

Previous research on a range of global pharmacist-led interventions reported that pharmacists lack confidence in their digital abilities. This perceived lack of preparedness was linked to a potential fear towards a responsibility shift, a slight tech-averseness in the profession, a strong preference for human interactions, and discomfort with new, ambiguous situations like the introduction of digital opportunities in the healthcare landscape (Rosenthal et al., 2010).

A more recent global study indicated that more pharmacists now recognize the potential of digital health and intend to learn more about it in order to integrate it into their daily practice (Benetoli et al., 2017).

The Benetoli study, however, showed that in 2016 pharmacists were somewhat skeptical about implementing digital health tools. Some of the main barriers were difficulty in establishing the boundaries of a professional relationship when adopting digital tools and the perceived fear of providing misleading information. As the ecosystem is in a transition phase and not all factors are clear as yet, these barriers are understandable in a profession like pharmacy. Nevertheless, education may eliminate some of the perceived barriers.

Pharmacy education addresses the competencies and skills through programs that teach elements of product expertise, pharmaceutical patient care, medication policy, quality care and research, and innovation, both at the undergraduate and the postgraduate levels (Rug et al., 2016).

In general, the study of pharmacy includes Science, Technology, Engineering, and Mathematics, collectively known as STEM. To many, these four disciplines form the basis for the skills needed to be successful in the evolving jobs of the future, as can be seen in QR Code 19.1.

QR Code 19.1

Future of jobs.

A New Fundamental Competency Proposed

Taking into consideration the advances in health technology as described in the previous parts of this book, it can be argued that a seventh competency should be added to the six competencies of the pharmacist. This seventh competency could be called *digital pharmacy literacy.*

The competency would link to all three knowledge domains and is defined as follows: *The pharmacist has expertise on digital healthcare technology in relation to optimizing patient outcomes of drug therapy and/or pharmaceutical interventions.*

The competency translates into skills that enable the pharmacist to

- develop, review, judge, and use digital health technology and data to optimize the management of adequate and safe drugs;
- counsel patients on digital health technology that improves the impact of medication use;
- analyze holistic data sets of both individual patients and broader populations to enable understanding of predictive analytics that support personalized care, prevention, and if needed population-based interventions; and
- translate analytic results into improved patient services.

As noted in Chapter 8 it will be beneficial for pharmaceutical care providers to gain understanding of which (emerging) data and data sets will be important in a future pharmacy business; which digital tools are required to converge suitable patient services that track the required data; how to collect, analyze, and visualize data; and how to translate the outcomes into benefits for patients.

Systematic implementation of this seventh domain can produce three positive results:

- Pharmaceutical care providers will be more aware of how technology influences their profession and will have a basic understanding of how to implement this technology to optimize pharmaceutical care.
- Pharmaceutical care providers will be able to select and use patient data sets to tailor individualized pharmaceutical care.
- Some providers will choose to specialize in pharmaceutical informatics or data science. They will become experts in big data analysis for population-based risk monitoring, stratification, and intervention optimization

The following sections provide more detail on how to operationalize this seventh competency domain.

Understanding the Ecosystem of Digital Health Technology

As outlined in previous chapters in this book, digital health technology is essential to augment pharmaceutical care providers and drive enhanced apothecary intelligence. Therefore at both the undergraduate level and the postgraduate level, being able to understand and select which digital (health) devices can make a central contribution to support and augment professional pharmaceutical care is of increasing importance.

Also, it will become more pivotal to be able to determine whether digital health content or support is genuine, as unfortunately false content is flooding the virtual space. Trained pharmaceutical care providers can consult patients to make decisions for reliable digital tools and thus can augment the trusted reputation that pharmaceutical care providers have globally.

In the business world, companies mastering digital excellence differ from less innovative ones in that the former's leadership is constantly investing in more digital tools and skills (Westerman et al., 2014). The difference in skills usually extends beyond technology, as digital transformation also requires changes in processes and thinking, as addressed in Part 4 of this book.

Thus, in order to master digital excellence, dedicated, ongoing education is imperative.

Data Consciousness

Being digital tool-savvy is one thing, but understanding how to use the data these tools produce is even more important. Nevertheless, in many countries computer science, data management, and information technology educational tracks are siloed from traditional pharmacy educational tracks.

Thus only pharmacy students with a clear affinity for technology and data topics will probably look for data science education during their academic education. They tend to find themselves back in departments like bioinformatics, health informatics, epidemiology, or even econometrics.

University of Buffalo's Jacobs School of Medicine and Biomedical Sciences, New York: Inspiration for Pharmacy

The medical school's Department of Biomedical Informatics trains doctoral and postdoctoral researchers in three major areas: *clinical informatics*, including sociotechnical and human-centered design, workflow analysis and cybersecurity; *translational bioinformatics*, including database management, pharmacogenomics, and predictive modeling; and *clinical research informatics*, including a big-data science training program, statistical machine learning, and data mining.

These training programs are designed to meet the growing need for investigators trained in biomedical computing, data science, and related information fields. Many universities around the world increasingly offer these hybrid academic programs, which prepare the students for valuable (new) positions in the medical and pharmaceutical arena.

On the other hand, although a number of universities have been introducing health data science master programs, many data scientists and (digital health) informatics students are educated with limited exposure to the professions that they will ultimately support once they join the labor market.

Thus, while many data scientists and data analysts tend to graduate with limited exposure to the true challenges in the pharmaceutical care journey, many data-savvy pharmacists tend to graduate with little access to information about the opportunities of healthcare technology, data analysis, and interpretation (for both individual patients and the broader population).

Once these graduates from different background enter the labour market, there is yet limited understanding of each other's competencies, so building effective combinatoric innovation (as in Chapter 2) will be a rather laggy process. Earlier cross-fertilization of digital and pharma knowledge can optimize this situation.

The solution seems simple. Gradually, we bring the fields closer together to allow cross-functional fertilization early in the university track and also in postgraduate curricula. There are already a number of examples where a hybrid approach could inspire pharmaceutical programs, as reflected in the example of Buffalo University in New York.

It will be important for both fields to become acquainted with continuous cross-functional approaches and to motivate interactions between personalities to bring together a variety of backgrounds, sparking comprehensive thinking patterns and building combined synergy. This synergy may drive creativity and better decision-making abilities, but above all shared understanding on how to optimize the pharmaceutical care pathway of the future.

It will not be necessary for practitioners in either field (pharmaceutical or data science and digital health informatics) to be expert in both fields in order to execute their role adequately in the future. Early awareness and understanding and being able to engage in dialogue about a digital solution in pharmacy will dramatically improve their position when they enter the labor market.

Specializing in Pharmacy Informatics

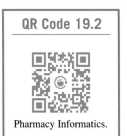

QR Code 19.2

Pharmacy Informatics.

In some countries a new academic track was formed to support candidates who want to specialize in informatics pharmacy jobs. These types of curricula are often called pharmacy informatics. For instance, the definition of the specialization proposed by the Canadian Association of Pharmacists is "the study of the interactions between people, work processes and health systems with a focus on pharmaceutical care and patient safety" (QR Code 19.2).

The Healthcare Information and Management Systems Society (HIMSS) defines pharmacy informatics as "the scientific field that focuses on medication-related data and knowledge within the continuum of healthcare systems—including its acquisition, storage, analysis, use and dissemination." Pharmacy informaticists take their knowledge of medication management and apply it to the design and development of discipline-specific systems and software. They can also be characterized as the interface between pharmacy and information technology.

The need for pharmacy informatics has been increasing and many educational systems are not organized sufficiently enough to provide interested students with all the content required in the field (Steckler et al., 2017).

Pharmacy informatics specialists typically work in pharmacy chains or managed care organizations, in hospitals, in payer environments, in academia, or in startups. With access to a broad set of pharmaceutical care data, these specialists develop, for example, digital clinical decision support systems, digital pharmaceutical care tools, or software that analyzes patient outcomes.

Although not every pharmacist needs to be a pharmacy informatics expert, every pharmacist needs to have an interest in the area, as many of us will work with zettabytes of data, as noted in Chapter 8.

General Skills Required for Pharmaceutical Care in the Digital Revolution

In 2015 the World Economic Forum (WEF) released an overview of skills considered as essential to thrive in the Fourth Industrial Revolution. It is expected that over one third of skills (35%) that were considered important in the 2015 workforce will have changed by 2020, according to the WEF (see QR Code 19.1).

Let us delve a bit further into a number of these skills and their relevance for pharmaceutical care providers.

Complex problem solving is expected to remain the most important asset that people can bring into a working environment. This is particularly relevant in the pharmaceutical care sector, as the academic fields of pharmacy and data science are becoming more and more integrated and half-time of pharmaceutical science knowledge is reduced more than ever. The analytic and biochemical nature of the education enables a pharmacist to reduce a problem to its core elements and to think critically and conceptually about what the solution might be.

In pharmaceutical care this means being able to reflect on changing ecosystems, analyze the healthcare system needs, define the new role and skillsets of pharmaceutical care providers, drive innovative processes by optimizing the PC design, integrate analytic and predictive technology, and so on.

With the avalanche of new medicines, *creativity* means new technologies and new ways of working, which is crucial for developing, staying abreast of, and benefiting from innovations. Although the algorithms and technologies described in Chapters 11 and 12 will enhance the work of pharmaceutical care providers, constructing these algorithms so that they are as creative and agile as humans will take a long time. In fact, it is even questionable whether robots will ever develop the creative and relational reasoning of humans. Identifying the best digital pharmaceutical care solutions requires out-of-the-box thinking, and educational frameworks should encourage providers to develop this skill by, for example, periodically thinking and working outside of their own area, continuously learning about mechanisms, and developing cross-functional approaches.

Emotional intelligence, which wasn't one of the top 10 skills identified by the WEF in 2015, will become a pivotal skill needed by pharmaceutical care providers (Gray, 2016). Emotional intelligence (EI) is the ability of individuals to recognize their own and other people's emotions, discern between different feelings and label them appropriately, use emotional information to guide thinking and behavior, and manage and adjust emotions to adapt to environments or achieve one's goal (Wikipedia, 2017c).

As addressed in this book's Foreword, EI is an essential skill that (at least at the time of this writing) separates humans from machines. Being able to read emotions, show empathy, understand feelings, and connect facts with emotions and react to them to guide interventions and solve issues are abilities unique to humans. Although facial expression and other behavioral analyses may provide important insights, it is expected to take at least decades before computers will be able to read true emotions and respond accordingly, if at all. In order for EI to thrive, qualities such as curiosity, empathy, adaptability, and emotional agility will need to be developed in such systems.

 Judgment and decision making will continue to be two of the most important skills enabling PCPs to adequately judge factors such as the value of digital tools, the ethical considerations of treatment choices, and the safety of artificial intelligence. Whether it is the jungle of apps, the rainforests of wearables, or the savannas of virtual reality, to truly make a balanced decision, digital health literacy needs to be augmented with discernment as to whether these data are unbiased, algorithms are programmed for benevolent outcomes, and last but not least how to synergize human factors with the results of big-data health analysis into something that is really meaningful for patients.

Connecting and coordinating with other healthcare system stakeholders was considered as an essential skill in 2015. Although technology can facilitate connecting technically, it is the human connective skill that will reduce factors such as silo-thinking and drive a shift towards making integrated pharmaceutical care plans and develop joint pathways to improved patient outcomes. Healthcare systems are under severe pressure globally and pharmaceutical stakeholders are a part of the puzzle that has to be solved. Only with a connected approach can sustainable and circular systems be developed, and in order to do so coordination and human connectivity skills are crucial.

Pharmaceutical care providers often face the daunting task of communicating with patients, employees, insurers, and physician office staff under time and resource restraints. The providers' educational backgrounds, levels of understanding, and preferred learning modes vary. This is why effective communication skills should continue to get sufficient attention in educational programs, as they are considered the ultimate prerequisite for people working together, achieving synergy, and integrating the different stakeholder's perspectives (Yao, 2016).

Serious Gaming to Enhance Skillsets

An interesting way to enhance the previously mentioned skills of the future may be through gaming. Serious gaming, as noted in Chapter 6, can be defined as the use of game principles for the purposes of learning, skill acquisition, and training. Although learners typically enjoy serious games over traditional lectures, serious games are effective not because they are games, but because of the cognitive and psychological processes involved when learners play them (Cain and Piascik, 2015).

One distinct advantage of gaming is the ability to establish a hypothetical "real" environment for learning in which the consequences of mistakes are minimized. Thus when undergraduate and postgraduate pharmacists are exposed to digital advances such as virtual reality, wearables, or chatbots; or to real-world data analysis and interpretation; or to future moral dilemmas, they have the opportunity to recognize the potential real-world needs of their future patients and learn how to adequately respond to those needs.

Unlike the vast majority of traditional educational methods, in game-based learning environments students receive dynamic and immediate feedback on their skills, knowledge, strategies, and so on. This adaptive feedback permits participants to learn from their previous failures, which is a vital feature of game-based learning. Learning from mistakes can be extremely powerful, as shown in Chapter 2, as it can boost the confidence of pharmacists and enable them to approach digital challenges with sureness in future endeavors.

The Future of the Pharmaceutical Care Job

Every now and then warnings pop up that automation and new technology will wipe out large numbers of middle-class jobs. However, these warnings have existed for many decades. When the agrimotor was developed farmers were afraid they would become redundant; however, there are still farmers, and some farmers effectively shifted to positions that had not existed prior to the introduction of the agrimotor.

The point is that skilled jobs are going to be in more demand, and unskilled jobs will change. For example, driving a car may not be a major source of employment a decade from now. But there will be new or other things that logically can't be automated, and unskilled labor is expected to move into those categories, just as many moved from agriculture to factories to the service economy.

How AI will affect the job market
Predicted net job creation by sector (2017–2037)

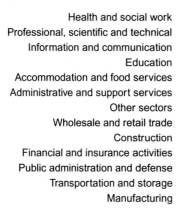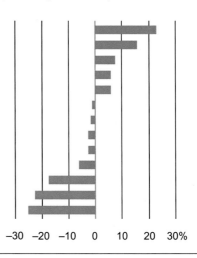

FIGURE 19.2

Job creation forecast in different industries. Reproduced from PwC (2018).

Figure 19.2 exemplifies how jobs are expected to be changed by artificial intelligence.

We expect a similar situation for pharmaceutical care providers. In a healthcare system under pressure due to aging and budget constraints (see Part 1 of this book), automating some tasks may provide more space for other (human, nonautomated) tasks, and the digital revolution will offer new roles as well.

Analyze Which Tasks Can Be Automated, and Which Tasks Cannot

Healthcare in general is not an industry where jobs can be easily automated. For example, in the United States healthcare is expected to have only a 30%–40% sensitivity for automation, which is strongly related to the fact that the care element is something machines cannot yet take over (McKinsey, 2018).

To understand the impact of the digital revolution on your own role, it makes sense to detail the tasks that belong to a certain competency framework and strive to identify which of those tasks are prone to automation versus which ones are much more difficult for machines to perform (the ones where the human factor is central).

Doing this analysis provides first of all insight into the areas where machines substitute some parts of certain functions, but it also provides new perspectives on the actual value of a role and how to valorize the role in the future.

Be Prepared for New Roles

 Even if the analysis ends up showing that your role can be automated in large part, another aspect has to be considered. It is a Marxian concept in which many roles will be obsolete due to automation, but as indicated earlier the reality has been that machines also complement labor, raising output in ways that lead to higher or at least other demands for labor and that interact with adjustments in the workforce.

That said, what are some potential new roles in pharmaceutical care? It is easy to imagine that pharmacy chains in the future will need a manager to oversee the quality of wearables, a digital therapeutic associate, or a pharmbot specialist.

In general, pharmaceutical care providers may need to obtain guidance from a digital apothecary intelligence leader or a virtual pharmacy reality officer. Moreover, roles like pharmacy data interoperability lead, digital health management team member, or adherence data expert will be the backbone of future pharmacy institutions.

The authors leave it up to the reader to imagine how these roles' job profiles will look, but trust in the fact that this way of thinking will spark our vision of how current pharmaceutical care roles can migrate to new ones.

In conclusion, half-time of knowledge is being reduced faster in the digital revolution, quickly changing the requirements of the educational biome for pharmaceutical care providers. However, given the professional standards of pharmaceutical care providers, their competencies and skills, and the fact that it will still take quite some time before machines are capable of performing the valued roles that humans perform, pharmaceutical care providers will not be usurped any time soon but will evolve and adapt to adjusted and new role descriptions.

In the last Part 4 of this book, we will deep-dive into activities to do today to be prepared for the digital day after tomorrow.

 This means for circular pharmaceutical care:

- Pharmaceutical education is expected to continue as a STEM+ education.
- Digital pharmacy literacy is proposed as the seventh knowledge domain of pharmacists.
- Not every pharmacist needs to be a pharmacy informatics expert, but every pharmacist should be interested in pharmacy informatics.
- Cross-fertilization between pharmacy and data science should start as early as possible in educational pathways to stimulate faster synergy in later working environments.
- General skills needed to excel in the digital revolution are expected to shift largely to human emotional intelligence, sound judgment, and excellent reasoning abilities; thus these skills need to receive sufficient attention in future educational tracks.
- Based on the digital evolution, new pharmaceutical care roles will develop, and at this point we can only guess what their formal titles will be.

An animation—kindly adopted by Pharmabrain—on the topic of Education for Digital Pharmaceutical Care can be found on www.pharmacare.ai.

Education.

How: What to do tomorrow as a pharmaceutical care leader

Digital by Design: Creating effective future oxygen supply

20

Claudia Rijcken

You must be the change you want to see in the world
M. Gandhi

Much as oxygen does in our physical environment, to energize other systems and structures, it is vital to analyze how to efficiently generate new sources of energy. To do so requires identifying areas that need improvement, areas that are open to change, adequate resources and tools, followed by seamless execution and agile adjustment.

In this chapter you will read about Digital by Design (DbD), which is a structured framework meant as a guide to effectively implement digital innovation into daily pharmaceutical care practices. DbD is accomplished in several phases that address the questions why, who, what, and how, followed by the do (production and implementation) and sustain phases.

In digital transformative processes, technological choices and strategies for their use are expected to match the results derived from up-front strategic analyses, as this information sets standards for how processes, products, and services are designed.

The principles of Quality by Design are useful in pharmaceutical care systems. Joseph M. Juran, a quality expert, first outlined this concept.

Designing for quality is one of the three universal processes of the Juran Trilogy, in which Juran describes what is required to achieve breakthroughs in new products, services, and processes. Juran believes that quality can be planned and that most quality crises and problems relate to the way in which quality is planned in the design process. In this respect, the principles of Quality by Design was introduced in pharmaceutical development as a systematic approach to achieving quality in pharmaceutical manufacturing by implementing six well-defined steps (Yu, 2008).

In digital transformative processes in pharmaceutical care, this framework may be referred to Digital by Design (DbD). DbD can be defined as a systematic approach to digital service development that begins with predefined objectives and emphasizes the target population and process understanding

Pharmaceutical Care in Digital Revolution. https://doi.org/10.1016/B978-0-12-817638-2.00020-1

and control, based on solid analysis and up-front risk management. In digital pharmaceutical care, this approach means that the likelihood of a digital solution's success is determined largely by the attention paid to digitization processes during the design phase.

DbD is not a statistical method, but an early structured framework to build digital perspectives into a service model. It is built on the basis of a solid understanding of the product and process by which it is developed, along with knowledge of the risks involved in designing the service and how best to mitigate those risks (see also Part 3 of this book).

DbD is best depicted as six crucial steps:

1. WHY: Identify true pharmaceutical care problem and the blue sky
2. WHO: Select the most relevant patient group
3. WHAT: Validate how the target population sees the blue sky
4. HOW: Choose the most suitable future solution (may be digital)
5. DO: Lead the (digital) transformation process
6. SUSTAIN: Check the new process and adjust, where required

FIGURE 20.1

Digital by Design in pharmaceutical care.

In the following sections, the six steps shown in Figure 20.1 are further explained.

WHY: Identify True Pharmaceutical Care Problem and the Blue Sky

To identify solutions with the highest likelihood for success, a defined problem and the desired result need to be made crystal clear by envisioning the best possible outcome (i.e., its future blue sky), balanced by the previously explained triple goal of achieving healthier populations, better treatment for patients, and more balanced costs. Whether the impetus for change is due to innovative goals or more resource efficiency, improved patient satisfaction, or changing healthcare policies, the current pharmaceutical care pathway will have to be adequately analyzed and potential bottlenecks in that pathway transparently brought to the table (QR Code 20.1).

In healthcare systems under pressure (as we discuss in Chapters 1, 3, and 4), up-front envisioning, where optimal patient outcomes can be created by a team of healthcare providers makes the most sense. After implementation of a solution, it becomes clear how a solid definition of the preferred and measurable outcome positively affects the process and the role that WHY plays in the process. For example, if pathway optimization for psoriasis is the focus, defining why all stakeholders see a PASI score of 100, which is above the more commonly used score of 90, as the preferred clinical outcome may be the first step. Or defining why a Quality of Life (QoL) improvement of 10 points on a Visual Analogue Scale (VAS) is more clinically relevant than an improvement of 5 points in a certain disease. Or why choosing to track PREMS outcomes may prevail over PROMS in a given optimization project (see Chapter 3 for more on this topic).

Also, when defining the WHY, preferably take into account aspects that may affect patients' needs, regulatory and legal boundaries, and potential corporate conditions; also, local team preferences and process optimization goals should be made explicit.

WHY Questions to ask in the WHY phase are, for example: Why would we want to change a current pathway? Why should we consider a digital solution? Why are patient outcomes suboptimal in the current pathway? Why should we improve patient convenience? Why is the safety of patients in potential danger? Why is the process organized in a unsustainable way, leading to otherwise avoidable waste or harm? Why is a blended care approach most feasible? Why is an increase in cost-effectiveness a potential outcome?

Posing open questions is preferred, and once analyzed in detail they can lead to well-defined, demarcated topics that, if feasible, can then be used in the next step: whom are we targeting?

The WHY phase often involves a labor-intensive, serious strategic management process that is analytical in nature and that requires formalized procedures in order to produce data and analyses that can then be used as input for strategic thinking.

One pitfall for many organizations is the time it takes to define a new strategy. It is important that an organization aligns its goals and the pace of its strategic process in a timely way; otherwise, the solution it derives might be obsolete the moment it is presented. Because the process requires knowledge of and experience with current pharmaceutical care pathways and an analytical, curious, and structured mindset to identify bottlenecks, it is important to identify the right talent and skills required to do the job in an accurate and timely way.

 The WHY process should lead, for instance, to a stated mission and a vision of how a blue-sky situation might look after the digital innovation project is completed and implemented.

WHO: Select the Most Relevant Patient Group

Now that the mission and vision of a digital transformation is formulated, the next DbD step is to determine who will benefit most from optimization of the process and whom to target in the first pilot. Every disease has its own type of treatment and determinants. The better those are understood up front, the easier it will be to a select a group that may benefit most from an outcome-based innovation pathway. Is it the elderly population, who are slightly tech-averse but may have the highest likelihood of satisfaction after a social robot helps them with their medication? Or is it Generation Z, who are hesitant to visit physical pharmacies but instead want to manage their healthcare needs online and thus may be happy to have a chatbot provide answers to the questions they ask?

 WHO   Questions to ask in the WHO phase are, for example: Who is most adversely affected by the current suboptimal process? Who is a stakeholder in the optimization process and therefore should be involved, for example, patients, physicians, payers, or governments? Who would be most happy with the improved outcomes and should we defined as the target population? Who will benefit financially from a cost-effectiveness improvement?

The WHO process should lead, for instance, to clear segmentation of the target population in scope and the stakeholders relevant to include in the digital service design.

WHAT: Validate How the Target Population Sees the Blue Sky

As noted in Chapter 5, the wishes and needs of patients should be addressed as early as possible in the Digital Pharmaceutical Care (DPC) equation. Assumptions on why the mission and vision matter, whether envisioned outcomes make sense for patients, and which group of people will benefit most should be validated in order to develop a service that truly meets the needs of the final customer.

To gain better insight on the requirements and expectations of patients or healthcare system stakeholders, a short proof-of-principle or proof-of-concept trial can be used. If that is not possible, validated survey techniques to determine patients' needs may be used. Focus groups, structured polls, interviews, and broader analytic searches for expectations of customers may provide more insight on how to connect the professional's ideal world with the expectations of other pharmaceutical care stakeholders, such as patients and payers.

 WHAT   Questions to ask in the WHAT phase are, for example: What do we think of our mission, vision, and expected outcome improvement plan; are we tackling a real problem? What is the blue-sky outcome for patients (e.g., clinical value or changed process)? Will this principle work in our specific case? What value will the solution offer to the end consumer? What impact can we expect on quality of life? What determinants of health are most affected by the digital service concept? What advantages will it give other stakeholders?

The WHAT process should lead, for instance, to an aligned perspective on what matters most to the target population and on the positive impact the digital service will have on improving the lives of those taking medications.

HOW: Choose the Most Suitable Future Solution

Once the reason for change is identified, the optimal outcome is clearly defined and validated, and the target population is identified, the basic strategies for changing a project are for the most part complete. Because in principle digital technology follows strategy, now is the time to determine whether and how a digital solution can help relieve the identified problem.

As noted earlier digital technology does not always provide the solution. For example, if the target population see its blue sky as being improvement of low-threshold, verbal explanations, then adjustments to the current care pathway should start with solid communication planning (rather than a digital solution).

In other situations analysis may reveal that measuring digital biomarkers at home increases the likelihood of identifying adverse effects earlier than does seeing patients in the community or hospital pharmacy, in which case digital therapeutic devices may be the most suitable option.

In the first case, the first three steps of the DdD model (WHY, WHO, WHAT) led to a nondigital solution that solved the problem; in the second case digitalization provided the answer.

In the HOW phase, technology should be regarded as an enabler, may be supportive, may be an outcome measurement tool, or may even be the game changer in a program. Choosing the best equipment to provide optimal patient solutions requires a thorough analysis of the technologies proposed in Part 2 of this book and their conditions for success.

To redesign an implementation plan so that it offers a new paradigm, the current pharmaceutical care process needs to be viewed from a process-engineering perspective. Process redesign analysis is a redesign of core processes with the purpose of finding and implementing breakthrough improvements to those processes (Persson, 1995).

Process Redesign in Healthcare

Kaiser Permanente (KP), a US-based managed care organization (MCO), recognized in the early 2010s an opportunity to rethink how to deliver care specifically related to patient experience and affordability. Under the project name Reimaging Ambulatory Design (RAD), the organization explored how and where healthcare will be delivered in the future, how technology will be leveraged, how social trends influence health behavior, and how people will engage in their own care.

RAD consists of three design principles, six strategies, dozens of tactics, and five platform solutions. Each platform solution includes a detailed patient experience framework that recasts the entire network delivery strategy with specific recommendations for the service model, operations, facility design, and technology.

It completely changed the way new healthcare ecosystems at KP are currently being built.

In previous literature pharmaceutical processes have been described typically as networks of processes (Romero, 2013). It is possible to take the full analytical approach and map the entire pharmaceutical process as a set of data points that experience transition into a next point and determine the efficiency or inefficiency of that transaction in a mathematical way. This analysis offers great insight as to where the most time, money, patient satisfaction, or treatment outcomes are lost. To conduct an analysis like this requires data analyst expertise, as noted in Chapter 19.

However, if this capability is not available, simply sequentially mapping the stepwise process of the patient pathway, as explained in Chapter 6, will be sufficient.

HOW

Questions to ask in the HOW phase are, for example: How does the current process look in a map? How could a digital solution lead to measurable improved outcomes? How is the literacy level of the target population that will use the digital solution and how are current adoption rates? How are advantages and disadvantages of various digital solutions positioned? How is the maturity level of the proposed digital solution and which data regarding privacy, quality, and security are publicly available? How can we test the solution? How do we assure agility and flexibility? How is the chosen digital solution interoperable with existing pharmacy applications? How is the capacity and scalability of the solution/platform? How could Kaggle help with identifying the best solution? How much money do we need to make the pilot happen? How does an implementation team look like? How do we set timelines?

Now is also the time to run a digital health compliance blueprint, as described in Chapter 17, as well as to consider the ethical aspects, as proposed in Chapter 18. When deciding to work with privacy-sensitive data flows or artificial intelligent solutions, in the design phase we need to consider potential ethical concerns and the prevailing moral values of good pharmaceutical care.

It is also important to realize that the HOW phase is not only about technology but is also about resources, research, and timing. Although the end-stage benefits will be huge, innovation in smaller teams may require a significant number of people, as well as a significant amount of time and money.

Another factor to determine in the HOW phase is the scalability of the project, that is, consider whether the application will be used only locally and if not whether it can be scaled up easily so that it can be used, for instance, in a regional pharmaceutical chain or even be scaled up to a global level. These factors determine the structure in which the digital tool must be developed, how the vendors work with and the stakeholders involved in the development process.

The HOW process should lead, for instance, to a sound, well-thought-out project plan, including timing, tools, people, stakeholders, and so on. Adequate project management expertise and support may be considered in this and the DO phase, regardless of the size of the organization.

DO: Lead the (Digital) Transformation Process

Now that the strategy, expected outcome, target population, and project plan are mapped, the project plan can be brought into seamless execution in the experimentation phase.

The well-known Chinese proverb, "A journey of a thousand miles begins with a single step," is applicable here. Too many dreams and plans slip away simply because people are afraid to take the initial step. Being courageous models the leadership needed to excite curiosity and the will to create new ideas. In Chapter 21 we expand on how to take on such a role and create a culture for success.

Also, being adaptive and open to change during the process is important. Mario Andretti, one of most successful racecar drivers in history, once said: "If everything seems under control, you're not going fast enough." Transformation is a volatile and unsettled phase. In this phase, the notion of brilliant failures (refer to Chapter 2) can help create a failure-and-risk-accepting attitude towards innovation.

How to Lead Digital Transformation

The World Economic Forum addressed four themes that will be of crucial importance to the digital transformation of healthcare over the next decade: smart care, care anywhere, empowered care, and intelligent healthcare enterprise (WEF, 2017). The relevance of these themes to pharmaceutical care are reflected in different settings within this book.

Pharmaceutical care providers, with their strong STEM+ competency profile (see Chapter 19) combined with digital health literacy, are perfectly suited to act as leaders in the four domains indicated by the World Economic Forum.

While Mario Andretti's comment might seem unnerving at first, it is most appropriate for leaders who aim to navigate the digital world. No race—or transformation—is risk-free; thus having the leadership and courage to make decisions that push the limits of an organization is a necessity (Arora et al., 2017).

Here are a few tips that can help in the DO phase:

- Learn as much as you can about digital health technologies that can optimize your pharmaceutical care pathways. B. F. Skinner has been credited with saying, "Education is what survives when what has been learned has been forgotten." A vision based on this kind of knowledge can drive ongoing, innovative insights.
- Learn as much as you can about how people operate and leverage the wisdom of the crowd. Externally, it will help you understand patient behavior and achieve a smooth adoption process. Internally, it will help build a highly performing team that is willing, flexible, and resolute enough to implement innovation.

- Keep advocating the WHY mission and path. It will help you push forward when things become difficult (as they always do at a certain point in change processes). Doing so will require reenvisioning the future again and again.
- In the execution phase take time to see the bigger picture and identify new opportunities within the process. Strive to inspire teams, and let them propose adjustments and improvements. Doing so may well motivate the team and can ultimately create an iterative, innovative, self-learning environment.

> **DO**

Questions to ask in the DO phase are, for example: Does the digital solution truly support patient outcomes? Does the changed process meet target group expectations? Do we move according to plan? Do patients adopt the digital service according to expectation? Do we need to adjust strategy based on ongoing insights? Do we need to communicate first successes or failures, by whom and to whom? Do we need to involve additional stakeholders or team-members?

The DO process should lead, for instance, to a proof-of-concept report, showing the value of the (digital) service implementation, validation of the hypothesis of better patient outcomes, and transparency in patient satisfaction, potential scalability, and financial sustainability.

SUSTAIN: Check the New Process and Adjust Where Required

The design phase sets the right measurement parameters, and in equal measure a disciplined pharmaceutical care professional follows up on the acquired insights and adjusts the process where needed.

Experimentation in Step 5 in the DO process tends to lead to a wealth of new data, transformed into insights, that reflect either a strong improvement in a new patient pathway or a potential need to adjust the primary digital innovation in order to achieve even better results in the second plan. Or it may lead to the conclusion that a new service was not beneficial, for instance, because of legal, adoption, quality, or other reasons.

A pilot that will not scale up can still be useful if the reasons for failure are shared in order to keep others from making the same errors. Thus even if you have a project that ends in this way, consider the value of brilliant failures; perhaps it could be useful in the format proposed in the future thought 1 in the final chapter of the book.

In cases of success the new digital service can be scaled up to bigger or even different target populations. Additional stakeholders may be involved, more resources added, and new communication plans considered, including social media. A success is only a success once people are become aware of it.

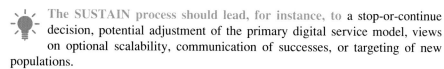

Questions to ask in the sustain phase are, for example: Did we meet the prespecified triple goals and do we wish to continue? Should we adjust parts of the services based on ongoing insights and target population expectations? Do tangible outcomes really show better patient satisfaction? For which populations could this digital tool offer a solution as well? Have projected outcomes been met within the expected timeframe? Which steps should be altered in order to produce better outcomes? Can circularity of the pharmaceutical pathway be made transparent, for example, by less medication waste, lower hospitalization rates, or better quality of life? How can we share what we learned with other stakeholders?

The SUSTAIN process should lead, for instance, to a stop-or-continue decision, potential adjustment of the primary digital service model, views on optional scalability, communication of successes, or targeting of new populations.

Considerations

The DbD concept is still in its infancy. Adopting a DbD framework may provide a more structured, innovative framework leading to improved patient outcomes. However, most important, gathering information and sharing insights garnered from the pilots will be imperative for future synergy among early adopters. Thus future thought 1 in the final discussion on sharing pilot experiences in MSOCs is an important step to consider in order to fuel our pharmaceutical care community with newly created oxygen.

The next Chapter 21 explains building a culture in order to successfully execute DbD frameworks.

This means for circular pharmaceutical care:

- DbD is a structured framework that facilitates effective implementation of digital innovation.
- WHY, WHO, WHAT, HOW, DO, and SUSTAIN are the essential steps for transforming the digital pharmaceutical care pathway in both corporate and small business environments.
- "A journey of a thousand miles begins with a single step." Just do it. With digital literacy, a professional analytical and ethical mindset, and a DbD-structured approach, the conditions are set for an optimal design process to start.
- DbD is still in its infancy, and active sharing of digital pharmaceutical care pilot experiences will support further development of the DbD paradigm.

Hayfields of high-performance cultural transformation

21

Paul Rulkens

We shape our buildings; thereafter our buildings shape us
Winston Churchill

Growing a hayfield is like building a high-performance culture: If you don't nurture it every day, it will quickly be overrun by weeds, and the beauty of the grasses will be soon overlooked.

In this chapter you will read about an actionable pathway that describes how digital pharmaceutical care providers can immediately start role modeling the essential behaviors to build a high-performance organization.

In a recent panel discussion about the future of healthcare, one of the panelists mentioned that artificial intelligence (AI) currently has a better track record of interpreting MRI images than its human radiologist counterparts, something that was noted in Chapter 11. It was concluded that in the near future we will divide radiologists into two groups. The first group consists of the radiologists who simply want their toys back and are doomed to defend an ever-shrinking turf of relevant expertise. The second group will consist of the radiologists who choose to expand their skills to be effective in those scenarios where human judgment, personal connection, and professional instinct trumps AI.

This is an interesting example of *the approaching train dilemma:* Imagine a train coming at us at a predictable trajectory and speed, and yet we find ourselves paralyzed, unable to react and therefore rely on hope to avert imminent disaster. If we know change is coming, what can pharmacy leaders and professionals start doing today to build the right organizational high-performance culture for the future?

Why Culture Drives Results

 In 1998 the struggling UK Olympic rowing team got a new coach. He quickly introduced a single rule for all athletes: Whenever you need to decide, ask yourself one question: *Will it make the boat go faster?* The athletes followed

Pharmaceutical Care in Digital Revolution. https://doi.org/10.1016/B978-0-12-817638-2.00021-3
253

the coach's lead and applied this mindset enthusiastically to everything they did. Two years later the team captured Olympic gold. By asking a simple question, the entire culture of the team changed. This example illustrates two things. First, an organizational culture may either drive exceptional performance or may pose the biggest hurdle for any future success. Second, the minimum effective behavior you show as a leader is the maximum behavior you can expect from others. Thus, by deliberately role modeling, a leader can influence the behaviors and culture of an entire organization.

The biggest myth about successfully preparing for the future is that availability of resources, understanding of cutting-edge technology, and fast application of new ideas are the main drivers of success. If this were the case, historically, big players in an industry or professional field would continue to maintain their dominant position when disruptive innovation enters their market. It is, however, very rare that established players make a successful transition to new business models or technologies. For example, Barnes & Noble, the bookselling giant, was quickly surpassed by the upstart Amazon when internet distribution of books took hold.

The same is true for the failed transition of Kodak to digital photography, or Nokia's inability to extend to the smart phone market. They had all the necessary resources available, yet still failed. This will be no different for the pharmaceutical business. We may have full access to the newest insights, technology, and resources, yet success is far from guaranteed. The difference between the successful pharmaceutical care providers and the less successful ones will be cultural: a difference in mindsets, beliefs, and behaviors. Therefore the most important factor for maximizing chances of success as a pharmaceutical care provider is to focus on building a future-oriented, high-performance organizational culture where new ideas can bloom. Fertile grounds beat better seeds every time. The six keys to build this high-performance culture are creating clarity around goals, practical ways to measure progress, a mindset of playing to win, an attitude to fall in love with clients, using power laws, and understanding how to let go in order to reach out.

The Need for Clarity, Connection, and Goals

Organizational results are downstream from organizational culture; therefore you will never get the new results that you want from the existing behaviors that you like. Only by changing the culture of an organization will you get different results.

Three elements are essential to start creating a future-oriented culture: vision, connection, and tangible goals. The most effective way to build a culture where innovation focus and future orientation are the norm is to deliberately build supportive language, metaphors, and stories to clearly support your new goals.

That's why a simple question such as, "Does it make the boat go faster," is so effective to improve performance. It creates a massive amount of clarity. It also provides the connection between individual decisions and the vision of what a desirable future looks like.

Next to having a vision and creating a connection, the third element to build a future-oriented organizational culture is to translate a vision into tangible goals. It has been said that life is about goals and that all else is just commentary. Often, bright organizations simply fail because of vague, unrealistic, or missing goals. Criteria for good goals are:

- **A clear statement of where you are, to where you want to be:** For example, it's important to be very specific about the revenue of your current innovative products or services, compared to the revenue of your future innovative products or services.
- **A feasibility check:** Has it been done before? If not, make your goal smaller. After all, often the most successful organizations are not the first movers, but the ones who enter the market shortly after the first movers. The latter tend to leverage the learnings of others: The iPod used existing technology in an attractive package to quickly dominate the portable music market.
- **A clear distinction between goals and alternatives:** For example, the goal can be to build a pharmacy business which is prepared for the future. Alternatives to achieve this goal may be the application of block chain, or AI, or wearables, etc. The simple rule is to keep your eyes on the ball and never confuse your actual goals with arbitrary alternatives to achieve your goals. If you do, you limit your options for success.
- **Practical ways to frequently measure progress on a goal:** Which data tell you that you are on your way to achieve your goals? Without checking your progress on a regular basis, you will have no way to steer the ship and avoid shipwreck.
- **Incorporation of behavioral components:** If you picture future success, you need to realize that you will not see how to do it, until you see yourself doing it. Which behaviors will help you most to support your goals? For example, if developing an AI solution is an important part of your goals, your organization must build trust and behave in such a way that more and more decision making is delegated to a system or a process.

How Distinctions Build a Culture Focused on the Future

Leaders who drive a cultural transformation make abundant use of behavioral distinctions to illustrate language, metaphors, and stories. A behavioral distinction describes the difference between good behavior and the best behavior. Two behavioral distinctions are essential for successful pharmaceutical care providers to lead digital transformation:

The First Important Distinction Is: Are You Playing to Win, or Are You Playing Not to Lose

Imagine two companies. One is playing to win, the other is playing not to lose.

If you are playing to win, you're doing the following:

- **Always looking for ways to make your existing business obsolete** with new technology, products, or services.
- **Focusing to dominate your marketplace niche.** You have developed a healthy allergy to average results and refuse to just hang on.
- **Willing to take controlled risks, quickly test ideas, embrace brilliant failures,** and aggressively expand on expected and unexpected successes.
- **Having a structural process in place to prevent your best people from leaving.**
- **Spending more money, time, and energy on innovation,** and less on bending the rules in your favor, such as lobbying for preferential treatment with lawmakers.
- **Building a business where your future services and products are very different from what you have today.**
- **Willing to confront your peers and invoke the ire of your competitors.** Attraction and repulsion are two sides of the same coin. When you move into uncharted territory, you will break current norms and standards, which are often venerated deeply by existing players. This means that you will encounter a healthy share of both cheerleaders and detractors. This is why, when it comes to high performance, the majority is always wrong (see QR Code 21.1).
- **Attracting the customers you serve best.** They typically value advanced products and new services over price. This enables you to step away from existing customers that are a poor fit for your new future business.

All of these behaviors will drive a culture of winning and enable your organization to quickly incorporate new products and services.

QR Code 21.1

Why the majority is always wrong.

The Second Important Distinction Is: Do You Fall in Love With Your Patients, or Fall in Love With Your Product or Processes?

If you fall in love with your patients, instead of falling in love with your products or services, you give patients what they need, not what they want. This is the difference between a handyman and an architect. When a part of a kitchen has broken down, people will go to a handyman to get it fixed. The handyman will give what the client wants. On the other hand, if the client goes to an architect, the architect may propose a completely new floor plan for the house. This may be exactly what the client needs.

ⓘ The value distance between what a client wants and what a client needs is huge. In pharmaceutical care, examples of the difference between somebody who gives people what they want versus what they need are providing extended services to help clients beyond mere treatment support, understanding expertise outside the pharmacy field, and the willingness to give clients access to this expertise.

How to Use Power Laws

The difference in performance between number one and number two in sports is often very small. The difference in prize money between number one and number two, however, is huge. This is called a power law: Small differences in achievement may translate into huge differences in rewards.

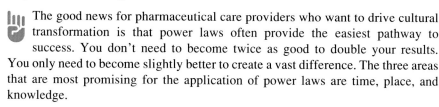 The good news for pharmaceutical care providers who want to drive cultural transformation is that power laws often provide the easiest pathway to success. You don't need to become twice as good to double your results. You only need to become slightly better to create a vast difference. The three areas that are most promising for the application of power laws are time, place, and knowledge.

- **Time** is your most important resource. You can't save it, stop it, or get more of it; and when it's gone, it's simply gone forever. Building a new future therefore starts with the highest and best use of your time. These are all the activities that lie at the intersection between your skills, your passion, and the value you create for others. Which part of the pharmaceutical care provider blueprint allows you to expand your existing skills, ties into your deep passion, and creates the most value for your future clients?
- **Place** is the second area where power laws can be applied. For example, you can apply AI in the most brilliant way possible, but if your environment simply does not trust the judgment of an algorithm, you will get nowhere. It's as futile as opening a McDonald's franchise next to an all-you-can-eat restaurant. What would be the place where you are surrounded by clients who actually love what you do?
- **Knowledge** is the third area susceptible to power laws. For example, if you are the only expert who knows how to shave off 10% of a pit stop time in a Formula One race, you command respect and a top salary. Ask yourself as a pharmaceutical care provider: Which piece of knowledge, if I decide to get it in the next few months, will really make a difference and set me apart from everyone else?

The Value of Strategic Quitting

When designing a new future, the biggest pitfall is to simply add new goals on top of existing goals and activities. Typically, this excessive loading leads to overwork and stress, resulting in frustration and a deep failure to execute (as explained in Chapter 2 as well); we call this an Expensive Old Organization. Instead, if you want to lead in digital transformation, one of the most important leadership behaviors is *strategic quitting*: You have to let go, in order to reach out. Before you start with a new project, ask yourself which activities you have to quit first (see QR Code 21.2 for a verbal explanation).

QR Code 21.2

Strategic quitting.

The area for pharmaceutical care providers where applying strategic quitting may be most effective is *irrelevant excellence*. Nothing is sadder than professionals becoming excellent at something that is rapidly becoming irrelevant. Define which part of your work will no longer have a place in your future business. Then plan to eliminate this part of your work as soon as possible.

How to Take the First Step and Maintain Momentum

After setting a goal to become a successful digital pharmaceutical care provider, the first step is to define exactly which behaviors will support you most to get there in the easiest way possible. Then role model these behaviors to transform your organizational culture. In summary, the six areas where new, consistent behaviors can make a huge impact are:

- Creating clarity around your medium- and long-term goals.
- Continuing efforts to measure progress on these goals.
- Playing to win: If the goals don't make you slightly uncomfortable, you're probably not thinking big enough.
- Falling in love with your patients: Ask yourself regularly how your goals will help to improve the condition of the client.
- Using the power laws of time, place, and knowledge.
- Letting go in order reach out. A constant focus on strategically quitting irrelevant activities will help you to free up time, money, and energy.

The way you spend your day defines the way you will spend your life. If after reading this book, you will execute three (small) actions every day to build the necessary high-performance culture to become a successful digital pharmaceutical care provider, you will have performed more than 1000 small actions after one year. This not only will have a dramatic impact on the culture of your organization, but will most certainly set you apart from most of your peers. Information is overrated and is useless without action. Motion beats meditation every time. What are you waiting for?

This means for circular pharmaceutical care:

- If this book has inspired you to chase a future of circular pharmaceutical care by implementing digital health technology, you need to be aware of which behaviors will enable you to succeed in that ambition.
- A six-item blueprint of goal-clarity, progress-measurement, playing-mindset, customer-orientation, power-laws, and letting-go may help to create a culture to increase the likelihood of success.
- By executing three (small) actions every day to build the necessary high-performance culture to become a successful digital pharmaceutical care provider, you will have performed more than 1000 small actions after one year.

Final discussion: Circular pharmaceutical care

Claudia Rijcken, Paul Iske, Rob Peters, Barry Meesters, Paul Rulkens, Wilma Göttgens

If you want a happy ending, that of course depends on where you stop the story.
Orson Welles

If you have read the preceding chapters in this book, you may be as inspired as the authors are about how a health-tech convergence can create opportunities to make apothecary intelligence better. Just as the giant sequoias keep growing and growing as they age, the digital forest is progressing exponentially and in the process is helping to prevent, diagnose, and treat diseases. It is also igniting patient-centric, "hammock" healthcare. Similar to how sequoias produce seeds for future growth, virtual reality, wearables, chatbots, and digital therapeutics are generating seeds of data of unimaginable size for further grow of pharmaceutical care.

In this chapter you will read about our final reflections on the nine future thoughts presented at the start of the book. We conclude with a discussion about the balanced conditions described in this book and how technology can help pharmacists are served by apothecary intelligence, establish circular and improve the lives of the patients they serve.

Without a doubt we are in a transition phase, and the future is not yet clear. As Lucien Engelen wrote in his book *Augmented Health(Care)*, "We are just at the end of the beginning." Engelen addresses the fact that there are still many unanswered questions, for example in the regulatory, legal, educational, and ethical sectors. Like Gerd Leonhard in the Foreword of this book, Engelen also notes what is probably our most important challenge: to maintain an appropriate balance between digital care and human care.

We started this book with nine future thoughts on the future for the pharmaceutical care landscape. Now we take a final look at their convergence.

1. **The transition to a circular pharmaceutical care model is a matter of education, attitude and process change.**

 In general, circular business models can have different emphases and various objectives, for example, to extend the life of materials, products, knowledge, or services; to use a "waste = food" approach to help recover materials; and to use closed-loop systems-thinking approaches in designing solutions.

Although the circularity concept is derived from economic ecosystems, service models can be circular as well. As noted in the book's introduction, circular pharmaceutical care is defined as a regenerative system where medication, tools, knowledge, and services are provided in closed loops or cycles, with the goal to continuously optimize patient outcomes, reduce waste, and avoid harm due to medication use.

This book describes patient expectations, environmental challenges, systems, technology, skills, behaviors, and boundaries around creating a circular pharmaceutical care model.

> What brought us into the current pharmaceutical model will not be enough to get us to the next phase.

It is to be expected that we will always be in need of the traditional values of pharmaceutical care and human judgment, empathy, and decision making. Also, it is highly unlikely that the digital informatics domain will lead pharmaceutical care for the next number of years. Pharmaceutical caregivers, however, may benefit from embracing a blended concept in which digital and human assets synergize, a concept which will be driven in large part by patient needs and expectations.

We are now in the midst of this transitional phase, where we find ourselves identifying how digitization can best serve the health and well-being of society. Such a transition phase requires a curious mindset, a flexible approach, and structured implementation. In other words, an awareness of the scope of the changes taking place.

This "helicopter view" means that educational systems have the opportunity to introduce the seventh pharmaceutical competency, "digital health literacy," as explained in Chapter 19. Only by igniting awareness of the growth of the digital health ecosystem can we prepare students such that they can convert the relevant innovation into knowledge that will augment their future roles.

It is not about immediately implementing all this knowledge. It is about critically reviewing existing situations and applying the four lenses of innovation (refer to Chapter 2) to determine which of the available tools can best enhance a personalized pharmaceutical care pathway.

It is about fueling an innovative attitude that searches for combinatoric pathways to apply existing knowledge in new environments.

And it is about judging where care can be digital and where care needs to be human in order to create the highest value for patients.

We are living in an era in which a wealth of data are being recorded, so from a health perspective we may be able to create cradle-to-grave health insights. This will enable us to visualize digital twins and conceptualize ideal treatment pathways, leading to ultra-personalized pharmaceutical care with a minimum of waste or harm. In fact, that is probably what this population sees as the sine qua non for future healthcare provision.

This circular approach takes data from living biomarker systems, which are meticulously analyzed within these pathways, resulting in a circular journey that takes on a life on its own. However, it takes time to de-silo healthcare systems, create interoperability and alignment, and shift behaviors towards new approaches. That said, brilliant achievements have already been made in these areas, and many examples are included in this book. With the right mindset and a healthy dose of persistence, we can take advantage of the big promises before us and step-by-step close the gaps in the pathway, as shown in Figure 1.

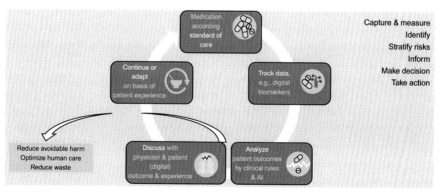

FIGURE 1

Circular pharmaceutical care.

Within a full circular model a pharmaceutical system invests in medications, digital biomarker analysis, patient coaching by humans, and achieves the best possible healthcare without waste.

This book covers the fundamental conditions needed for exponential success towards the circular model.

2. Health data are useless unless converted into value-adding knowledge that drives action.

We often say that computers are smart, but at other times we call them stupid because they can only answer questions that are most often formulated by humans. No computer has been developed as yet that can absorb data from both biotic and abiotic sources and that can perform adequate, unsupervised reasoning of that data. Thus we are obliged to develop systems that correctly digest the zeta bytes of data we are generating on the Internet of Everything and Everyone (IEE) and that can effectively handle waste-reduction goals with the data.

As we mention multiple times throughout this book, creating knowledge from the vast amount of available health data is essential for driving personalized patient care, whether it be information we have some awareness of or things we cannot yet imagine.

This level of knowledge can help us improve healthcare and change processes and behaviors where needed. However, it isn't enough to track data and create analytical systems or to know how to achieve a circular pharmaceutical model; these things become meaningful only through actions that truly optimize healthcare.

Here a knowledge phenomenon appears: over time the knowledge behind an innovative system loses some of its relevance.

To understand this phenomenon, consider some of the first examples of mobile technology. The early pioneers manually collected information that subsequently provided the scientific knowledge that led to the first radio common carrier (RCC). The RCC systems became obsolete with the arrival of cellular systems that support mobile phones (which made us always reachable, something that at one time people could not have imagined). Now we live with a "if you are not wired, you are fired" mentality, and internet and smart health technologies have infused the fundamental technology behind the first mobile phones.

In some ways these changes apply to pharmacy software systems. These systems were developed decades ago to collect prescription data, patient characteristics, and other vital information needed to achieve adequate medication management. Globally, the adoption rate of these systems is huge, and many, if not all, pharmacies could no longer function without them.

Most pharmaceutical care providers are familiar with storing data on patient demographics, distributed medicines, prescription details, claims titles, and pharmaceutical care in pharmacy software. Such data are converted into information that now is considered as the sine qua non for care. The data warrant the high-quality pharmaceutical care that we have in many countries, but the systems as such have lost some of their innovative character.

In fact, certain types of data in current pharmacy software systems may become obsolete. For example, when blockchain technologies make it possible for patients to directly reimburse commercial payers, the middle-man role now in pharmacy systems may no longer be required.

However, with the digital technologies discussed in Chapters 9–16, pharmacy software systems offer great possibilities for augmentation that will help personalize future patient experiences. New data exchange requests will be posed by patients eager to share their health data to enhance medication insights. These new opportunities will require a willingness to change software and make systems flexible and interoperable and to influence patients' expectations about the use of such systems

Connecting the new digital health world with existing pharmacy records will generate new information, that – once digested accurately – can augment a pharmaceutical care pathway, which is where highest-value, personalized healthcare can be created.

 3. Patient-centric pharmaceutical care is a blend of medication expertise, holistic data analysis, hammock healthcare, and the unique qualities of the human heart.

Many countries are facing the prospect of a perfect healthcare storm in which the demand for care outweighs the resources available for that care. An aging population with multiple morbidities and the population's increasingly complex requirements for care are stretching limited budgets and pushing prices and reimbursements down (as explained in Chapter 1). In addition, many healthcare systems do not have the staff needed to provide precision-level pharmaceutical care, leading to suboptimal quality in current processes.

You may recall the patient Jeanny discussed in Chapter 7. Jeanny's home is an example of integrated technology that allows the prevention and optimal treatment of diseases in a home environment, meaning that Jeanny was allowed the comfort of "hammock" care (a metaphor for super-convenient homecare). The range of treatments that can be delivered outside hospitals is increasing substantially, thus emphasizing the potential to extend pharmaceutical care services to home environments.

Therefore future pharmaceutical care may be envisioned as hybrid service centers of digital and human care.

Centralized pharmaceutical care will be provided in highly specialized care centers where patient dashboards store risk stratification and pattern recognition trends that are monitored by pharmaceutical professionals. The quality of the data and their privacy and security will be governed and ensured through the principles presented in Chapter 17 and the Appendix. Those patients with significant deviations will be contacted digitally or invited for a human consultation, depending on the type of care required.

Face-to-face dialogue with professionals will be crucial regarding concerns and services such as medication adherence, explanation of the additive value of digital therapeutics for drug treatment, and immersive coaching on the impact of life events. Patients may also prefer to gather at low-threshold community pharmaceutical care centers to engage in social interactions or to make use of educational technologies that centralized care centers offer (e.g., a broad range of augmented reality videos on a medication's mechanism of action, lifestyle behaviors, or functions of the human body, as described in Chapter 13).

Thus when patients prefer human care above robotic support, this right can and should always be granted, as explained in Chapter 18.

> All alternative care pathways need to guarantee measurable, appropriate, and personalized interactions with a pharmaceutical care practitioner.

For those who do not want to visit a physical facility, digital options such as chatbots, care robots, augmented reality glasses, or wearables may be offered, as discussed in Part 2 of this book. Technology may help people with impairments retain autonomous management of their medications, even in housebound situations. In such cases both digital and home visit pharmaceutical services can enhance care experiences and optimize patient outcomes.

Flexibility in blended care is essential, as not all diseases can be treated in the same way or not all patients are housebound; thus personalized approaches are needed in this model.

Governments and payers are called upon to stimulate and incentivize blended care approaches by jointly defining conditions and expected outcomes and subsequently building value-based healthcare models around these systems of care (as discussed in Chapters 3 and 4).

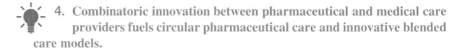 **4. Combinatoric innovation between pharmaceutical and medical care providers fuels circular pharmaceutical care and innovative blended care models.**

We describe in this book how combinatoric innovation creates multidisciplinary value by connecting parties with diverse skills and ideas so that they can explore and discover how they can create value together.

> This is why in a joint innovative approach, with pharmaceutical care providers and physicians collaborating, patients and healthcare systems are both in a more advantageous position.

Although the educational background and perspectives of the two professions differ, there is significant overlap and synergy in providing care that is experienced as good by patients.

Previous research has shown positive results on collaboration between the two professions to optimize the treatment of specific diseases. Also, recent research showed that physicians identified enhanced clinical outcomes, access to medication knowledge, and creation of a multidisciplinary model for learners as the top benefits of incorporating pharmacists into teams. These findings were similar to the perceptions of pharmacists, with the exceptions being that physicians were more concerned about space limitations and pharmacists noted that a physician's acceptance to pharmaceutical consulting sometimes was difficult (Williams et al., 2018).

Currently, as regulation allows, in many countries the functions delegated or shared between physicians and pharmaceutical care providers more often include authorizing refills or adjusting doses. Future team approaches may for example benefit from joint identification of digital treatment and synergistic treatment pathways. This means that together the physician/pharmacist team executes the Digital by Design pathway discussed in Chapter 20, selects from the technologies in Part 2 of this book, and shares responsibilities for developing blended care pathways.

Because the process of joint innovation is nonlinear, this requires mutual trust and is to a certain extent unpredictable. Therefore it often cannot be captured in short-term outcomes and requires a long-term commitment to develop and change cultures (as described in Chapter 21).

For clarity in a potential entropic process, pharmacists and physicians may consider establishing a collaborative digital innovation agreement (CDIA).

Such an agreement specifies, for example, biannual goals for digital health innovation, how these goals value patient outcomes, the conditions and measures for success, the roles and responsibilities of each provider, and so on.

Having a transparent CDIA may also facilitate jointly negotiating adequate payer reimbursement for the development and delivery of blended care models, reimbursement that many healthcare providers currently see as a major hurdle. Medical and pharmaceutical digital health provisions are not an either-or situation; are not an either-or situation, they augment each other.

Thus, as well as certified digital medical solutions being reimbursed, also digital pharmaceutical solutions are expected to be integrated in hospital and community pharmacy claims systems.

A combined effort toward receiving this reimbursement situation may expedited adoption of innovative blended care models.

 5. Not all pharmaceutical care providers need to be data scientists, but every pharmaceutical care provider needs to have some interest in data science.

This book shows how individual health technologies disrupt treatment pathways. As previously mentioned, more important than the individual digital tools is the expected super-convergence of these tools. For pharmacists hammock healthcare likely will mean a convergence of data on genomics, home robotics, health apps, chatbots, augmented reality, and digital therapeutics. All these tools will deliver data that will work together in an ecosystem or platform that, once analyzed and implemented in service models adequately, can improve the lives of people taking medication.

Exponentially adopting digital technologies in combination with improved understanding of causal relationships between, for example, life patterns and medication tolerance will enable pharmaceutical care providers to take on a Tesla-like role.

Teslas are electric vehicles, and to a great extent their motors can be maintained remotely by smart analysis of data and reprogramming. Actually, drivers are remotely signaled when software issues need repair, before they get stuck in a "dead" car.

In analogy with Tesla, in future blended pharmaceutical care processes with focus on prevention, patients can be proactively contacted before medication-related exacerbation of a disease even takes place (e.g., due to adverse events). Such a warning system will become critical for safety optimization, as is the remote warning system in a Tesla.

To augment the judgment and decision-making role in such a prevention-oriented safety system, stakeholders will have to learn how to deal with the information derived from data and how to interpret that information in a way that is best for an individual patient.

Even when future AI systems explain up front how they make decisions, human understanding of the potential bias, security risks, and data anomalies is required to make critical safety decisions, including whether to follow the advice of an AI system (see Chapter 11 for more information on this topic).

Therefore in Chapter 19 we emphasize the need for all pharmaceutical care providers to develop a certain level of digital savviness. Educational systems are to be incentivized to facilitate and motivate this digital health literacy. This knowledge will enable professionals to acquire apothecary intelligence (see Chapter 11), which includes interpreting data in decision-supporting models, understanding how to build an outcome-based program as explained in Chapter 3, and acting as a trusted adviser to both peer healthcare providers and patients in precision medicine interventions.

Also, a thorough understanding of the data is essential to make ethically sound decisions, which only humans can do.

The big challenge will be to develop AI programs with goals that are aligned with those of humans (which we refer to as benevolent AI in Chapter 11). As Max Tegmark explains in his book *Life 3.0,* that in order to let AI make our life better, we need to teach AI what our goals are, we need to make AI adopt those goals, and most importantly, we need to drive AI to retain our goals (Tegmark, 2017). Pharmaceutical care providers understand what matters most to patients and can enhance this information with outcomes of health data analysis. AI can help by providing personalized suggestions, but only if the algorithms are digesting the data in an appropriate way. Therefore pharmaceutical care providers need to understand what their digital health tools and dashboard are consulting them and how they retrieve that knowledge. This is why we propagate that the pharmacist of the future has a certain amount of data science knowledge in order to execute the human judgment role of optimal personalized care adequately.

6. Future pharmaceutical care providers are STEM+ professionals, data analytics translators, as well as trusted service providers, who offer digital care if possible and human care where needed.

Future pharmaceutical care providers may be best visualized as blended care orchestrators. Through their medication expertise and professional attitude, pharmacists guide patients ethically and effectively through a blended, personalized value chain. With digital literacy and cradle-to-grave data, pharmacists will consult healthcare system partners and collaborate with medication manufacturers and payers to enable effective outcome-based payment models.

Being a pharmacist is not just a job. In addition to being an academic professional with matching expectations, it entails a complex package of different skills, as we discuss in Chapter 19, where we describe pharmacy as a STEM+ education. Pharmacists offer analytical, pharmaceutical triage services based on thorough product expertise and disease understanding, smart digital data analysis on broad digital biomarkers, excellent human communication skills, and solution-oriented creativity.

Thus the future academic disciplines for care-providing pharmacists appear to be in life sciences and mathematics as well as humanities and social sciences.

In a 2018 online poll (see Chapter 5) at least half, if not more, of the 10 elements patients identified as part of good care are driven by excellence in humanistic and social skills. Ask people why a certain health service is their favorite, and they will hardly ever say "because it is the most efficient one." Efficiency is often said to be for processes and computers. But when asked about the best experienced healthcare provision, people will most often go in the direction of "because I felt understood, people listened, it was affectionate, there was a sincere interest or an empathic approach."

Whereas human science and mathematical expertise may be augmented by algorithms, empathy, compassion, and trust—essential when caring for someone—are words that are difficult to convert into abiotic vehicles like computers.

Given the changing needs in a data and digital driven society, tasks of pharmacists with a pharmaceutical care practice may evolve into those shown in Table 1.

Table 1 Changing Tasks for Pharmaceutical Care-Oriented Pharmacists

	2019	2024 and Beyond
Medication characteristics expert	High	High
Trusted healthcare system partner	Moderate to high	High
Integrated health data expert	Partially	High
Behavioral support role	Moderate	High
Medication management scope	Descriptive analytics	Predictive algorithms
Patient outcomes accountable	Partially	High
Ethical assessment role	Significant	High
Manufacturing expert	Depends on role	Depends on role
Location of care	Predominantly physical	Blended
Distribution expert	Depends on role	Depends on role

7. **Digital health compliance blueprints, Digital by Design frameworks, and high-performance cultural transformations are convenient enablers of digital pharmaceutical care.**

Most of us don't like changes, but everybody likes improvements. The degree to which the pharmaceutical care environment is subject to change is the degree to which we need to warrant that these changes actually improve the system so that we do not wind up with an old, expensive system, as explained in Chapter 2.

Within transformative processes, such as the one we describe in this book, there are a number of conditions that increase the likelihood for success in the long term. John Kotter, emeritus professor of Harvard Business School, has extensively researched those conditions. The conditions include having a sense of urgency, having a powerful guiding coalition, having a vision clearly and often communicated, and having a plan to create short-term wins, as well as avoiding a premature declaration of victory and embedding change in organizational cultures.

You can find information on all these elements in this book, but here we focus on the necessity of removing (internal) obstacles like anger over compliance, stress due to complex processes, and fear of cultural transformations.

Improved regulatory literacy, taking a structured approach, and building cultural savviness can help reduce uncertainty in innovation processes and thus facilitate the design and adoption of innovations.

By taking the structured blueprint approach proposed for digital health compliance in Chapter 17, regulations and laws can enable early understanding of what is required to develop appropriate digital health services that deserve patients' trust. Use of the Digital by Design framework (Chapter 20), which includes steps that do not allow gaps in the development of an optimal patient solution, embeds digital health technology into a continuous strategy that meets the criteria of circular care. These new approaches may be best suited for a community pharmacy culture that provides exceptional care and that is prepared for continuous change according to the principles discussed in Chapter 21.

Even when some or all obstacles as described above are removed, there is still the refrain, "success is success only if it is communicated effectively."

When building empirical experience and expertise, early adopters of innovation may decide to share digital adoption successes broadly, early and transparently with patients.

For example, consider adopting an initiative like "Ask me about digital," which was introduced by Bertalan Mesko in June 2018. The ultimate goal of this initiative is to facilitate doctor-patient communications through the power of technology by displaying an "Ask me about digital" sticker at the doctors' office or wearing a badge with the same expression.

Using such a symbol in a pharmaceutical care environment could show patients that the pharmaceutical care provider

- is educated in digital health matters related to good pharmaceutical care;
- is open to responding to questions and recommendations about online pharmaceutical content as well as the use of digital health devices;
- indicates clearly and explicitly which digital channels and data are used in communication with patients; and
- always follows the pharmaceutical professional standards.

Such an communication combined with an open mindset for innovation may engage more patients earlier in a digital care journey and improve the digital reputation of the pharmaceutical care provider involved.

8. Core values and virtues of pharmaceutical care practitioners should serve as the beacons through which patients feel comfortable in making well-informed, autonomous medication choices.

In the fast-developing world of digital health, computers are increasingly becoming a digital pharmaceutical brain. However, the ethical standards for assessing how this digital brain functions are still in their infancy (you can find a number of examples throughout the book, particularly in Chapter 18). This lack of transparent ethical standards often results in patients worrying about the way their health data are being used, about the validity of autonomously generated treatment choices, and about the right to be treated by a human care provider. In an environment where laws, norms, market forces, and the architecture of systems are still under development, values are the anchors for assessing what is and what is not good care.

In this dynamic period of change, professional values are the pharmaceutical care practitioners' compass for guiding patients through complex uncertainties.

As indicated, pharmacists' core values can be defined as being committed to patients' well-being, maintaining pharmaceutical expertise, acting socially responsible, caring in an appropriate way, and showing professional autonomy. Pharmacists have always enjoyed a reputation of professional predictability and trust, and they have the opportunity to be seen as having the skills essential to assure patients about the role digital health applications can play in their health care.

Values and ethics in pharmaceutical care can be accessed by either a deontological (or consequentialism, being focused on the intention) or a teleological approach (focused on the outcome, the end justifies the means).

For instance, as a teleological consideration, consider the case of flight safety improvements, where the risk of terror attacks might be enough to justify large-scale data collection about travelers' migration patterns and also experiments based on AI applications.

On the other hand, clinical interventions are hard to justify on teleological grounds (think of the horrific history of medical experimentation on unsuspecting human subjects), and ethics must be weighed on the basis of intentions rather than potential patient outcomes.

Ethical standards for digital health may become as important at shaping healthcare care systems as technological standards have been since the 1980s.

However, in the absence of available standards, making an adequate deontological assessment for digital health dilemmas requires a balanced virtue-based ethics approach.

Pharmaceutical care practitioners may consult patients to assess what they consider as good care and then let this information determine whether a digital tool can support individuals' beliefs about their well-being. Possible questions for practitioners are: will the technology address individual patient preferences in a compliant and secured way? Is the technology transparent on how it deals with data? Are there any side effects when using the technology (e.g., a nocebo effect)? Can patients become dependent on the digital tool?

A decision has to be balanced with other professional values as well, which reflects the great complexity of this responsibility.

In ethical questions, an answer is almost never a dichotomic statement.

Many steps must be taken to ensure that the overall condition of a patient is improved, and not to the benefit of any particular party. Human and social skills are of the utmost importance for really determining core patient preferences. These are certainly essential skills for pharmaceutical care practitioners; these skills cannot be automated by digital technology and are fundamental values that professionals bring to healthcare systems.

 9. Keeping the balance is the crux for achieving circular pharmaceutical care.

In its discussion of the forestry of digital health options, this book reveals one major red line that crosses through every chapter: only by maintaining the balance between digital and human pharmaceutical care, we can achieve circularity in medication treatment pathways, enhance patient-centric services and benefit optimally from augmented apothecary intelligence.

In the Anthropocene epoch we mined the earth and introduced many innovations that focused only on the short term. Now we must deal with plastic in oceans, melting poles, and extreme weather conditions. We mined trees and destroyed forests. Species have disappeared, landslides occur much more often, and populations are forced to migrate to different areas to survive.

This is what happens once innovation is introduced in an imbalanced way.

It is basically the consequence of a nonholistic view of the concept of value, which is in its pure definition a combination of financial capital, societal capital (social and ecological), and intellectual capital (knowledge, information, systems, processes, customer relationships).

In principle, disturbing balance is not a bad thing; actually, it demonstrates the progress of mankind. Historically, disturbances by geological, political, or technological revolutions sparked creativity and in many cases increased prosperity. In 1800 more than 40% of the world's newborns died before the age of five. Now, only fewer than 5% of children die before the age of five. Moreover, since 1990, on average, 130,000 fewer people have been in extreme poverty every day.

Perhaps 20 years from now we will laugh about 2019 as being a time when we still had to take control of own healthcare, had to go to hospitals, and had to wait in long lines for medications. With the help of the technologies we discuss in this book, it is predicted somewhere by the year 2039 a super-convergence of smart devices will enable us to live long and healthy lives right in our homes; and who knows, perhaps one day technology will even makes us immortal.

Some visionaries claim that this process will be exponential. A balanced approach may facilitate us to live with the technology that will change the way we provide healthcare.

We second the opportunities that technology will bring. Moving care into homes, making better informed decisions, coming closer to what really matters for the individual—that is, ultraprecision medical support as the panacea for 2039.

But humans don't hard-code pharmaceutical decisions like technology may do.

Technology may advise and augment and can act as a tool, an assistant, or maybe even a peer. But the balanced decision needed in complex medication regimens requires a human decision based on a holistic patient profile and medical and pharmaceutical care expertise. For instance, in palliative care dialogues, a patient—feasible for participation in a last-resort oncology clinical study—may ask a pharmaceutical care provider: what would you advise me based on available science and what would you do in my situation? That will never be a question for a machine because the answer requires professional understanding as well as human empathy.

Also, defining good care and an individually succeeded life will never be determined by a mathematical equation. Genotype, phenotype, culture, and so many more human circumstances determine what people regard as happiness, joy, and empathy; and this requires a flexible and agile perspective, one that must be handled with care and balance in order to create the highest likelihood of a truly personalized patient treatment.

Final Words

By taking strategically chosen cuttings and using the best possible breeding techniques, parts of the rainforests in Brazil have been regenerated; forest ecosystems have been retained in Asia; and timber in Uganda has been rehabilitated.

Thus a circular approach has enabled to bring back life in areas where the balance was once disturbed.

In this scenario forestry has become back in synergy with mankind and innovative knowledge has been used to offer sustainable solutions for local populations.

The combinatoric synergy of digital and human pharmaceutical care offers similar opportunities to further improve a patient's life, provided a balanced path is chosen.

That is what pharmaceutical care in digital revolution is about:

Blending human and digital pharmaceutical care to establish apothecary intelligence.

We wish you an inspirational way forward when balancing all opportunities to build apothecary intelligence in new pharmaceutical forests!

| Education | Inspiration | Dialogue | Action |

List of abbreviations

AAN	Artificial Neural Networks
ADHD	Attention Deficit Hyperactivity Disorder
AI	Artificial Intelligence
AI	Apothecary Intelligence
AMD	Age-related Macular Degeneration
API	Application Programming Interfaces
APP	Australian Privacy Principles
AR	Augmented Reality
ASCO	American Society for Clinical Oncology
BAT	Baidu, Alibaba, and Tencent
BBC	British Broadcasting Corporation
BCE	Beliefs, Concerns, and Expectations
BCI	Behavior Change Interventions
BCT	Behavioral Change Technique
BIDMC	Beth Israel Deaconess Medical Center
BMC	Business Model Canvas
BMI	Body Mass Index
BSB	Broader Societal Benefits
BYOhD	Bring Your Own health Device
CAGR	Compound Annual Growth Rate
CAR-T	Chimeric Antigen Receptor-T
CDA	Clinical Document Architecture
CDIA	Collaborative Digital Innovation Agreement
CDER	Center for Drug Evaluation and Research
CDISC	Clinical Data Interchange Standards Consortium
CDSS	Clinical Decision Support System
CDM	Chronic Disease Management
CE	Conformité Européene
CAR-T	Chimeric Antigen Receptor T-Cell
CIA	Confidentiality, Integrity and Availability
CMA	Continuous Medication Availability
COPD	Chronic Obstructive Pulmonary Disease
COPPA	Children's Online Privacy Protection Act
CPA	Certified Public Accountant
CQOE	Culture of Quality and Organizational Excellence
CRISPR	Clustered Regularly Interspaced Short Palindromic Repeats
CRP	C-Reactive Proteine
DbD	Digital by Design
DHI	Digital Health Intervention
DL	Deep Learning

DPC	Digital Pharmaceutical Care
DTx	Digital Therapeutic
ECG	Electrocardiograph
EI	Emotional Intelligence
EFPIA	European Federation of Pharmaceutical Industry Associations
EHR	Electronic Health Record
EMA	European Medicines Agency
EMR	Electronic Medical Record
EPR	Electronic Pharmacy Record
ER	Emergency Room
EU	European Union
FACT	Fairness, Accuracy, Confidentiality, Transparency
FAIR	Findable, Accessible, Interoperable, Reusable
FAMGA	Facebook, Amazon, Microsoft, Google, Apple
FDA	Food and Drug Administration
FHIR	Fast Healthcare Interoperability Resources
FIP	International Pharmaceutical Federation
GAS	Goal Attainment Scaling
GDP	Good Distribution Practice
GDPR	General Data Protection Regulation
GP	General Practitioner
GPD	Gross Domestic Product
GRC	Governance Risk and Compliance
GPS	Global Positioning System
HCP	Health Care Provider
HCV	Hepatitis C Virus
HIB	Health Impact Bond
HIMSS	Healthcare Information and Management Systems Society
HIPAA	Health Insurance Portability and Accountability Act
HL7	Health Level Seven
HTA	Health Technology Assessment
ICD	International Classification of Diseases
ICER	Institute for Clinical and Economic Review
ICHOM	International Consortium for Health Outcomes Measurement
ICT	Information and Communication Technology
IDC	International Data Corporation
IEC	International Electrotechnical Commission
IEE	Internet of Everything and Everyone
IoH	Internet of Health
IoT	Internet of Things
IoMT	Internet of Medical Things
IoPT	Internet of Pharma Things
IMDRF	International Medical Device Regulators Forum

ICHOM	International Consortium for Health Outcomes Measurement
IHI	Institute for Healthcare Improvement
IP	Internet Protocol
ISMS	Information Security Management System
ISO	International Organization for Standardization
KP	Kaiser Permanente
LDL	Low Density Lipoprotein
LMIC	Low and Middle-Income Countries
MCO	Managed Care Organization
MDR	Medical Device Regulations
MDSAP	Medical Device Single Audit Program
MEM	Micro-Electromechanical System
ML	Machine Learning
MPR	Medication Possession Ratio
MR	Mixed Reality
MRB-QoL	Medication-Related Burden Quality of Life
MSOSC	Massive Simultaneous Online Social Communities
MTM	Medication Therapy Management
NAS	New Active Substance
NExT	New Experiences and Technologies
NHS	National Health Service
NIST	National Institute of Standards and Technology
NL	The Netherlands
NLP	Natural Language Processing
NLP	Neuro Linguistic Programming
NOAC	New Oral AntiCoagulant
OBF	Outcome-Based Financing
OECD	Organisation for Economic Co-operation and Development
OWASP	Open Web Application Security Project
PBRSA	Performance-Based Risk-Sharing Arrangement
PC	Pharmaceutical Care
PCP	Pharmaceutical Care Provider
PCS	Pharmaceutical Care Stakeholder
PDC	Proportion of Days Covered
PGHD	Patient Generated Health Data
PHA	Personal Health Application
PHI	Protected Health Information
PIL	Patient Information Leaflet
PIP	Poly Implant Prothèse
PPC	Pharmaceutical Patient Care
PREM	Patient Reported Experience Measures
PROM	Patient Reported Outcome Measures
QoL	Quality of Life

RAD	Reimaging Ambulatory Design
RCC	Radio Common Carrier
RCTs	Randomized Controlled Trials
RFID	Radio Frequency Identification
RWD	Real World Data
RWE	Real World Evidence
RPA	Robotic Process Automation
ROI	Return of Investment
SaMD	Software as a Medical Device
SEO	Search Engine Optimization
SMPC	Summary of Manufacturing and Product Chart
SMS	Session Manager Subsystem
SOP	Standard Operating Procedure
SPC	Summary of Product Characteristics
SPoC	Single Point of Contact
SPoT	Single Point of Truth/Single Point of Trust
STEM	Science, Technology, Engineering, Mathematics
TEDI	Technology Enhanced Drug Impact
TGA	Therapeutics Goods Administration
UK	United Kingdom
US	United States
VAS	Visual Analogue Scale
VHBC	Value-Based Healthcare
VPA	Virtual Personal Assistant
VR	Virtual Reality
VUI	Voice-User Interface
WEF	World Economic Forum
WHO	World Health Organization

Appendix: Overview of Laws, Legislation, and Standards Referred to in Chapter 17

Rob Peters, Barry Meesters

This appendix is an addendum to Chapter 17. In that chapter we present the elements required to create a compliance blueprint (see Figure A.1) and the related laws, legislation, and standards. In this appendix we provide a more detailed view on the four pillars that determine the legislative landscape.

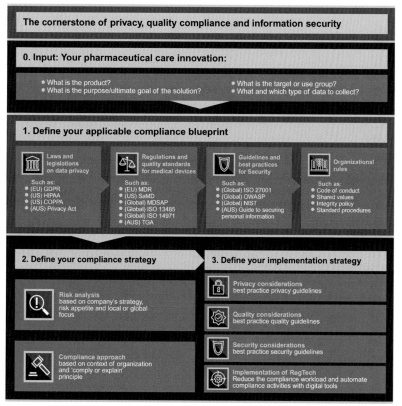

The cornerstone of privacy, quality compliance and information security

0. Input: Your pharmaceutical care innovation:
- What is the product?
- What is the purpose/ultimate goal of the solution?
- What is the target or use group?
- What and which type of data to collect?

1. Define your applicable compliance blueprint

Laws and legislations on data privacy
Such as:
- (EU) GDPR
- (US) HIPAA
- (US) COPPA
- (AUS) Privacy Act

Regulations and quality standards for medical devices
Such as:
- (EU) MDR
- (US) SaMD
- (Global) MDSAP
- (Global) ISO 13485
- (Global) ISO 14971
- (AUS) TGA

Guidelines and best practices for Security
Such as:
- (Global) ISO 27001
- (Global) OWASP
- (Global) NIST
- (AUS) Guide to securing personal information

Organizational rules
Such as:
- Code of conduct
- Shared values
- Integrity policy
- Standard procedures

2. Define your compliance strategy

Risk analysis based on company's strategy, risk appetite and local or global focus

Compliance approach based on context of organization and 'comply or explain' principle

3. Define your implementation strategy

Privacy considerations best practice privacy guidelines

Quality considerations best practice quality guidelines

Security considerations best practice security guidelines

Implementation of RegTech Reduce the compliance workload and automate compliance activities with digital tools

FIGURE A.1

The steps in a compliance blueprint.

279

The information in this appendix focuses only on the most common regulations related to privacy, quality, and security. More information on the organizational rules is included in Chapter 17.

General Comments on the Compliance Blueprint
Variations in Legislation Among Countries

Because local laws and regulations vary significantly among countries, we are not able to refer to all of them. For example, to show the affect that legislation can have in an individual country, we refer to the NHS Choices website for information on healthcare solutions in the United Kingdom. The NHS created a library that provides an overview of the topics a digital health developer needs to consider (Developer NHS UK, 2018). The NHS is also providing a much broader overview related to recommendations and standards in specific areas. We recommend that the reader finds out whether such an overview exists in their country as well.

Completeness of References

Please note that the following legislation and guidelines are not all-conclusive, as we describe only the most common legislation in the United States, the EU, and Australia in 2018. Although these countries are considered frontrunners in regulatory requirements and digital innovations, there are interesting materials in other countries as well.

The overview we set out here focuses on the most relevant, future-proof legislation for the next 5 years (2019–24). Most probably, amendments or addendums to these laws will be released after this book is published; therefore we recommend that one will always check on the most recent regulations.

More Details on Laws and Legislation on Data Privacy

Chapter 17 refers to the following privacy laws and regulations:

- **EU privacy regulation:** General Data Protection Regulation (GDPR)
- **US privacy regulation:** Health Insurance Portability and Accountability Act (HIPAA)
- **US privacy regulation:** Children's Online Privacy Protection Act (COPPA)
- **Australian privacy regulation:** Privacy Act: Australian Privacy Principles

In the overview below, we deep-dive further in granular details of each individual regulation to data privacy.

EU Privacy Regulation: General Data Protection Regulation

The European Union's General Data Protection Regulation 2016/679 strengthens and unifies data protection for all people living in the EU (Wikipedia, 2017d). As its name suggests the GDPR functions as a law across all EU member states. The Data Protection Bill is accepted by the United Kingdom as well, which implies that the United Kingdom will follow the GDPR's principles. The GDPR, which was passed in 2016, became effective in May of 2018.

 The GDPR is not dependent on interpretations by local governments or other authorities, but local laws and regulations on data, including medical data, can apply as well.

The GDPR covers all personal data defined "as any data from which a living individual is identified or identifiable, whether directly or indirectly." GDPR applies to all organizations established within or outside the EU that process EU residents' personal data.

A number of individual categories of personal data specifically related to health information, and thus relevant for pharmaceutical care interactions, are shown in Figure A.2.

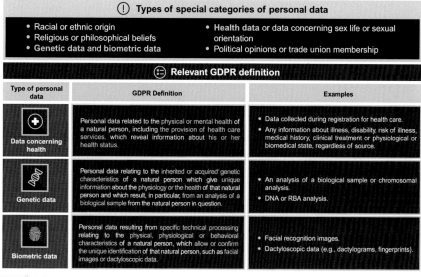

Special categories of personal data.

Pharmaceutical care stakeholders in EU-regulated countries must comply with the GDPR the moment protected health information is involved, just as their counterparts in the United States and Australia must do with HIPAA and the Privacy Act, respectively.

US Privacy Regulation: Health Insurance Portability and Accountability Act (HIPAA)

US HIPAA Privacy rules ensure confidentiality and security of protected health information (PHI) the moment the information is transferred, received, handled, or shared. The rules apply to healthcare providers and organizations and all their business associates, and should help these groups develop and follow procedures related to the appropriate handling of PHI data, which includes, for example, paper, electronic, and *verbal* versions (CDHCS, 2017).

Under HIPAA patient data is referred "protected health information (PHI)," which is similar to the GDPR's "sensitive personal data." This applies to all healthcare data. HIPAA defines PHI as any individually identifiable "past, present, and future information about mental and physical health and the condition of an individual, the provision of healthcare to an individual, and information related payments for healthcare."

⚠ Under HIPAA, the act is applicable to predefined (called covered) entities (such as a healthcare provider, physician, insurance company, and healthcare clearing house) and business associates. Conversely, GDPR applies to *all* organizations established within or outside the EU that process EU residents' personal data.

US Privacy Regulation: Children's Online Privacy Protection Act (COPPA)

The moment a digital solution is developed for or can be used by children under the age of 13 and is developed for use in US jurisdictions it falls under COPPA requirements.

The US Federal Trade Commission issued this act specifically to regulate and enforce the online collection of personal information about children under the age of 13 years.

The primary goal of COPPA is to give parents control over what information is collected online about their children. The act specifies what a healthcare provider (e.g., a pharmacist) must include in the mandatory privacy policy and how to seek verifiable consent from a parent or guardian before collecting personal information about children under the age of 13 years.

This consent form is extensive and can be provided in different ways, such as (1) a consent form signed by a parent, (2) credit card signatures, (3) a call from a parent to authorized personnel collecting the consent, or (4) by checking a parent's identification documents.

Furthermore, it is clearly defined which additional security measures must be taken and what the guidelines are for online marketing towards children's indications.

Under GDPR the specific obligations related to processing data of children are included by topic in the regulation. Similar to COPPA, the GDPR also defines children as a separate category of people who need specific protection from unauthorized processing of data.

Australian Privacy Regulation: Privacy Act: Australian Privacy Principles

The original Privacy Act was passed in 1988 and went into effect in 1989. This Privacy Act has been changed several times, with the last change resulting in the Information Privacy Act 2014, which became effective in January 2018 (ACT, 2018). The primary objectives of this act are to

- promote protection of the privacy of individuals;
- recognize that the protection of the privacy of individuals is balanced with the interests of public sector agencies in carrying out their functions or activities;
- promote responsible and transparent handling of personal information by public sector agencies and contracted service providers; and
- provide a way for individuals to complain about an alleged interference with their privacy.

Australia instituted the Health Records (Privacy and Access) Act in 1997, and the latest version became effective in April 2016 (ACT, 2016). The main purposes of this dedicated act are to

- provide privacy rights in relation to personal health information;
- maintain integrity of records containing personal health information; and
- provide access to personal health information contained in health records.

Under the Privacy Act of Australia, the Australian Information Commissioner issued several guidelines and documents to promote the understanding and awareness of the Australian Privacy Principles (APPs). As of May 2018 Australian authorities had defined a total of 13 separate APPs from open and transparent management of personal information (APP 1) to the correction of personal information (APP 13). The content and mandatory requirements of these APP guidelines can be found at www.oaic.gov.au/agencies-and-organisations/app-guidelines.

More details on Regulations and Quality Standards for Medical Devices

Chapter 17 noted the following relevant regulations and quality standards for medical devices as being relevant when working with digital pharmaceutical care solutions:

- **US medical software regulation:** Software as a Medical Device (SaMD)
- **Australian medical regulation:** Therapeutic Goods Administration (TGA)

- **Global Medical Device Single Audit Program** (MDSAP)
- **Global ISO 13485, medical devices**—Quality Management System—Requirements for regulatory purposes
- **Global ISO 14971, medical devices**—Application of risk management to medical devices
- **EU medical software regulation:** Medical Device Regulation (MDR)

US Medical Software Regulation: Software as a Medical Device (SaMD)

The FDA makes a distinction between wellness and healthcare devices. The FDA does not regulate general wellness products, as strict as healthcare devices the moment they are intended for general use only and present a very low risk to users' safety. However, due to the increasing gray area between the wellness and healthcare applications entering the pharmaceutical care sector, we will focus first briefly on the criteria for wellness devices.

Wellness Devices

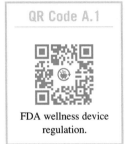

QR Code A.1

FDA wellness device regulation.

In the Cure Act the FDA describes a general wellness product as a device that helps maintain or encourage a general state of health and healthy lifestyle or that associates the role healthy lifestyle choices play in reducing the risk or impact of certain chronic diseases or conditions. To help clarify whether a pharmaceutical care innovation can be classified as a wellness product (and thus will not have to follow the regulations applied to medical devices), the FDA has provided a framework for such products, as shown in QR Code A.1 (FDA, 2016).

However, as in many guidelines, there is room for interpretation, and the FDA strives to continuously improve those that it provides. The most recent version was issued in December 2017 (FDA, 2018a). This update specified and categorized activities that fall under the definition of wellness device:

Devices that do the following are classified as wellness devices:

- Provide administrative support for a healthcare facility;
- Maintain or encourage a healthy lifestyle;
- Serve as an electronic patient record; and
- Transfer and store data, convert formats, and display data and results.

Software as a Medical Device (SaMD)

Since 2017 the United States' definition of Software as a Medical Device has been, "software intended to be used for one or more medical purposes that perform these procedures without being part of a hardware medical device" (FDA, 2017).

The guidelines set under the authority of the FDA define Software as a Medical Device as (FDA, 2002):

- software used as a component, part, or accessory of a medical device;
- software that is itself a medical device;
- software used in the production of a device; and
- software used in implementing the device manufacturer's quality system.

The FDA approval process and requirements are somewhat stricter on most topics compared with the European regulations. Once the new Medical Device Regulation becomes effective in Europe in 2020, US and European regulations will be more closely aligned.

FDA PreCert

 In 2017 the FDA launched the Software Precertification Pilot Program (FDA, 2017). After reviewing management systems for software design, validation, and maintenance, the goal of the program is to determine whether an organization meets software development quality standards.

The program focuses on precertification of software manufacturers that have demonstrated a culture of quality and organizational excellence and that incorporate data from all appropriate sources. The FDA evaluates organizational excellence based on five Culture of Quality and Organizational Excellence (CQOE) principles:

- **Product quality:** Includes the development, testing, and maintenance necessary to deliver SaMD products at the highest level of quality.
- **Patient safety:** Involves providing a safe patient experience and emphasizing patient safety as a critical factor in all decision-making processes.
- **Clinical responsibility:** Includes conducting clinical evaluations and ensuring that patient-centric issues, including labeling and human factors, are appropriately addressed.
- **Cybersecurity responsibility:** Involves protecting cybersecurity and proactively addressing cybersecurity issues through active engagement with stakeholders and peers.
- **Proactive culture:** Incorporates a proactive approach to surveillance, assessment of user needs, and continuous learning.

There are questionnaires for each of these principles, and the outcomes from the questionnaires are used to determine quality-related PreCert scores. If a score is sufficiently high an applicant can be precertified by the FDA. The results also may indicate other areas for further development in the precertification process.

In 2018 initial participants like Apple, Fitbit, and Johnson & Johnson will pilot the process. The FDA published a full working model for the software precertification program in June 2018 (FDA, 2018c).

It is noteworthy that the precertification process and recent approaches of the FDA are risk-based (we discuss such risk-based approaches in Chapter 17).

To understand more about the software precertification program model, please refer to the FDA's Digital Health Software Precertification (PreCert) Program (FDA, 2018c).

Australian Medical Regulation: Therapeutic Goods Administration (TGA)

In Australia the Therapeutic Goods Administration (TGA) governs the quality of pharmaceutical and medical devices. The TGA, as part of the Department of Health, safeguards and enhances the health of the Australian community through effective and timely regulation of therapeutic goods.

Australia's approach is similar to the approach in Europe and the United States. The TGA is also using a risk-based approach, as regulations related to labeling and packaging, import and export rules and legislation, legislative instruments, and safety requirements are set in different standards, which are described on the TGA website (TGA, 2018).

Global Medical Device Single Audit Program (MDSAP)

The International Medical Device Regulators Forum (IMDRF) states that a global approach in auditing and monitoring of the manufacturing of medical devices (which could affect digital health software as well) could improve patient safety and optimize international scale up. The MDSAP program allows a single regulatory audit of a manufacturer's quality management system, which should satisfy the requirements of multiple regulatory jurisdictions.

These audits are conducted by auditing organizations authorized by the participating regulatory authorities to audit under MDSAP requirements.

The program became operational as of January 1, 2017, and currently affects the United States, Canada, Brazil, Japan, and Australian manufacturers of medical devices.

Since January 1, 2019, Health Canada accepts only MDSAP certificates from medical device manufacturers, instead of certificates related to quality systems as before. It is expected that additional markets and organizations, such as the World Health Organization (WHO) and the EU will adopt the MDSAP program as well (Deloitte, 2017a, b).

Global ISO 13485, Medical Devices—Quality Management Systems—Requirements for Regulatory Purposes

The International Organization for Standardization (ISO) comprises well-known and globally recognized specifications, guidelines, and frameworks.

In 2017 the organization recognized 163 countries. The ISO is the world's largest developer of voluntary international standards and facilitates world trade by providing common standards among nations. Over 20,000 standards have been set, covering everything from manufactured products and technology to food safety, agriculture, and healthcare.

ISO 13485 is the global standard for medical device quality management systems. Regardless of their size and type, the moment organizations are involved with medical devices, the ISO 13485 standard becomes applicable, which is obviously the case for organizations providing pharmaceutical patient care. ISO 13485 is designed to be used by organizations involved in the design, production, installation, and delivery of medical devices and related services.

ISO 13485 is related to the MDSAP described earlier in this appendix. One aspect of MDSAP follows the standard of ISO 13485 that specifies requirements for a quality management system for medical devices. That is, ISO 13485 requires the pharmaceutical care stakeholder to demonstrate whether the quality system of the company or institute is effectively implemented and continuously maintained and improved.

ISO 13485 facilitates an effective quality management system, including the following key aspects:

- **Management responsibility:** Focuses on promotion and creating awareness of management's responsibility to comply with regulatory requirements and to have an effective and continuously maintained and improved quality management system.
- **Product safety:** Provides guidance for controls to ensure product safety in the quality management system and working environment.
- **Risk management:** Focuses on risk management activities during product development.
- **Requirements:** Provides guidance for requirements related to inspection, traceability, documentation, validation, and verification of effectiveness of corrective and preventive actions within the quality management system related to medical devices.

Compliance with ISO 13485 under the Medical Device Regulation is often seen as one of the major requirements to prove the implementation of a good and effective quality management system.

Global ISO 14971, Medical Devices: Application of Risk Management to Medical Devices

This standard (ISO 14971) specifies a process to identify the hazards associated with medical devices (including digital health software) in all stages of their lifecycle. When developing a digital health innovation, the main items relevant to ISO 14971 for pharmaceutical care stakeholders are as follows:

- **Process:** Establish a process to manage and control the risks associated with your organization's medical devices.
- **Management:** Make sure that top management demonstrates commitment to medical device risk management.

- **Qualifications:** Make sure that the people who perform risk management tasks have the knowledge and experience that are required to carry out the tasks that have been assigned to them.
- **Risk management plan:** Establish a risk management plan for each particular medical device under consideration, in use, or development.

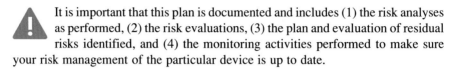 It is important that this plan is documented and includes (1) the risk analyses as performed, (2) the risk evaluations, (3) the plan and evaluation of residual risks identified, and (4) the monitoring activities performed to make sure your risk management of the particular device is up to date.

EU Medical Software Regulation: Medical Device Regulation (MDR)

The MDR is being developed to establish a robust, transparent, predictable, and sustainable regulation for medical devices, including software that qualifies as a medical device. The new regulation will become effective in 2020.

The definition of a medical device in the MDR is any instrument, apparatus, appliance, software, implant, reagent, material, or other article to be used, stand-alone or in combination, for human beings for one or more of the following medical purposes:

- diagnosis, prevention, monitoring, prediction, prognosis, treatment of alleviation of disease
- diagnosis, monitoring, treatment, alleviation of, or compensation for, an injury or disability

As noted in Chapter 17 categorization goes from class I (low risk) up to class III (high risk).

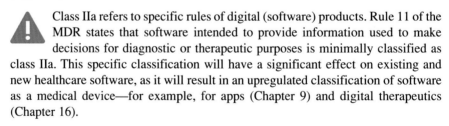 Class IIa refers to specific rules of digital (software) products. Rule 11 of the MDR states that software intended to provide information used to make decisions for diagnostic or therapeutic purposes is minimally classified as class IIa. This specific classification will have a significant effect on existing and new healthcare software, as it will result in an upregulated classification of software as a medical device—for example, for apps (Chapter 9) and digital therapeutics (Chapter 16).

The basis for the MDR is the European Medical Device Directive (due since 1993). Many incidents such as the PIP breast implant scandal (BBC, 2013) and the many digital solutions that have come to the market, increased the urge for the medical device regulation to be updated and be regarded as the standard quality baseline for the EU.

Healthcare software will have an important place in the new MDR. Stand-alone healthcare software will be recognized as medical devices, resulting in more medical software (such as mobile applications) being classified as medical devices.

Pharmaceutical care solutions with software implications are recommended to take into account new MDR classification and requirements immediately from the development phase on.

More Details on Guidelines and Best Practices for Security

In Chapter 17 we wrote about how to support organizations in defining and implementing security measures and the general, globally accepted standards, guidelines, and best practices relevant for digital health compliance, such as

- ISO/IEC 27001 Information security management system (ISMS);
- Open Web Application Security Project (OWASP);
- National Institute of Standards and Technology (NIST); and
- Guide to securing personal information in Australia.

Let us deep-dive somewhat further into each of these individual standards and guidelines.

ISO/IEC 27001 Information Security Management

This standard is the one best-known in terms of providing requirements for an accurate and effective information security management system (ISMS). An ISMS is a systematic approach to managing sensitive company information in the most secure way. This risk-based system covers different topics and areas, such as people, processes, and IT systems. The standard is part of the ISO/IEC 27000 group, which focuses entirely on keeping information assets secure. There is not a specific focus on healthcare organizations; however, individual health organizations can certify and thus give customers a reliable insight in their quality level of security. As of 2018 the ISO 27001 certificate is not an obligation. However, many governments, and on a general European level, are already preparing cybersecurity laws that affect many businesses, including the health and life science sector.

Open Web Application Security Project (OWASP)

The Open Web Application Security Project (OWASP) is a worldwide nonprofit organization focused on improving the security of software (in general) (OWASP, 2018). The organization is providing practical information about application security to individuals, corporations, universities, government agencies, and many other organizations. OWASP is issuing software tools and knowledge-based documentation on how to improve security on a daily basis. The information is open-sourced available, and all materials can be downloaded.

 All software developers are supposed to know the best practices under OWASP. The organization published the *"Top 10 Most Mobile Risks"* and *"Top 10 Most critical Web Application Risks,"* including the procedures to follow to mitigate those risks (OWASP, 2018).

National Institute of Standards and Technology (NIST)

NIST (NIST, 2018) is a nonregulatory government agency that develops standards and guidelines for technology companies and also for federal agencies, to comply with several security legislation and requirements. Furthermore, NIST standards and guidelines assist in protecting information systems through cost-effective security measures and programs (see QR Code A.2). Several national governments require that companies must comply with the NIST standards, although they are not actually legislation (but are accepted as guidelines in information security) (Lord, 2018).

In many cases complying with NIST guidelines and recommendations will support being compliant with other regulations such as HIPAA. Also, complying with NIST standards means that the focus is not only on the security of a product but also on the security level of an entire organization.

Australia: Guide to Securing Personal Information

In Australia guidance to secure personal data is mainly available under the data privacy legislative framework.

Under this guide, information security involves taking appropriate measures and setting in place technical or organizational structures required to protect information that is not intended to be made publicly available.

As soon as handling personal information comes into the picture, a plan must be made on how to protect personal information during different product stages or a product's entire lifecycle (see Figure A.3).

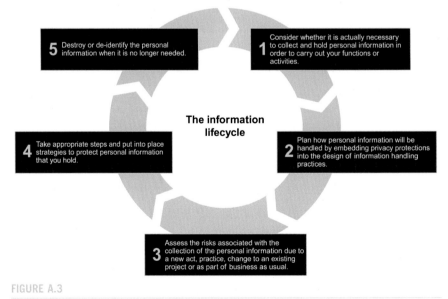

FIGURE A.3

Australian personal data security lifecycle. From OAIC (2018).

The guidance has similar aspects as the European Guidance with focus on principles such as data minimization, privacy by design and the use of risk analysis.

We refer to the full detailed text under the guide (OAIC, 2018). In Australia it also become mandatory, as of 2018, to report data breaches related to health information (OAIC, 2017).

References

Academy of Medical Sciences, 2017. Enhancing the Use of Scientific Evidence to Judge the Potential Benefits and Harms of Medicines. Available at: https://acmedsci.ac.uk/file-download/44970096 [Accessed 15 April 2018].

Accel+Qualtrics, 2017. The Millennial Study. Available at: https://www.qualtrics.com/millennials/ [Accessed 7 July 2018].

Accenture, 2017. Accenture Survey Highlights Healthcare Data Breaches Among English Consumers. Available at: https://www.news-medical.net/news/20170426/Accenture-survey-highlights-healthcare-data-breaches-among-English-consumers.aspx [Accessed 20 December 2017].

Accenture, 2018. 2018 Consumer Survey on Digital Health. Available at: https://www.accenture.com/t20180306T103559Z__w__/us-en/_acnmedia/PDF-71/accenture-health-2018-consumer-survey-digital-health.pdf.

ACT, 2016. Health Records (Privacy and Access) Act 1997. Available at: http://www.legislation.act.gov.au/a/1997-125/current/pdf/1997-125.pdf.

ACT, 2018. Information Privacy Act 2014. Available at: http://www.legislation.act.gov.au/a/2014-24/current/pdf/2014-24.pdf.

Aitken, M., 2016. Outlook for Global Medicines through 2021. Quintiles IMS, Parsippany.

Akili, 2018. Programs. Available at: https://www.akiliinteractive.com/programs-products/ [Accessed 13 December 2018].

Alignbiopharma, 2017. Technology Standards in Development. Available at: https://www.alignbiopharma.org [Accessed 7 September 2017].

Alleman, S.S., et al., 2016. Matching adherence interventions to patient determinants using the theoretical domains framework. Front Pharmacol. 7, 429. Available at: https://doi.org/10.3389/fphar.2016.00429.

AngelMed Guardian System, 2018. Available at: http://www.angel-med.com/?option=com_content&view=article&id=26&Itemid=8 [Accessed 23 August 2018].

APhA, 1995–2018. Principles of Practice of Pharmaceutical Care. Available at: https://www.pharmacist.com/principles-practice-pharmaceutical-care [Accessed 18 May 2018].

Argonaut, 2018. Argonaut Project. Available at: http://argonautwiki.hl7.org/index.php?title=Main_Page [Accessed 24 August 2018].

Arora, A., Dahlstrom, P., Groover, P., Wunderlich, F., 2017. A CEO Guide for Avoiding the Ten Traps That Derail Digital Transformations. Available at: https://www.mckinsey.com/business-functions/digital-mckinsey/our-insights/a-ceo-guide-for-avoiding-the-ten-traps-that-derail-digital-transformations [Accessed 28 December 2017].

Atluri, V., Cordina, J., Mango, P., Velamoor, S., 2016. How Tech-Enabled Consumers are Reordering the Healthcare Landscape. Available at: http://www.mckinsey.com/industries/healthcare-systems-and-services/our-insights/how-tech-enabled-consumers-are-reordering-the-healthcare-landscape [Accessed 13 July 2017].

Australia PSA, 2016. National Competency Standards Framework for pharmacists in Australia 2016. Available at: https://www.psa.org.au/wp-content/uploads/2018/06/National-Competency-Standards-Framework-for-Pharmacists-in-Australia-2016-PDF-2mb.pdf.

Babylon, 2018. A Comparative Study of Artificial Intelligence and Human Doctors for the Purpose of Triage and Diagnosis. Available at: https://assets.babylonhealth.com/press/BabylonJune2018Paper_Version1.4.2.pdf.

Badowski, M., Michienzi, S.R., 2017. Examining the implications of analytical and remote monitoring in pharmacy practice. Available at: https://www.pharmaceutical-journal.com/research/examining-the-implications-of-analytical-and-remote-monitoring-in-pharmacy-practice.

BBACH, 2017. The European Code of Conduct for Research Integrity (Revised Version). Available at: https://ec.europa.eu/research/participants/data/ref/h2020/other/hi/h2020-ethics_code-of-conduct_en.pdf.

BBC, 2013. Q&A: PIP Breast Implants Health Scare. Available at: http://www.bbc.com/news/health-16391522 [Accessed 13 June 2018].

Benetoli, A., Chen, T.F., Schaefer, M., Chaar, B., Aslani, P., 2017. Do Pharmacists Use Social Media for Patient Care? Int. J. Clin. Pharm. 39 (2), 364–372. Available at: https://doi.org/10.1007/s11096-017-0444-4.

Bentahar, A., 2017. 2017 Will be the Year of Voice Search. Available at: https://www.forbes.com/sites/forbesagencycouncil/2017/01/03/2017-will-be-the-year-of-voice-search/#2040f4cf12c5 [Accessed 10 August 2017].

BIDMC, 2016. Artificial Intelligence Achieves Near-Human Performance in Diagnosing Breast Cancer. Available at: https://www.sciencedaily.com/releases/2016/06/160620085204.htm [Accessed 4 June 2018].

Boni, M., 2017. Transforming eHealth Into a Political and Economic Advantage. Available at: https://ec.europa.eu/digital-single-market/en/news/transforming-ehealth-political-and-economic-advantage [Accessed 13 July 2018].

Bostrom, N., 2014. Superintelligence, Paths, Dangers, Strategies. Oxford University Press, Oxford.

Boudreax, E., et al., 2014. Evaluating and selecting mobile health apps: strategies for healthcare providers and healthcare organizations. Transl. Behav. Med. 4 (4), 363–371. https://doi.org/10.1007/s13142-014-0293-9.

Brookings, 2017. Impact Bonds for Health. Available at: https://www.brookings.edu/wp-content/uploads/2017/11/impact-bonds-for-health_slides_20171212.pdf.

Brown, K., 2017. The Future of Pharmaceuticals is Printing Custom Drugs. Available at: https://gizmodo.com/the-future-of-pharmaceuticals-is-printing-custom-drugs-1818846684 [Accessed 22 October 2017].

Byambasuren, B., et al., 2018. Prescribable mHealth apps identified from an overview of systematic reviews. NPJ Digit. Med. 1 (12). Available at: https://doi.org/10.1038/s41746-018-0021-9.

Cain, J., Piascik, P., 2015. Are Serious Games a Good Strategy for Pharmacy Education? Am. J. Pharm. Educ. 79 (4), 47. https://doi.org/10.5688/ajpe79447.

Canada CCocEip, 2017. Competencies of Pharmacy Professionals. Available at: http://www.cccep.ca/pages/competencies_of_pharmacy_professionals.html?page=accreditation [Accessed 22 October 2017].

CDHCS, 2017. What is HIPAA? Available at: http://www.dhcs.ca.gov/formsandpubs/laws/hipaa/Pages/1.00WhatisHIPAA.aspx [Accessed 4 July 2018].

CE, 2018. CE marking. Available at: https://ec.europa.eu/growth/single-market/ce-marking_nl [Accessed 17 June 2018].

Celler, B., et al., 2017. Impact of at-home telemonitoring on health services expenditure and hospital admissions in patients with chronic conditions: before and after control intervention analysis. JMIR Med. Inform. 5 (3), e2. Available at: https://doi.org/10.2196/medinform.7308.

Chesbrough, H., 2003. Open Innovation: The New Imperative for Creating and Profiting from Technology, first ed. Harvard Business Review, Boston.

Choudhry, N.K., et al., 2017. Effect of reminder devices on medication adherence: the REMIND randomized clinical trial. JAMA Intern. Med. 177 (5), 624–631. Available at: https://doi.org/10.1001/jamainternmed.2016.9627.

Christensen, C., 2009. The Innovator's Prescription. McGraw-Hill, New York.

Christensen, C., 2016. The Innovators' Dilemma. Harvard Business Review Press, Boston.

Christensen, C., Waldeck, A., Fogg, R., 2017. The Innovation Health Care Really Needs: Help People Manage Their Own Health. Available at: https://hbr.org/2017/10/the-innovation-health-care-really-needs-help-people-manage-their-own-health [Accessed 24 December 2017].

Cipolle, R.J., Strand, L.M., Morley, P.C., 2004. Pharmaceutical Care Practice: The Clinician's Guide. McGraw-Hill, New York.

Cipolle, R., Strand, L., Morley, P., 2012. Pharmaceutical care practice. In: Pharmaceutical Care Practice. McGraw-Hill, New York.

Cognizant, 2016. Medication Adherence in the Real World. Available at: https://www.slideshare.net/cognizant/medication-adherence-in-the-real-world-63632949 [Accessed 3 May 2018].

Comstock, J., 2016. Walgreens Pill Reminder, Activity Tracking Both Improved Medication Adherence in Study. Available at: http://www.mobihealthnews.com/content/walgreens-pill-reminder-activity-tracking-both-improved-medication-adherence-study [Accessed 23 June 2018].

Couch, 2018. Are Patients Receiving Value in Terms of Health Literacy? Available at: https://www.prnewswire.com/news-releases/study-finds-almost-half-of-patients-skip-medication-300647249.html [Accessed 2 August 2018].

Council on Credentialing in Pharmacy, 2010. Scope of contemporary pharmacy practice. J. Am. Pharm. Assoc. 50 (2), e35–e69. Available at: https://doi.org/10.1331/JAPhA.2010.10510.

Council-of-Europe, 1997. The Oviedo Convention: Protecting Human Rights in the Biomedical Field. Available at: https://www.coe.int/en/web/bioethics/oviedo-convention [Accessed 10 October 2018].

Cutler, R., et al., 2018. Economic impact of medication non-adherence by disease groups: a systematic review. BMJ Open 8 (1), e016982. Available at: https://doi.org/10.1136/bmjopen-2017-016982.

Cyjax, 2017. What is GDPR, Why it is Needed and How to Prepare. Cyjax, London.

Dangi, R., 2017. Medication Adherence: Systems, Technologies and Global Markets. BCC Research.

Das, R., 2017. Does Blockchain Have a Place in Healthcare? Available at: https://www.forbes.com/sites/reenitadas/2017/05/08/does-blockchain-have-a-place-in-healthcare/#431787c1c31e [Accessed 28 July 2017].

Datatyilsynet, 2018. Data Protection by Design and by Default. Available at: https://www.datatilsynet.no/en/regulations-and-tools/guidelines/data-protection-by-design-and-by-default/ [Accessed 30 June 2018].

De Gier, J., Bouvy, M., Egberts, A., De Smet, P., 2013. Handbook Pharmaceutical Care (Handboek Farmaceutische Patientenzorg). Prelum, Houtem.

Deepmind, 2018. Deepmind. Available at: https://deepmind.com [Accessed 2 August 2018].

DEL, 2017. European Ethical Code for Data Donation. Available at: https://www.oii.ox.ac.uk/research/projects/a-european-ethical-code-for-data-donation/ [Accessed 4 October 2018].

Delogne, M., 2018. New PatientsLikeMe Studies Reveal How Patients Experience and Define "Good" Health Care. Available at: http://news.patientslikeme.com/press-release/new-pat ientslikeme-studies-reveal-how-patients-experience-and-define-good-health-care [Accessed 1 June 2018].

Deloitte, 2015. Enterprise Compliance and Life Sciences Compliance Advisory. Deloitte, London.

Deloitte, 2017a. Monitoring a Regulatory Convergence. Deloitte.

Deloitte, 2017b. Personalized Health: The Healthcare of Tomorrow is Coming Closer. Deloitte, Amsterdam.

Deloitte DCoHS, 2017. Pharma and the Connected Patient, How Digital Technology is Enabling Patient Centricity. Deloitte.

Derrington, D., 2017. AI for Health and Healthcare. Available at: https://www.healthit.gov/sites/default/files/jsr-17-task-002_aiforhealthandhealthcare12122017.pdf.

Developer NHS UK, 2018. Safe, Legal and Secure. Available at: https://developer.nhs.uk/library/save-legal-secure/ [Accessed 3 July 2018].

Dieleman, J., et al., 2016. National spending on health by source for 184 countries between 2013 and 2040. Lancet 387 (10037), 2521–2535. Available at: https://doi.org/10.1016/S0140-6736(16)30167-2.

Dima, A.L., Dediu, D., 2017. Computation of adherence to medication and visualization of medication histories in R with AdhereR: towards transparent and reproducible use of electronic healthcare data. PLoS ONE 12 (4), e0174426. Available at: https://doi.org/10.1371/journal.pone.0174426.

Douglas, H., 2009. Science, Policy and the Value-Free Ideal, first ed. University of Pittsburgh Press, Pittsburgh.

DPA, 2015. Conclusions DPA investigation Nike + Running app. Autoriteit Persoonsgegevens, Amsterdam, The Netherlands. Available at: https://autoriteitpersoonsgegevens.nl/sites/default/files/01_conclusions_dpa investigation_nike_running_app.pdf.

DTX Alliance, 2017. DTX Solutions. Available at: https://www.dtxalliance.org/dtx-solutions/ [Accessed 11 December 2017].

Duhigg, C., 2012. The Power of Habit: Why We Do What We Do in Life and Business. Random House, New York.

Dunn, J., 2017. It Looks Like Apple Has Some Work to do if it Wants Siri to be as Smart as Google Assistant. Available at: http://www.businessinsider.com/siri-vs-google-assistant-cortana-alexa-knowledge-study-chart-2017-6?international=true&r=US&IR=T [Accessed 31 July 2017].

Ebri, 2018. Consumer Engagement in Health Care Among Millennials, Baby Boomers, and Generation X: Findings from the 2017 Consumer Engagement in Health Care Survey. Available at: https://www.ebri.org/pdf/briefspdf/EBRI_IB_444.pdf.

e-Estonia, 2017. We Have Built a Digital Society and So Can You. Available at: https://e-esto nia.com [Accessed 29 August 2017].

EFPIA, 2016. The Pharma Industry in Figures—R&D. Available at: https://www.efpia.eu/pub lications/data-center/the-pharma-industry-in-figures-rd/new-chemical-or-biological-enti ties/ [Accessed 31 July 2017].

EFPIA, 2018a. Towards Outcome-based Healthcare—The EFPIA Vision. EFPIA, Brussels. Available at: https://www.efpia.eu/news-events/the-efpia-view/blog-articles/towards-outcomes-based-healthcare-the-efpia-vision/ [Accessed 10 August 2018].

EFPIA, 2018b. Value of Medicines. Available at: https://www.efpia.eu/about-medicines/use-of-medicines/value-of-medicines/ [Accessed 3 July 2018].

Elsberg, M., 2014. Zero. van Holkema & Warendorf, Amsterdam.

EMA, 2016. Revised Framework for Interaction Between the European Medicines Agency and Patients and Consumers and Their Organisations. EMA, London. Available at: https://www.ema.europa.eu/documents/other/revised-framework-interaction-between-european-medicines-agency-healthcare-professionals-their_en.pdf.

EMA, 2018. EMA Reviewing Medicines Containing Valsartan From Zhejiang Huahai Following Detection of an Impurity. Available at: https://www.ema.europa.eu/en/news/ema-reviewing-medicines-containing-valsartan-zhejiang-huahai-following-detection-impurity-some [Accessed 27 August 2018].

eMarketer, 2016. Mobile Phone, Smartphone Usage Varies Globally. Available at: https://www.emarketer.com/Article/Mobile-Phone-Smartphone-Usage-Varies-Globally/1014738 [Accessed 6 September 2017].

Engelen, L., 2018a. Augmented Health(care), first ed. Lightning Source, UK.

Engelen, 2018b. Patients Included. Available at: https://patientsincluded.org [Accessed 18 November 2018].

Est van, R., Gerritsen, J., Kool, L., 2017. Human Rights in the Robot Age. Parliamentary Assembly of the Council of Europe, France.

EU, 2017. Attitudes Towards the Impact of Digitisation and Automation on Daily Life. Available at: https://ec.europa.eu/digital-single-market/en/news/attitudes-towards-impact-digitisation-and-automation-daily-life [Accessed 1 August 2017].

EU, 2018a. 2018 Reform of EU Data Protection Rules. Available at: https://ec.europa.eu/commission/priorities/justice-and-fundamental-rights/data-protection/2018-reform-eu-data-protection-rules_en [Accessed 4 June 2018].

EU, 2018b. General Data Protection Regulation. 2016/679. Available at: https://eur-lex.europa.eu/legal-content/EN/TXT/?uri=celex:32016R0679 [Accessed 5 June 2018].

Eurofound, 2018. Health and Well-Being at Work. Available at: https://www.eurofound.europa.eu/topic/health-and-well-being-at-work [Accessed 5 July 2018].

Eyal, N., 2014. Hooked. Penguin Books, London.

FDA, 2002. General Principles of Software Validation; Final Guidance for Industry and FDA Staff. Available at: https://www.fda.gov/downloads/MedicalDevices/.../ucm085371.pdf.

FDA, 2016. General Wellness: Policy for Low Risk Devices. Available at: https://www.fda.gov/downloads/MedicalDevices/DeviceRegulationandGuidance/GuidanceDocuments/ucm429674.pdf.

FDA, 2017. Digital Health Software Precertification Pilot Program. Available at: https://www.fda.gov/downloads/Training/CDRHLearn/UCM569275.pdf.

FDA, 2018a. Changes to Existing Medical Software Policies Resulting from Section 3060 of the 21st Century Cures Act. Available at: https://www.fda.gov/downloads/MedicalDevices/DeviceRegulationandGuidance/GuidanceDocuments/UCM587820.pdf.

FDA, 2018b. 2018 Safety Alerts for Human Medical Products. Available at: https://www.fda.gov/Safety/MedWatch/SafetyInformation/SafetyAlertsforHumanMedicalProducts/ucm590808.htm [Accessed 7 February 2019].

FDA, 2018c. Digital Health Software Precertification (Pre-Cert) Program. Available at: https://www.fda.gov/MedicalDevices/DigitalHealth/DigitalHealthPreCertProgram/default.htm [Accessed 1 June 2018].

FDA, 2018d. FDA Permits Marketing of Artificial Intelligence-Based Device to Detect Certain Diabetes-Related Eye Problems. Available at: https://www.fda.gov/newsevents/newsroom/pressannouncements/ucm604357.htm [Accessed 15 June 2018].

Finkle, J., 2016. J&J Warns Diabetic Patients: Insulin Pump Vulnerable to Hacking. Technology News, October 4, 2016. Available at: https://www.reuters.com/article/us-johnson-johnson-cyber-insulin-pumps-e/jj-warns-diabetic-patients-insulin-pump-vulnerable-to-hacking-idUSKCN12411L [Accessed 17 May 2018].

FIP, 2009. FIP Community Pharmacy Section—Vision 2020. FIP, The Hague. Available at: https://www.fip.org/CPSvision/data/FIP%20Vision%202020.pdf.

FIP, 2012. A Global Competency Framework. FIP, The Hague. Available at: https://www.fip.org/files/fip/PharmacyEducation/GbCF_v1.pdf.

FIP, 2013. Pharmacist Ethics and Professional Autonomy: Imperatives for Keeping Pharmacy Aligned with the Public Interest. Available at: https://www.fip.org/www/uploads/database_file.php?id=358&table_id= [Accessed 12 October 2018].

Fogg, B., 2003. Persuasive Technology. Morgan Kaufmann Publishers, San Francisco.

Fortune, 2016. 2017, Why Drug Costs Will Keep Rising In. Available at: http://fortune.com/2016/12/19/healthcare-drug-costs-2017-predictions/ [Accessed 16 January 2018].

Fox, G., et al., 2017. Why People Stick With or Abandon Wearable Devices. Available at: https://catalyst.nejm.org/stay-abandon-wearable-devices/ [Accessed 20 December 2017].

Frank, R., 2016. ISO/TC 307. Available at: https://www.iso.org/committee/6266604.html [Accessed 15 August 2017].

Future of Life Institute, 2017. Asilomar AI Principles. Available at: https://futureoflife.org/ai-principles/ [Accessed 31 July 2018].

Future of Life Institute, 2018. Future of Life Institute. Available at: https://futureoflife.org [Accessed 11 October 2018].

Ga4gh, 2018. Global Alliance for Genomics and Health. Available at: https://www.ga4gh.org/aboutus/ [Accessed 20 October 2018]

Gallup, 2016. Americans Rate Healthcare Providers High in Honesty and Ethics. Available at: http://www.gallup.com/poll/200057/americans-rate-healthcare-providers-high-honesty-ethics.aspx [Accessed 30 August 2017].

Gandhi, R., Nayak, S., Franzblau, M., 2018. Healthcare 2020. Infosys Limited, India.

Gartner, 2018. Wearables Hold the Key to Connected Health Monitoring. Available at: https://www.gartner.com/smarterwithgartner/wearables-hold-the-key-to-connected-health-monitoring/ [Accessed 15 August 2018].

Gibson, R., 2015. The Four Lenses of Innovation. Wiley, New Jersey.

Ginsburg, G., Phillips, K., 2018. Precision medicine: from science to value. Health Affairs 37 (5), 694–701. Available at: https://doi.org/10.1377/hlthaff.2017.1624.

Graafland, M., 2014. Serious games in surgical education. Available at: https://pure.uva.nl/ws/files/2222491/152796_12.pdf.

Graber, M., 2013. The incidence of diagnostic error in medicine. BMJ Qual. Saf. 22 (suppl 2), ii21–ii27. Available at: https://doi.org/10.1136/bmjqs-2012-001615.

Grace, K., et al., 2018. When will AI exceed human performance? Evidence from AI experts. J. Artif. Intell. Res. 62, 729–754. Available at: https://doi.org/10.1613/jair.1.11222.

Gray, A., 2016. 10 Skills You Need to Thrive in the Fourth Industrial Revolution. Available at: https://www.weforum.org/agenda/2016/01/the-10-skills-you-need-to-thrive-in-the-fourth-industrial-revolution/ [Accessed 3 August 2017].

Gronde, v. d. T., Uyl-de Groot, C., Pieters, T., 2017. Addressing the challenge of high-priced prescription drugs in the era of precision medicine: a systematic review of drug life cycles, therapeutic drug markets and regulatory frameworks. PLoS ONE 12 (8), e0182613. Available at: https://doi.org/10.1371/journal.pone.0182613.

Health-RI, 2017. Health-RI. Available at: https://www.health-ri.org [Accessed 28 December 2017].

Heidbuchl, H., Vrijens, B., 2015. Non-vitamin K antagonist oral anticoagulants (NOAC): considerations on once- vs. twice-daily regimens and their potential impact on medication adherence. Europace 17 (4), 514–523. Available at: https://doi.org/10.1093/europace/euu311.

Heldenbrand, S., et al., 2016. Assessment of medication adherence app features, functionality, and health literacy level and the creation of a searchable Web-based adherence app resource for healthcare professionals and patients. J. Am. Pharm. Assoc. 56 (3), 293–302. Available at: https://doi.org/10.1016/j.japh.2015.12.014.

HL7, 2018. HL7. Available at: https://www.hl7.org [Accessed 30 May 2018].

HL7-FHIR, 2018. HL7-FHIR. Available at: https://www.hl7.org/fhir/ [Accessed 1 August 2018].

Huckman, R., Stern, A., 2018. Why Apps for Managing Chronic Disease Haven't Been Widely Used, and How to Fix It. Available at: https://hbr.org/2018/04/why-apps-for-managing-chronic-disease-havent-been-widely-used-and-how-to-fix-it [Accessed 20 September 2018].

Hussein, M., Brown, L.M., 2012. PDB59 cost-effectiveness analysis of medication therapy management in patients with type 2 diabetes in community pharmacy/ambulatory care settings: results from a decision-analytic Markov model. Value Health, 15(4), p. A181. Available at: https://doi.org/10.1016/j.jval.2012.03.980.

IBM, 2018. Watson. Available at: https://www.ibm.com/watson/health/ [Accessed 12 August 2018].

ICHOM, 2017. ICHOM. Available at: www.ichom.org [Accessed 18 October 2018].

IDC, 2018. Data Age. Available at: https://www.seagate.com/files/www-content/our-story/trends/files/idc-seagate-dataage-whitepaper.pdf.

IHI, 2017. Triple Aim. Available at: http://www.ihi.org/Engage/Initiatives/TripleAim/Pages/default.aspx [Accessed 10 August 2017].

Intersoft Consulting, 2019. Art. 12 GDPR: Transparent information, communication and modalities for the exercise of the rights of the data subject. Available at: https://gdpr-info.eu/art-12-gdpr/ [Accessed 7 February 2019].

IPH, 2018. Institute of Positive Health. Available at: https://iph.nl [Accessed 19 May 2018].

Irish Institute of Pharmacy, 2017. Professional Competencies of Pharmacists. Available at: https://iiop.ie/professional-competencies [Accessed 21 October 2017].

Iske, P., 2016a. Combinatoric Innovation, Navigating a Complex World, first ed. www.kno-com.com, Amsterdam.

Iske, P., 2016b. Institute of Brilliant Failures. Business Contact, Amsterdam.

ISO, 2018. ISO. Available at: www.iso.org [Accessed 30 June 2018].

Iuga, A., McGuire, M., 2014. Adherence and health care costs. Risk Manag. Healthc. Policy 7, 35–44. Available at: https://doi.org/10.2147/RMHP.S19801.

Kardas, P., Lewek, P., Matyjaszczyk, M., 2013. Determinants of patient adherence: a review of systematic reviews. Front. Pharmacol. 4, 91. Available at: https://doi.org/10.3389/fphar.2013.00091.

Kashgary, A., et al., 2017. The role of mobile devices in doctor-patient communication: a systematic review and meta-analysis. J. Telemed. Telec. 23 (8), 693–700. Available at: https://doi.org/10.1177/1357633X16661604.

Kenyon, C., et al., 2018. Controller adherence following hospital discharge in high risk children: a pilot randomized trial of text message reminders. J. Asthma 13, 1–9. Available at: https://doi.org/10.1080/02770903.2018.1424195.

Keulartz, J., et al., 2004. Ethics in technological culture: a programmatic proposal for a pragmatist approach. Sci. Technol. Hum. Values 29 (1), 3–29. Available at: https://www.jstor.org/stable/1558004.

Kitson, P., et al., 2018. Digitization of multistep organic synthesis in reactionware for on-demand pharmaceuticals. Science 359 (6373), 314–319. Available at: https://doi.org/10.1126/science.aao3466.

KNMP, 2012. Charter Professionalism of the Pharmacist. KNMP, The Hague. Available at: https://www.knmp.nl/professie/professioneel-handelen/handvest-van-de-apotheker-1/charter-professionalism-of-the-pharmacist.

KNMP, 2016. Pharmacist Competency Framework & Domain-specific Frame of Reference for the Netherlands. Available at: https://www.knmp.nl/downloads/pharmacist-competency-frameworkandDSFR-Netherlands.pdf.

Lawton, R., et al., 2016. Using the Theoretical Domains Framework (TDF) to understand adherence to multiple evidence-based indicators in primary care: a qualitative study. Implement Sci. 11, 113. Available at: https://doi.org/10.1186/s13012-016-0479-2.

Lord, N., 2018. What is NIST compliance?. Available at: https://digitalguardian.com/blog/what-nist-compliance [Accessed 21 August 2018].

MacIntyre, A., 1985. After Virtue, second ed. Duckworth, London.

Mack, H., 2017. Study: Texting to Improve Medication Adherence Shows High Engagement. Available at: http://www.mobihealthnews.com/content/study-texting-improve-medication-adherence-shows-high-engagement [Accessed 4 July 2018].

Madsen, L., 2014. Data Driven Healthcare. Wiley, New Jersey.

Marr, B., 2018a. How Much Data do We Create Every Day. Available at: https://www.forbes.com/sites/bernardmarr/2018/05/21/how-much-data-do-we-create-every-day-the-mind-blowing-stats-everyone-should-read/#433924f260ba [Accessed 30 June 2018].

Marr, B., 2018b. Why The Internet of Medical Things (IoMT) Will Start to Transform Healthcare in 2018. Available at: https://www.forbes.com/sites/bernardmarr/2018/01/25/why-the-internet-of-medical-things-iomt-will-start-to-transform-healthcare-in-2018/#623a1e874a3c [Accessed 22 August 2018].

Mayo, C., et al., 2017. Big data in designing clinical trials: opportunities and challenges. Front. Oncol. 7, 187. Available at: https://doi.org/10.3389/fonc.2017.00187.

McKinsey, 2018. Automation potential and wages for US jobs. Available at: https://public.tableau.com/profile/mckinsey.analytics#!/vizhome/AutomationandUSjobs/Technicalpotentialforautomation [Accessed 22 July 2018].

Mercy-Virtual, 2018. Mercy Virtual Hospital. Available at: http://www.mercyvirtual.net/about/ [Accessed 15 July 2018].

Microsoft, 2018. Project Innereye. Available at: https://www.microsoft.com/en-us/research/project/medical-image-analysis/ [Accessed 22 August 2018].

MIT Media Lab, 2018. Medrec. Available at: https://medrec.media.mit.edu [Accessed 15 December 2018].

Mitchell, E.M., 2016. Concentration of health expenditures in the U.S. Civilian Noninstitutionalized Population, 2014. In: Statistical Brief (Medical Expenditure Panel Survey (US)) [Internet]. Agency for Healthcare Research and Quality (US), Rockville, MD (2001—Statistical Brief no. 497). Available at: https://www.ncbi.nlm.nih.gov/books/NBK425792/.

Mittelstad, E., Floridi, L., 2018. The Ethics of Biomedical Data. Springer, New York.

Mohammed, M., et al., 2018. Development and validation of an instrument for measuring the burden of medicine on functioning and well-being: the Medication-Related Burden Quality of Life (MRB-QoL) tool. BMJ Open 8, e018880. Available at: https://doi.org/10.1136/bmjopen-2017-018880.

Mordorintelligence, 2017. European Telemedicine Market—Growth, Trends and Forecasts (2016–2021). Available at: https://www.mordorintelligence.com/industry-reports/euro pean-telemedicine-market-industry [Accessed 3 September 2017].

Morrisey, E., Corbett, T., Walsh, J., Molloy, G., 2016. Behavior change techniques in apps for medication adherence. Am. J. Prev. Med. 50 (5), e143–e146. Available at: https://doi.org/ 10.1016/j.amepre.2015.09.034.

Network World, 2008. Chapter 1: Overview of Network Security. Available at: https://www. networkworld.com/article/2274081/lan-wan/chapter-1–overview-of-network-security. html [Accessed 7 July 2018].

Neura, 2017. 2017 Report on Digital Health and Medication Adherence. The Neura, Sunnyvale.

NIST, 2018. NIST. Available at: https://www.nist.gov/ [Accessed 19 July 2018].

Noah, et al., 2018. Impact of remote patient monitoring on clinical outcomes: an updated meta-analysis of randomized controlled trials. NPJ Digit. Med. 1 (20172). Available at: https:// doi.org/10.1038/s41746-017-0002-4.

OAIC, 2017. Guide to mandatory data breach notification in the my health record system. Available at: https://www.oaic.gov.au/agencies-and-organisations/guides/guide-to-man datory-data-breach-notification-in-the-my-health-record-system [Accessed 22 December 2017].

OAIC, 2018. Guide to Securing Personal Information. Available at: https://www.oaic.gov.au/ agencies-and-organisations/guides/guide-to-securing-personal-information [Accessed 7 February 2019].

OECD, 2013. What Future for Health Spending? OECD Economics Department Policy Notes, No. 19, June 2013. Available at: https://www.oecd.org/economy/health-spending.pdf.

OECD, 2017. Health at a glance 2017: OECD indicators. OECD Publishing, Paris. Available at: https://doi.org/10.1787/19991312.

Osterwalder, A., Pigneur, Y., 2010. Business Model Generation, first ed. Wiley, New Jersey.

Ourworldindata, 2018. Life Expectancy 2013. Available at: https://ourworldindata.org/ life-expectancy [Accessed 1 August 2018].

OWASP, 2017. Security by Design. Available at: https://www.owasp.org/index.php/Security_ by_Design_Principles [Accessed 30 June 2018].

OWASP, 2018. The OWASP Foundation. Available at: https://www.owasp.org/index.php/ Main_Page [Accessed 30 June 2018].

Parkinson, M., 2018. Health Apps: Working Smarter, Not Just Harder. Available at: http:// www.pharmatimes.com/magazine/2018/julyaugust_2018/health_apps_working_smarter, _not_just_harder [Accessed 1 August 2018].

Partnership on AI, 2018. Partnership on AI. Available at: https://www.partnershiponai.org/# [Accessed 11 October 2018].

PCNE, 2013. Position Paper on the Definition of Pharmaceutical Care 2013. PCNE, Zuidlaren. Available at: https://www.pcne.org/news/14/the-pcne-definition-of-pharmaceutical-care-position-paper [Accessed 14 June 2018].

Persson, G., 1995. Logistics process redesign: some useful insights. Int. J. Logist. Manag. 6 (1), 13–26. Available at: https://doi.org/10.1108/09574099510805224.

Pew Research Center, 2017. 6-Key-Findings-On-How-Americans-See-The-Rise-Of-Automation. Available at: http://www.pewresearch.org/fact-tank/2017/10/04/6-key-findings-on-how-americans-see-the-rise-of-automation/ [Accessed 6 April 2018].

Pew Research Center, 2018. Millennials Stand Out for Their Technology Use, But Older Generations Also Embrace Digital Life. Available at: http://www.pewresearch.org/fact-tank/

2018/05/02/millennials-stand-out-for-their-technology-use-but-older-generations-also-embrace-digital-life/ [Accessed 1 August 2018].

Pharmacy Council NZ, 2015. Competency Standards for the Pharmacy Profession. Available at: https://enhance2.psnz.org.nz/assets/downloads/group_three/reflection/Standards_2015_FINAL.pdf.

PHMRA, 2018. Cost and Value of Medicines. Available at: https://www.phrma.org/advocacy/cost-and-value [Accessed 20 August 2018].

Piwek, L., Ellis, D., Andrews, S., 2016. The Rise of Consumer Health Wearables: Promises and Barriers. Available at: https://doi.org/10.1371/journal.pmed.1001953 [Accessed 10 July 2017].

Poplin, R., et al., 2018. Prediction of cardiovascular risk factors from retinal fundus photographs via deep learning. Nat. Biomed. Eng. 2, 158–164. Available at: https://doi.org/10.1038/s41551-018- 0195-0.

Porter, M., 2006. Redefining Health Care. Harvard Business School Publishing, Boston.

Porter, M., Lee, T., 2013. The Strategy That Will Fix healthcare. Available at: https://hbr.org/2013/10/the-strategy-that-will-fix-health-care [Accessed 3 August 2018].

PRnewswire, 2016. Telehealth Market Tot Show Over 27 CAGR Growth to 2021. Available at: http://www.prnewswire.com/news-releases/telehealth-market-to-show-over-27-cagr-growth-to-2021-led-by-north-america-604784566.html [Accessed 27 August 2017].

PwC, 2018. AI will impact employers before it impacts employment. Available at: https://www.pwc.com/us/en/services/consulting/library/artificial-intelligence-predictions/employer-impact.html [Accessed 15 August 2018].

Razakki, S., et al., 2018. A Comparative Study of Artificial Intelligence and Human Doctors for the Purpose of Triage and Diagnosis. Available at: https://marketing-assets.babylonhealth.com/press/BabylonJune2018Paper_Version1.4.2.pdf.

Rea, P., et al., 2016. Corporate Ethics Can't Be Reduced to Compliance. Available at: https://hbr.org/2016/04/corporate-ethics-cant-be-reduced-to-compliance [Accessed 13 October 2018].

Research2Guidance, 2017. mHealth App Economics 2017. Available at: http://www.uzelf.org/wp-content/uploads/2017/12/R2G-mHealth-Developer-Economics-2017-Status-And-Trends.pdf.

Rockhealth, 2018. Healthcare Consumers in a Digital Transition. Available at: https://rockhealth.com/reports/healthcare-consumers-in-a-digital-transition/ [Accessed 25 August 2018].

Roeser, S., Hillerbrand, R., Sandin, P., Peterson, M. (Eds.), 2012. Handbook of Risk Theory. Springer Science + Business Media B.V., New York.

Romeo, S., Corey, T., 2017. Internet of Health—Beecham Research Report. Available at: https://internetofbusiness.com/wp-content/uploads/2017/05/IoHEALTH-Market-Brief-17-Final.pdf.

Romero, A., 2013. Managing medicines in the hospital pharmacy: logistics inefficiencies. Lect. Notes Eng. Comput. Sci. 2, 1120–1125. Available at: http://www.iaeng.org/publication/WCECS2013/WCECS2013_pp1120-1125.pdf.

Rosenthal, M., Austin, Z., Tsuyuki, R., 2010. Are pharmacists the ultimate barrier to pharmacy practice change? Can. Pharm. J. 143 (1), 12–15. Available at: https://doi.org/10.3821/1913-701X-143.1.37.

Ross, A., 2016. The Industries of the Future. Simon & Schuster, New York.

Rug, UU, LUMC, KNMP, 2016. Pharmacy-specific Frame of Reference and Competency Standards Framework for Pharmacists [Dutch]. Available at: https://www.knmp.nl/downloads/domeinspecifiek-referentiekader-en-raamplan-farmacie-2016.pdf.

Sanyal, C., et al., 2018. Economic Evaluations of eHealth Technologies: A Systematic Review. PLoS ONE 13 (6), e0198112. Available at: https://doi.org/10.1371/journal.pone.0198112.

Schatsky, D., Piscini, E., 2016. Blockchain Reaches Beyond Financial Services With Some Industries Moving Faster. Available at: https://www2.deloitte.com/us/en/pages/about-deloitte/articles/press-releases/deloitte-survey-blockchain-reaches-beyond-financial-ser vices-with-some-industries-moving-faster.html [Accessed 14 August 2017].

Silva, J., et al., 2018. Emerging applications of virtual reality in cardiovascular medicine. J. Am. Coll. Cardiol. Basic Trans. Sci. 3 (3), 420–430. Available at: https://doi.org/10.1016/j.jacbts.2017.11.009.

Singapore MoH, 2017. Competency Standards for Advanced Pharmacists. Available at: http://www.healthprofessionals.gov.sg/docs/librariesprovider3/forms-publications/compe tency-standards-for-pharmacists-in-advanced-practice-2017-(web-version).pdf.

Snyder, C., Dorsey, E., Atreja, A., 2018. The best digital biomarkers papers of 2017. Digital Biomarkers 2, 64–73. Available at: https://doi.org/10.1159/000489224.

South African Government, 2017. Competency Standards For Pharmacists in South Africa. Available at: https://www.gov.za/nr/node/779355 [Accessed 20 October 2017].

Stanford, 2017. Harnessing the Power of Data in Health. Available at: https://med.stanford.edu/content/dam/sm/sm-news/documents/StanfordMedicineHealthTrendsWhitePaper2017.pdf.

Statista, 2018. Global Connected Wearable Devices. Available at: https://www.statista.com/statistics/487291/global-connected-wearable-devices/ [Accessed 29 July 2018].

Steckler, T., Brownlee, M., Urick, B., Farley, M., 2017. Pharmacy informatics: a call to action for educators, administrators, and residency directors. Curr. Pharm. Teach. Learn. 9 (5), 746–749. Available at: https://doi.org/10.1016/j.cptl.2017.05.003.

Steger, M.F., 2009. Meaning in life. In: Oxford Handbook of Positive Psychology. Oxford University Press, Oxford.

Sullivan, F., 2016. Vision 2025—The Future of Healthcare. Available at: http://www.frost.com/sublib/display-report.do?id=K0EB-01-00-00-00 [Accessed 1 August 2017].

Tailor, K., Steedman, M., Sanghera, A., 2017. Pharma and the Connected Patient. Available at: https://www2.deloitte.com/content/dam/Deloitte/global/Documents/Life-Sciences-Health-Care/gx-lshc-pharma-and-connected-patient.pdf.

Tao, D., et al., 2015. A meta-analysis of the use of electronic reminders for patient adherence to medication in chronic disease care. J. Telemed. Telec. 21 (1), 3–13. Available at: https://doi.org/10.1177/1357633X14541041.

Tarantola, C., 2017. The Top Medication Reminder Apps for Patients. Available at: https://www.pharmacytimes.com/contributor/christina-tarantola/2017/12/the-top-medication-reminder-apps-for-patients [Accessed 13 June 2018].

Taskforce PCPCC, 2012. Integrating comprehensive medication management to optimize patient outcomes. Available at: https://www.pcpcc.org/sites/default/files/media/medmanagement.pdf.

Tegmark, M., 2017. Life 3.0. Random House, New York.

TGA, 2018. Therapeutic Goods Administration. Available at: https://www.tga.gov.au/ [Accessed 30 June 2018].

The Circle, 2017. [Film] Regisseur: James Ponsoldt.

The Economist, 2017. A Digital Revolution in Health Care is Speeding Up. Available at: https://www.economist.com/business/2017/03/02/a-digital-revolution-in-health-care-is-speeding-up?etear=scnfbsponsoredrymanhealthcare [Accessed 12 July 2017].

The Work Foundation, 2018. Fitforwork. Available at: http://www.theworkfoundation.com/fit-for-work/ [Accessed 15 December 2018].

Thompson, C., 2016. How Does the Blockchain Work: A Simple Explanation. Available at: https://medium.com/the-intrepid-review/how-does-the-blockchain-work-for-dummies-explained-simply-9f94d386e093 [Accessed 28 July 2017].

Totalhealth, 2014. Public Health Information Too Complicated for Over 60%. Available at: http://www.totalhealth.co.uk/blog/public-health-information-too-complicated-over-60 [Accessed 28 August 2017].

Turner-Stokes, L., 2009. Goal attainment scaling (GAS) in rehabilitation: a practical guide. Clin. Rehabil. 23 (4), 362–370. Available at: https://doi.org/10.1177/0269215508101742.

UCLA Health, 2017. Patient Responsibilities. Available at: https://www.uclahealth.org/patient-experience/patient-responsibilities [Accessed 1 August 2017].

UHC, 2017. Managing Diabetes Through Prevention and Care. Available at: https://www.uhc.com/health-and-wellness/health-topics/diabetes/managing-diabetes [Accessed 11 December 2017].

van Beusekom, M.M., et al., 2016. Low literacy and written drug information: information-seeking, leaflet evaluation and preferences, and roles for images. Int. J. Clin. Pharm. 38 (6), 1372–1379. Available at: https://doi.org/10.1007/s11096-016-0376-4.

Vrijens, B., Urquhart, J., White, D., 2014. Electronically monitored dosing histories can be used to develop a medication-taking habit and manage patient adherence. Expert Rev. Clin. Pharmacol. 7 (5), 633–644. Available at: https://doi.org/10.1586/17512433.2014.940896.

Vrijens, B., et al., 2012. A new taxonomy for describing and defining adherence to medications. Br. J. Clin. Pharmacol. 73 (5), 691–705. Available at: https://doi.org/10.1111/j.1365-2125.2012.04167.x.

Waldrop, M., 2017. Virtual reality therapy set for a real renaissance. Proc. Natl. Acad. Sci. USA 114 (39), 10295–10299. Available at: https://doi.org/10.1073/pnas.1715133114.

Wang, T., et al., 2018. The Emerging Influence of Digital Biomarkers on Healthcare. Available at: https://rockhealth.com/reports/the-emerging-influence-of-digital-biomarkers-on-healthcare/ [Accessed 12 August 2018].

Wasserman, E., 2015. Theranos feels FDA's wrath over proprietary testing device. FierceBiotech. Available at: https://www.fiercebiotech.com/medical-devices/theranos-feels-fda-s-wrath-over-proprietary-testing-device [Accessed 7 February 2019].

WEF, 2015. Technological Tipping Points Report 2015. Available at: http://www3.weforum.org/docs/WEF_GAC15_Technological_Tipping_Points_report_2015.pdf.

WEF, 2017. Building the Healthcare System of the Future. Available at: http://reports.weforum.org/digital-transformation/building-the-healthcare-system-of-the-future/ [Accessed 29 April 2018].

Weng, S. et al., 2017. Can machine-learning improve cardiovascular risk prediction using routine clinical data? PLoS ONE 12 (4), e0174944. Available at: https://doi.org/10.1371/journal.pone.0174944.

Westerman, G., Bonnet, D., McAfee, A., 2014. Leading Digital: Turning Technology Into Business Transformation. HBR Press, Boston.

WHO, 2003. Adherence to Long-Term Therapies: Evidence for Action. WHO, CH. Available at: https://www.who.int/chp/knowledge/publications/adherence_report/en/ [Accessed 18 October 2017].

WHO, 2010. Telemedicine, Opportunities and Developments in Member States. WHO, Geneva. Available at: https://www.who.int/goe/publications/goe_telemedicine_2010.pdf.

WHO, 2014. The Case for Investing in Public Health. WHO, Geneva. Available at: http://www.euro.who.int/__data/assets/pdf_file/0009/278073/Case-Investing-Public-Health.pdf.

WHO, 2017. Medication Without Harm. WHO, Geneva. Available at: https://www.who.int/patientsafety/medication-safety/en/ [Accessed 2 September 2018].

WHO, 2018. Classification of Digital Health Interventions v1.0. Available at: https://www.who.int/reproductivehealth/publications/mhealth/classification-digital-health-interventions/en/ [Accessed 18 November 2018].

Wicklund, E., 2015. Using the Survey as a Patient Engagement Tool. Available at: http://mobihealthnews.com/news/using-survey-patient-engagement-tool [Accessed 7 April 2018].

Wikipedia, 2017a. Augmented Reality. Available at: https://en.wikipedia.org/wiki/Augmented_reality [Accessed 28 August 2017].

Wikipedia, 2017b. Blockchain. Available at: https://en.wikipedia.org/wiki/Blockchain [Accessed 16 August 2017].

Wikipedia, 2017c. Emotional Intelligence. Available at: https://en.wikipedia.org/wiki/Emotional_intelligence [Accessed 14 August 2017].

Wikipedia, 2017d. GDPR. Available at: https://en.wikipedia.org/wiki/General_Data_Protection_Regulation [Accessed 7 July 2018].

Wikipedia, 2018a. Artificial Intelligence. Available at: https://en.wikipedia.org/wiki/Artificial_intelligence [Accessed 16 August 2018].

Wikipedia, 2018b. Digital Therapeutics. Available at: https://en.wikipedia.org/wiki/Digital_therapeutics [Accessed 27 July 2018].

Wikipedia, 2018c. Machine Learning. Available at: https://en.wikipedia.org/wiki/Machine_learning [Accessed 29 June 2018].

Wikipedia, 2018d. Robot. Available at: https://en.wikipedia.org/wiki/Robot [Accessed 1 April 2018].

Wikipedia, 2018e. The Hippocratic Oath. Available at: https://en.wikipedia.org/wiki/Hippocratic_Oath [Accessed 19 October 2018].

Wilkinson, D., et al., 2016. The FAIR guiding principles for scientific data management and stewardship. Sci. Data 3, 160018. Available at: https://doi.org/10.1038/sdata.2016.18.

Williams, C., et al., 2018. Physician perceptions of integrating advanced practice pharmacists into practice. J. Am. Pharm. Assoc. 58 (1), 73–78. Available at: https://doi.org/10.1016/j.japh.2017.10.014.

Xiao, C., Choi, E., Sun, J., 2018. Opportunities and challenges in developing deep learning models using electronic health records data: a systematic review. J. Am. Med. Inform. Assoc. 25(10), 1419–1428. Available at: https://doi.org/10.1093/jamia/ocy068.

Yao, M., 2016. 4 Leadership Skills Every Young Pharmacist Should Master. Available at: https://today.mims.com/topic/4-leadership-skills-every-young-pharmacist-should-master [Accessed 10 August 2017].

Yeoman, G., et al., 2017. Defining patient centricity with patients for patients and caregivers: a collaborative endeavour. BMJ Innov. 3, 76–83. Available at: https://doi.org/10.1136/bmjinnov-2016-000157.

Yu, L., 2008. Pharmaceutical quality by design: product and process development, understanding, and control. Pharm. Res. 25 (4), 781–791. Available at: https://doi.org/10.1007/s11095-007-9511-1.

Index

Note: Page numbers followed by *f* indicate figures, *t* indicate tables, and *b* indicate boxes.